Microbiology
for the Allied
Health Professions

Microbiology
for the Allied Health Professions

SECOND EDITION

Adrian N. C. Delaat, A.R.T.

Coordinator, Laboratory Medicine Education
Provincial Laboratory and X-Ray Services Division
Manitoba Health Services Commission
Winnipeg, Manitoba, Canada

LEA & FEBIGER PHILADELPHIA

1979

Library of Congress Cataloging in Publication Data

Delaat, Adrian N. C.
    Microbiology for the allied health professions.

    Bibliography: p.
    Includes index.
    1. Medical microbiology. I. Title.
[DNLM: 1. Microbiology. QW4 D33lm]
QR46.D38 1979   616.01   78-5731
ISBN 0-8121-0612-1

Published in Great Britain by Henry Kimpton Publishers, London
PRINTED IN THE UNITED STATES OF AMERICA

Print No. 4 3 2 1

PREFACE

Choosing a microbiology text for students of the allied health professions is not an easy task. Although various books are available on the subject, none seems to fulfill the particular needs of the allied health professionals. Many microbiology texts offer an array of general information useful to the average undergraduate who has not yet selected a specialty, but mention little of the information most pertinent to health professionals. Other texts are directed to the medical student, who is more interested in clinical data than in technique, and consequently, these books contain much about disease syndromes and their management but little about the technical aspects of microbiology. Finally, there are several highly specialized texts that go far beyond the needs and comprehension of the average student of the allied health field.

The primary purpose of this book is to present the practical and elementary theoretic aspects of medical microbiology to the average high school graduate. As such, it offers a gentle exposure to what is often considered to be a difficult subject. I sincerely hope that it will whet the students' appetite for this fascinating subject, nourish them to the extent that they develop a healthy attitude toward microbiology, yet not stifle their enthusiasm with a diet too rich in content.

The first edition of this book was well received by members of the allied health professions. This response confirmed my belief that a book of this depth and breadth filled a need of these professionals. Thus, the second edition has been prepared with the same goals in mind as the first edition, but with the benefit of adding up-to-date information and culling out the inevitable mistakes. The classification of bacteria and the chapter organization in this edition have been completely rearranged to conform with that of the eighth edition of *Bergey's Manual of Determinative Bacteriology*. Such an arrangement should assist serious students in following up laboratory work related to identifying bacteria. New tables and charts that provide guides to the identification of organisms appear throughout the text; these revisions were made necessary by the new approach to classification and by the development of new information and techniques.

Compared to the first edition, more emphasis has been placed on the pathogenicity of various microbes. The information contained in the chapter on "Diseases Caused by Microbes" in the first edition has been enlarged to the extent that it now constitutes two substantial chapters: "Infectious Diseases" and "The Control of Infectious Diseases." The chapter on "Quality Control" was changed dramatically to reflect more clearly the current practices in that field. Outdated methods have been deleted and new ones incorporated.

Many contributed to the compilation of this book. I invite criticism and comment. Credit must go to my students who emphasized the need for a book such as this and who helped me to bring the various aspects into proper perspective, and to several colleagues who gave freely of their time and talents to critique early drafts and manuscripts. Dave Morrissey did the drawings for Chapter 22 and several others, Dorothy DiRienzi of Lea & Febiger was a most competent copy editor, and my wife Louise continued in her willing support.

Winnipeg, Canada   Adrian N. C. Delaat

CONTENTS

Part I
GENERAL MICROBIOLOGY

chapter 1

Introduction

"Read not to contradict and confute, nor to believe or take for granted, but to weigh and to consider."

These words by the sixteenth century philosopher, Sir Francis Bacon, aptly describe what should be the credo of the modern microbiologist. Few branches of the natural sciences have seen such rapid change as has the discipline of microbiology. The literature on hand, therefore, is full of apparent contradictions. Although the student may be baffled by such contradictions, he should not be alarmed by their existence. When he realizes that such contradictions stem from the rapid evolution of the discipline of microbiology, the keen student will welcome them as necessary evils, and will soon learn that the discipline is an interesting and rewarding area of study. Only recently has microbiology begun to emerge as a true and undisputed science. Before it reaches the stage of an exact science, many more contradictions will be committed to print. Therefore, if some statements in this text appear strange in comparison with other texts, please do not discard the statement as a fallacy. Consider: Is the statement of an earlier or later vintage than the one it contradicts? What is the context in which the statement is used? Does only hypothesis, or do proven experimental data back up the statement? Finding answers to such questions will not always be easy. By attempting to understand the principles involved rather than by memorizing the facts as stated, the student will soon find his way through the maze of statements and be able to sort out the proven fact from the postulated hypothesis. Only by raising further questions will the student become a participant in, rather than a spectator of, the discipline under study.

At the outset of your study of microbiology, I would like to allay two widespread misconceptions: First, not all microorganisms are harmful. On the contrary one only has to think of those organisms responsible for the making of cheese, wines, drugs, and many other useful products to refute this common belief. In fact, the beneficial microorganisms far outnumber the harmful ones.

Secondly, working with microorganisms, even with pathogens, is far less hazardous than driving a car. Of course, we must learn to respect certain dangers that are inherent in working with infectious material, just as drivers have to respect and obey traffic laws to ensure safety on the road. Most traffic accidents are caused by careless drivers and not by road hazards; so too, careless workers cause most accidents in the laboratory.

Your instructor will undoubtedly brief you on safe practices in the laboratory. It is your task to heed his instructions in order to protect yourself, your fellow workers and your community.

The simplest definition of microbiology is: "the science that studies microscopic organisms." This definition, of course, is too general and requires further clarification. By microscopic organisms we mean all living things that cannot be seen by the unaided eye. Microbiology involves a study of many aspects of the other life sciences. Because of its tremendous scope, various branches of microbiology have developed, each serving a specific interest. Bacteriology is the study of bacteria and rickettsiae; virology, the study of viruses; mycology, the study of yeasts and molds; parasitology, the study of parasitic animals.

These specialties have been subdivided even further. Many specialities devote most of their efforts to small groups of special organisms or to a certain area of study. For example, a plant bacteriologist limits his main interest to bacteria associated with plants; a veterinary virologist studies viruses that cause diseases in animals; and a brewmaster specializes in the study of yeasts related to the fermentation process. We could go on and on.

As a member of the allied health professions, you would, of course, be mainly interested in those organisms that cause disease in man—the pathogens. This area of microbiology is known as medical microbiology. Medical microbiology can be defined as the study of infectious diseases and their laboratory diagnosis. As such, medical microbiology includes the study of the treatment, control and prevention of infectious diseases. This elaboration brings us to two other sciences, immunology and epidemiology. Immunology is the study of the mechanisms by which the body reacts to "foreign" invaders. Epidemiology is the study of the distribution, spread and control of diseases.

By now you realize that medical microbiology is an extremely diverse field. In order to guide you through the maze of information about this subject in an intelligent and orderly fashion, this book has been divided into four parts.

Part I provides an introduction to the basic principles, theories and terminology of microbiology in general.

Part II deals specifically with various groups of microbes that are of medical interest. This systematic presentation allows you to study the microbes piecemeal, so to speak.

Part III introduces you to diagnostic microbiology, which involves the collection and analysis of specimens in order to detect and identify microbes. Because it is impossible to present a diagnostic approach that suits every need, this section should be considered a general guide rather than a blueprint.

Part IV presents the specific methods, media and reagents that are referred to in the preceding chapters.

To further develop your interests, you should seek to coordinate your studies with practical exercises. Practice these exercises shortly after you have studied each area. This will help you to understand the subject better and will also make you appreciate the difficulties constantly encountered by all microbiologists.

FURTHER READING

1. Stanier, R. Y., Doudoroff, M., and Adelberg, E. A.: *The Microbial World*, 3rd ed., Englewood Cliffs, N. J.: Prentice-Hall, 1970.
2. Wolk, C. P.: Physiology and cytological chemistry of blue-green algae, Bact. Rev., 37:32–101, 1973.

chapter 2
Brief History of Microbiology

It is difficult to state when microbiology actually began. Did it begin with the first description of microbial disease? If so, we must go back to the early Chinese scriptures. Did it begin with microscopy? Then, we must go back to the earliest lens grinders. We shall elect the latter as the beginning of microbiology.

2-1 THE DEVELOPMENT OF MICROSCOPY

Roger Bacon, a Franciscan monk, was the first to use two or more lenses as an aid to magnification in 1267. His lenses were reportedly of poor quality. During the middle of the sixteenth century, Hans Jansen perfected the art of lens making. Somewhat later, Robert Hooke brought lenses into practical use although it was not until late in the seventeenth century that anything resembling a microscope was devised. Antony van Leeuwenhoek, caretaker of the city hall in Delft, Holland, fancied the grinding of lenses as a hobby, and he built them into delicate instruments.

7

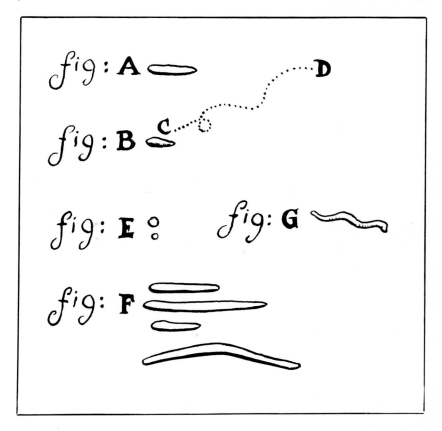

Fig. 2-1. These drawings of microorganisms from the human mouth were made by Antony van Leeuwenhoek in 1683. The dotted line, *C–D*, depicts the path of motion of the organism shown in drawing *B*.

Furthermore, he utilized these instruments to study an almost unlimited variety of specimens (see Fig. 2–1), and thus he discovered microbes of all descriptions. Moreover, he devised a few simple experiments to prove that hot water killed some of his "little beasties." Leeuwenhoek lived from 1635 to 1723, perfecting his microscopes so that the best would magnify up to 270 times.

In the following century, Ernst Abbe (1840–1905) developed a useful condenser, and Edison invented the electric light. Utilization of these two developments allowed magnifications of up to 1200 times, which is still the limit of the modern compound microscope utilizing ordinary light. During the 1920s, the use of ultraviolet light permitted slightly higher levels of magnification.

The greatest stride forward in microscopy, however, came in the 1930s with the invention of the electron microscope. Perfection of this instrument presently allows us to utilize working magnification of 30,000 to 90,000 times.

2-2 THE ORIGIN OF LIFE

Around 350 B.C., Aristotle wrote: "Animals sometimes arise in soil, sometimes in plants, and sometimes in other animals." Even today, some tribal cultures still believe that bees originate from the horns of bullocks buried in the mud. In the second half of the seventeenth century, Redi set out to prove that all living things have parents and that the theory of spontaneous generation was false. Redi simply covered spoiling meat with cheesecloth, thereby preventing flies from depositing eggs on the meat and hence the emergence of flies from the meat. While Redi's experiment refuted the belief that flies could originate spontaneously from putrid meat, it far from destroyed the idea of spontaneous generation altogether. Surely, proponents of that theory claimed, the microbes originate spontaneously.

Lazarro Spallanzani (1729–1799), on reading about Redi's work, was one of the few who believed that all living things, even the microbes, must have parents. In order to prove his belief, Spallanzani carried Redi's experiment one step further. He boiled mutton gravy and showed that, as long as the boiled gravy was kept sealed from the air, no microbes would originate from it.

A controversy developed between Spallanzani and an Irish priest named Needham who, together with Count Buffon, claimed that Spallanzani's experiment had destroyed a "vegetative force" and "elasticity of air" which were necessary for the appearance of microbes. The notions of vegetative forces and air elasticity were finally disproved in similar experiments by Schroeder and von Dush in 1854, who used cotton plugs, and by Louis Pasteur, who used swan-neck flasks.

The important thing to remember is that even today many "facts" are derived from hypothetic statements that have little or no supportive evidence. Even if it is derived from careful experimentation and brilliant deduction, any scientific "fact" may be refuted in time by the emergence of new evidence.

2-3 THE DISCOVERY OF THE NATURE OF FERMENTATION

Charles Caignard la Tour, 1777-1859, was the first person to detect budding yeasts in ferments. He referred to them as living objects capable of acting upon sugars through some effects of their vegetation.

Louis Pasteur, 1822–1895, was an artist, philosopher and scientist. To his sisters he once wrote: "To will is a great thing, for action and work usually follow will, and work is almost always followed by success." Reviewing Pasteur's life, one must admit he certainly worked and met with more than a little success. An eminent scientist at an early age, he was confronted with the problems of a much-troubled wine industry. In trying to solve the mysteries of souring wines, he asked himself a few simple questions: What initiates chemical changes in fruit juices? What maintains this reaction? Are bacteria (yeasts) the *cause* or the *product* of fermentation?

Pasteur was unable fully to answer all these questions. He did, however, establish microbiology as a science by discovering that:

  a. Some microbes grow only in the presence of air (aerobes).
  b. Some grow in the absence of air* (anaerobes).
  c. Only aerobes spoil wine.
  d. Ferments are not produced spontaneously.
  e. Ferments arise from within living organisms.
  f. Each ferment is produced by a special microbe.
  g. Fermentation proceeds without air.
  h. Heating at low temperatures prevents future spoiling.

From these conclusions, pasteurization became a household word, and the brewing industry a profitable business once more.

Pasteur is credited with discovering the nature of fermentation. However, Moritz Traube, in 1858, suggested the existence of enzymes, and Edward Buchner, in 1897, was the first to discover an enzyme, zymase.

2-4 THE PURE CULTURE CONCEPT

Spallanzani had already isolated single bacteria in capillary tubes in his attempts to demonstrate their mode of reproduction. Methods of culturing microbes, however, remained in a rather primitive state of development until Robert Koch (1843–1910) brought order to the chaotic laboratory methods employed prior to the 1860s. First, Koch developed staining methods by which bacteria placed on glass slides could be visualized more clearly.

---

*This in itself was an incredible discovery. Until then, it was believed that oxygen was one of the primary requirements for all life-forms.

His major contribution, however, was the development of a suitable solid medium on which mixtures of bacteria could be grown and, more importantly, kept in isolated colonies. Prior to Koch, methods of providing pure cultures consisted of "fishing out" single bacteria from broth cultures, which often contained many different bacteria in large numbers. One would have to be a pretty good fisherman to land a "clean catch" or a pure culture by such technique. Koch realized that one would have to use a solid medium to simplify the isolation of different cultures. His first solid medium consisted of sliced boiled potatoes. On these he could grow several bacteria that would develop into distinct "spots" on the surface of the slices. Koch referred to such "spots" as colonies, and colonies are presently defined as the descendants of a single organism growing in isolation from others and displaying certain distinct characteristics. Thus, a colony always constitutes a pure culture containing only one type of organism.

The use of potato slices allowed only a limited number of different bacteria to grow. Koch experimented with all sorts of solidifying agents that could be incorporated into suitable media for the more fastidious organisms. Gelatin proved quite successful, but it would melt at temperatures of 25°C and above and was also broken down by those organisms that produce gelatinase.

With the aid of his assistant, Koch discovered that the seaweed-extract agar was used by natives of Java in much the same way as he utilized gelatin. Agar has the added benefit that only very few bacteria can break it down and, more important, it has a melting point above 90°C and a solidifying point of about 42°C. Thus, agar can be incorporated into boiled broths, which can then be cooled to the point at which products such as blood and protein, which are spoiled by high temperatures, can be added, and the medium can be poured into Petri dishes before it reaches the solidification point of the agar. The development of suitable solid media probably did more for the advancement of bacteriology than any other single development.

2-5 THE GERM THEORY OF DISEASE

Early Greek writings ascribe certain diseases to worms too small to be seen. In 1546, Hieronymus Fracastorius advanced the theory of the "contagion," a substance capable of passing a disease on from man to man. Marcus von Plenciz developed this theory further and postulated that different microbes could cause different diseases. Again, Robert Koch proved these theories to be correct.

Following the isolation of the anthrax bacillus and the subsequent transmission of anthrax to previously healthy animals, Koch stated these postulates:

    a. In order for an organism to be incriminated as an etiologic agent of disease, the suspect organism must be found in every case of the disease.

    b. Secondly, the organism must be isolated in pure cultures from every case of the disease.

    c. Thirdly, the pure culture must be capable of producing the same disease in susceptible animals.

    d. Finally, the same organism must be isolated from the sick animals.

Only when all these facts had been established was Koch willing to accept that a specific organism was the actual cause of a disease. Since not all workers have taken Koch's advice, we probably still attribute certain diseases to organisms that are not the responsible agents.

2-6 FURTHER DEVELOPMENTS

It is impossible to give a true account of all the important historical developments of microbiology within the limits of this book. However, throughout this text, you will find references to early developments, particularly in sterilization, virology, and immunology. As was pointed out in Chapter 1, many areas of study have sprouted from microbiology. Where the future will take us is anyone's guess. By being aware of what has gone before, we should have a better appreciation of that to come.

FURTHER READING

1. Bernal, J. D.: *The Origin of Life*. London: Weidenfeld & Nicholson, 1967.
2. Brock, T. D.: *Milestones in Microbiology*. Englewood Cliffs, N. J.: Prentice-Hall, 1961.
3. Dobell, C.: *Antony van Leeuwenhoek and his Little Animals*. Dover Publ. Inc., 1932 (reprinted 1960).
4. Lechevalier, H. A. and Solotorovsky, M.: *Three Centuries of Microbiology*. New York, McGraw-Hill Book Company, 1965.
5. Vallery-Radot, R.: *The Life of Pasteur*. New York: Dover Publ. Inc., 1901 (reprinted 1960).

chapter 3
The Microbiologist's Tools

The tools and instruments used in microbiology are relatively simple when compared to those used by some scientists in other disciplines. An elementary understanding of thermo-regulating instruments, centrifuges, and pH meters and a fair understanding of microscopy provide the basic technical knowledge required to function as a useful participant in a "micro lab."

3-1 OVENS AND INCUBATORS

Both ovens and incubators work on the same principle. They are simply cabinets supplied with a built-in heater, which allows us to obtain higher temperatures inside the cabinet than those outside. The temperature is regulated by means of a thermostat. A thermostat is usually composed of a bimetallic strip that operates an electrical switch connected to a heating device. If two metals of different expansion rates are welded together (see Fig. 3–1), heat

13

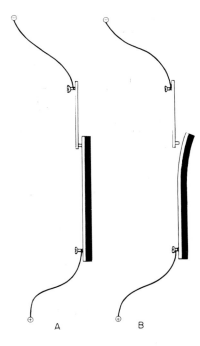

Fig. 3–1. A bimetallic strip thermostat. *A* allows current through to the heater; *B* cuts the current supply.

will cause one of them to expand more than the other, causing the entire strip to bend. When the strip is linked to an electrical switch, the circuit will be broken and the heater will turn off until the temperature drops sufficiently for the metal strip to take its original form. The difference between ovens and incubators lies simply in the temperature obtainable within. An instrument able to withstand temperatures of 100°C or more is usually referred to as an oven. Although we will use only the term incubator for the sake of simplicity, we imply the inclusion of ovens as well.

There are two basic types of incubators—the *gravity convection type* and the *mechanical convection type*. In the gravity convection type of incubator, the air is circulated by convection currents produced by heated air only. These convection currents are inadequate to circulate the heated air throughout the chamber when the temperature is to be raised only slightly above that of the outside temperature. The larger the incubator, the more serious this shortcoming becomes. In mechanical convection current types, the air is circulated by a fan.

An important point often neglected by careless workers is the loading of incubators. If packages to be sterilized or cultures to be incubated are placed in containers that do not permit proper airflow, the warmup period required will greatly impede the efficiency of the instrument. Remember that few media are better insulators than air (see also Chapter 4).

Another point to remember is that microorganisms grow best in a humid atmosphere. The more expensive incubators are supplied with built-in humidifiers that can be set to maintain a predetermined humidity. With the more conventional models, the technologist must periodically fill a beaker or pan of water which, when placed inside the incubator, will help maintain a suitable atmosphere.

The final and probably most important point is to check the temperature of all thermo-equipment daily.

3-2 WATERBATHS

A waterbath is essentially a pan with immersible heating coils. The coils are usually covered with a grid that has a dual purpose: it prevents direct contact between the coils and the objects to be incubated, and it promotes a more even distribution of convection currents. A good waterbath is the most sensitive incubator obtainable. When a waterbath is suitably insulated and has a tight fitting cover, a more stable temperature can be maintained than that with any other incubator. Under optimal conditions, temperatures can be controlled within a range of 0.5° C of the required temperature. The cover of a waterbath also serves a dual purpose. Besides helping to maintain the required temperature, the cover also reduces the rate of evaporation. When relatively high incubating temperatures are required, the rate of evaporation increases. Water of condensation will collect on the inside of the lid. To prevent this water from dripping into the test tubes, the lid should be constructed to allow proper drainage to the sides of the bath.

Tap water is hard in most areas. When used in a waterbath, it often causes scaling and subsequent corrosion of the bath. To prevent scaling, distilled water should be used at all times. To reduce contamination with algae and bacteria, 1 ml of a 10% zephiran solution may be added to every gallon of water added to the waterbath.

Temperature and water level checks should be made daily,

especially before long absences. Nothing sobers one up after a long weekend at the lake more quickly than the sight of a burned-out waterbath. Many technicians seem to forget that the water is the actual incubating medium. Obviously, the requisite incubating temperatures will not be reached when the level of the bath is lower than that of the reagents in the test tubes being incubated.

3-3 REFRIGERATORS AND FREEZERS

Every laboratory requires ample refrigeration facilities for storage of media, sera and other perishable reagents. Freezers are required for more prolonged storage of sera and more delicate reagents such as enzymes.

Since household refrigerators contain both a refrigeration and a freezing compartment, they suffice in the smaller laboratory. A few points to be remembered about refrigerators and their efficient use:

a. Automatically defrosting units cost little more than ordinary units and, in the long run, save both time and reagents.
b. Locate the unit away from hot air ovens, radiators, hot water pipes and similar objects.
c. Periodically clean and disinfect the unit's interior with a 0.1% zephiran solution.
d. Never store ether and other volatile, inflammable materials in an ordinary refrigerator. A spark from the motor might cause an explosion.

3-4 CENTRIFUGES

A centrifuge is an instrument designed to speed up the separation by gravity of solid particles suspended in liquids. The rate at which particles settle as sediments in liquids depends on several factors:

a. The size of the particle
b. The weight of the particle
c. The density of the liquid
d. The viscosity of the liquid
e. The gravitational force

In a centrifuge, the gravitational force (G) is increased mechanically. The degree of increased gravitational force is measured by a relative centrifugal force (RCF expressed in G) as follows:

$$RCF = 1.118 \times 10^{-5} \times R \times rpm^2$$

(R equals the radius of the centrifuge in centimeters; rpm, the number of revolutions the centrifuge makes every minute). Hence, a centrifuge with a radius of 20 cm and a speed of 4000 rpm will produce an RCF of approximately 1800 G, or particles in suspension spun at that speed will settle 1800 times faster than when left on the bench. In practice, a few more factors play a role in efficient centrifugation:

    a. The time of centrifugation
    b. The temperature required to maintain viability of the products being centrifuged. Refrigerated centrifuges should be used for products that deteriorate easily in the heat liberated from friction of the centrifuging tubes.

Generally, bacteria settle at about 2000 to 4000 G, yeasts at about 1000 to 2000 G, viruses at 50,000 to 150,000 G, and erythrocytes in saline solution at about 500 to 1000 G. In most instances, these figures apply for a simple benchtop centrifuge accommodating the ordinary 15-ml centrifuge tube, and they may be simplified further as follows:

Erythrocytes in serum	1500 rpm	20 minutes
Erythrocytes in saline solution	1500 rpm	10 minutes
Yeast cells in saline solution	1500 rpm	10 minutes
Bacteria in saline solution	3000 rpm	10 minutes

Naturally, the higher speeds needed for viruses to settle require a more sophisticated instrument.

The following are a few basic hints on operating a simple centrifuge:

    a. Tubes must always be placed in pairs. Each pair must be accurately balanced and both tubes of each balanced pair must be placed diametrically opposite one another.
    b. Be sure that the rubber cushions are in position at the bottom of the bucket or sleeve.
    c. Be sure that the tube is long enough to rest on the cushion and is not supported by its weaker rim.
    d. Be sure that the plug or stopper is sufficiently tight so it will not be forced into the liquid while spinning.
    e. Be sure that the buckets are placed properly on their hinges.
    f. Use the safety head, closing lid, or both.
    g. Start the motor gradually, pausing periodically before increasing the speed.

h. Allow the centrifuge to come to a full stop on its own, unless a built-in brake system is supplied.

i. Read the operating instructions for the specific model before using the instrument.

3-5 THE MEASUREMENT OF pH

Basically, pH can be defined as an internationally recognized measure of acid intensities of liquids. Acid intensities are most simply expressed as the concentrations of free hydrogen ions (H^+) in solution.* Some hydrogen compounds, such as hydrochloric acid (HCl), will dissociate rapidly and completely. Others, such as acetic acid (CH_3COOH) dissociate more slowly and incompletely. Others still, such as disodium hydrogen phosphate ($Na_2 HPO_4$) and potassium dihydrogen phosphate ($KH_2 PO_4$), resist pH changes because they try to maintain the status quo regarding free hydrogen ions in solution. These latter compounds are called buffer salts. More specifically, a *buffer* is a solution of a weak acid and one of its salts, or a weak base and one of its salts. A *base* is a compound that dissociates in water to release hydroxide ions (OH^-).

Water dissociates into both hydrogen and hydroxide ions. It is neither an acid nor a base, because H^+ and OH^- dissociate in equivalent concentrations. Pure water is therefore known as a neutral solution. Its H^+ concentration is 0.000,000,1 of a mole,† or 10^{-7} of a molar solution. This log number is used to express the pH value. At pH 7.0, a solution is neutral; at less than 7.0, acid; when higher than 7.0, alkaline. At pH 6.0, a solution is 10 times more acid than at 7.0; at 5.0, 100 times; at 4.0, 1000 times, and so on. At pH 8.0, a solution is 10 times more alkaline than at 7.0, and so on.

Temperature, the presence of other reactants, and the concentration of ions themselves also affect the pH value to some extent. For example, a solution may have a pH of 7.4 at room temperature, but 7.1 at 85°C. This variation, of course, is due to the rate of dissociation of solutes in the solution, which increases when the temperature is raised.

To the novice microbiologist, the niceties of ion dissociation theories are irrelevant. What is far more important is an understand-

---

*In actual fact, free hydrogen ions do not exist. They occur as hydrated protons called hydronium ions.
†A molar solution is an aqueous solution containing the same number of grams per liter as the molecular weight number of the solute.

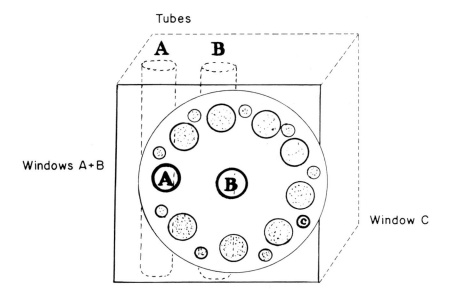

Fig. 3–2. The Lovibond comparator.

ing of the means and methods by which pH can be measured and adjusted. For this purpose, two apparatuses are available, either the comparator block or the pH meter.

THE LOVIBOND COMPARATOR*

This comparator consists of a cubic bakelite box with two receptacles for test tubes (A and B) on top and three "windows" in front (see Fig. 3–2). Inside the box, one finds a disc with a series of standardized colored glass "panes" arranged in a circle. By rotating the disc, each pane appears in front of window A. The colors of the panes are standardized to correspond with various pH values of a given indicator. The pH value corresponding with the pane appearing in window A may be read off from window C. To measure the pH of solutions containing different indicators, different discs are required.

---

*British Drug House.

To measure the pH of a given solution, one proceeds as follows:

a. Place 5 ml of the solution in each of two tubes, A and B.
b. Place tube A in the receptacle to the left.
c. To tube B add the required amount of indicator solution and place the tube in the other receptacle.
d. Rotate the disc while comparing the colors in both windows, A and B, until a match is obtained.
e. Read the pH from window C when this match is perfect. A "near" match will result in an accurate pH value of ±0.1 units.

THE pH METER

A more accurate pH value may be obtained by employing an electrode pH meter. Several such instruments are on the market, some sensitive enough to measure pH values of ±0.001. A pH meter consists of a pair of electrodes that are sensitive to H+ concentrations and are connected to an electrical circuit measuring the electromagnetic forces, and a potentiometer which indicates the measurements. The most common pH meters employ a glass electrode coupled with a calomel electrode as a standard.

Since each instrument requires specific operational steps, refer to manufacturers' pamphlets for detailed instructions. However, a few general rules apply to all pH meters:

a. Be careful when handling the electrodes. The glass electrode membrane is delicate and breaks upon the slightest impact with glass beakers or other hard objects.
b. Be sure that the calomel electrode is filled with the appropriate salt solution (usually saturated potassium chloride).
c. Allow the instrument time to warm up.
d. Frequently standardize the instrument against approved standards in a wide range of pH values.
e. Wash the electrodes with distilled water between each measurement.
f. Keep the electrodes immersed in water when the instrument is not in use.

ADJUSTMENT OF pH

The ability to measure pH, whether using a comparator or a pH meter, would have little value if one were not able to adjust the pH to the desired level. How is the pH adjusted?

When using the comparator, place the tubes in each receptacle as indicated previously. Instead of trying to match the color in each window by rotating the disc, rotate the disc so that the required pH value can be read from window C. If the colors in windows A and B match, the solution under test has the required pH value. If a match is not obtained, determine whether the pH value is to be raised or lowered, and add either 0.1 N HCl or 0.1 N NaOH in small measured amounts until a match is obtained.* By calculating how much 0.1 N acid or base had to be added to the 5 ml of test solution in order to obtain a proper pH value, one can determine how much 1.0 N acid or base has to be added to the remaining volume of solution. Similarly, one can utilize a pH meter to determine the pH value and the amount of acid or base solution that must be added to obtain the proper pH.

3-6 THE MICROSCOPE

A microscope may be defined as an optical instrument designed to magnify images of small objects. Its efficient use requires some basic knowledge of its parts and some measure of skill and training. However, so many different types of microscopes are presently on the market that no single model can be chosen to represent all types. Therefore, the following is an account of basic principles of microscopy as they apply to the light microscope. The compound microscope and some definitions and basic principles of less conventional microscopic methods, such as fluorescence, phase contrast, and electron microscopy, are also discussed.

GENERAL PRINCIPLES OF MICROSCOPY

When light rays pass obliquely from one medium into another, they bend depending on the angle of entry and the difference in optical density of the two media (optical density is more appropriately referred to as refractive index, RI). This phenomenon is illustrated in Fig. 3–3. At the top of this figure, light rays pass perpendicularly through plane glass. Here, the direction of the rays remains unchanged even though the refractive index of glass (1.5) is greater than that of air (1.0). When light rays enter the same glass at an angle, they are refracted toward an imaginary line, X–Y. This line, X–Y, represents the path the rays would take were they to enter the glass perpendicularly, and will hereafter be referred to as

---

*A liter of solution containing one gram equivalent mass of an acid or base is a 1 N solution.

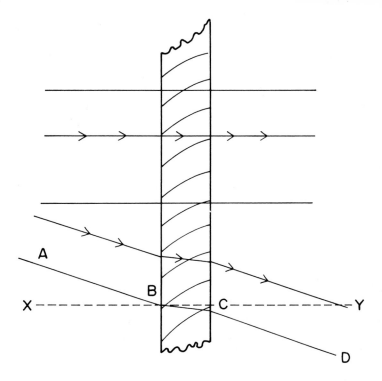

Fig. 3–3.   Basic light refraction.

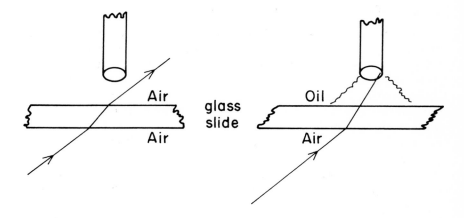

Fig. 3–4.   Correction of refraction by oil.

the "norm." Upon leaving the glass, the rays refract away from the norm, as shown by line A–D (see Fig. 3–3).

In the practice of microscopy, we make use of these simple principles when we apply immersion oil* to a specimen on a slide. Oil, at 1.51, has almost the same RI as glass. Therefore, if the space between the object and the objective lens is bridged with oil, the path of the light rays will be corrected to permit better resolution (see Fig. 3–4).

Resolution. Resolution is the ability of a lens to reveal detail. More precisely, it is the ability of a lens or a system of lenses to reveal closely adjacent structural details as separate and distinct. Resolution is also known as the resolving power of a lens or system of lenses. Resolution is restricted by two factors:

a. The wavelength of the light, λ.
b. The numerical aperture (NA) of the lens, i.e.,

$$\text{Resolution} = \frac{\lambda}{2\,\text{NA}}$$

Numerical Aperture. What is numerical aperture? The NA is an optical constant for any single lens; it refers to the ability of a lens to gather light rays projected toward it. It may be defined as the product of the RI of the medium outside the lens (n) and the sine of half the angle of the cone of light absorbed by the objective (u), or, $\text{NA} = n(\sin u)$. Since the sine of an angle is opposite over hypotenuse, sin u may be expressed as half the diameter of the lens over the distance from the periphery of the lens to the object when in focus (see Fig. 3–5).

From this, it follows that when the focal distance is reduced, the NA will have to be increased (see Fig. 3–6).

It should also follow that when oil is not used as in Fig. 3–4, the focal length will have to be reduced in order to allow light rays to enter the lens. This necessitates the use of a lens with a higher NA, which is attained by the use of oil instead of air.

Are you still with me? If you are, you may have noticed the referral to "when in focus" a few lines back; if not, simply remember that the higher the NA, the more the lens will reveal.

Focus. What do we really mean by "focus"? To better understand focus, we must enlarge our discussion of refraction (see Fig. 3–3). When light rays enter a curved glass, the rays are refracted. Because not all rays enter a curved glass at the same angle, various

---

*Oils containing PCBc (polychlorinated biphenyls) may be hazardous and should not be used when they may come in contact with the skin.

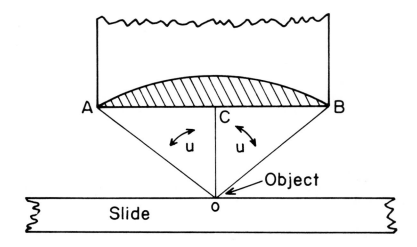

Fig. 3–5.   The numerical aperture is one times AC over AO.

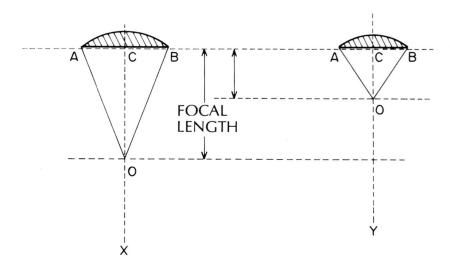

Fig. 3–6.   The NA must vary in x and y. If AC = 4 and AO = 10, then the NA
is 0.4, x. If AC = 4 and AO = 5, then the NA is 0.8, y.

degrees of refraction occur. These variables can be compounded by curving a glass in opposite directions on each side.

Thus, we can produce convex, or positive lenses, by which light rays are concentrated at a focal point, and concave or negative lenses, by which light rays are scattered (see Fig. 3–7). [It is of interest to note the change in "norm" (X–Y) upon entry and departure of a particular type of light ray from each type of lens.]

When using a convex lens, we should note that there are two focal points, or focal planes, A and B, one on each side of the lens (see Fig. 3–8). An object placed in one plane, A or B, will result in a clear image at the other plane, and only there. In other words, an object placed at A will only be in focus at B. You will also note that the image has been inverted (Fig. 3–8). The two points A and B are called conjugate foci and will vary when the object is moved closer to or farther from the lens (Fig. 3–9).

Moving the object, A, closer to the lens will result in a larger image being formed farther away. The object can be brought in so

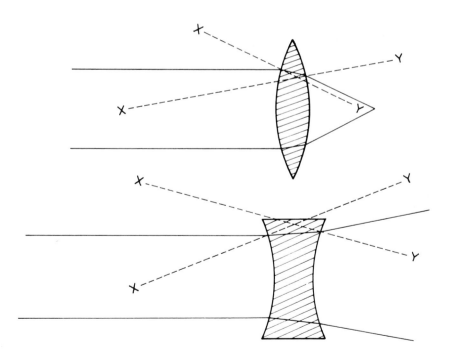

Fig. 3–7.   Refraction by a convex lens (above) and a concave lens (below).

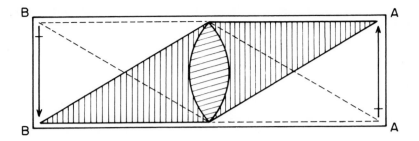

Fig. 3–8. The two focal planes of a convex lens, A–A and B–B.

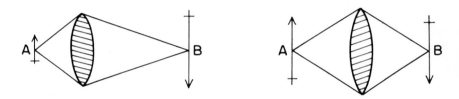

Fig. 3–9. Different focal points of the same lens, with the object in different planes.

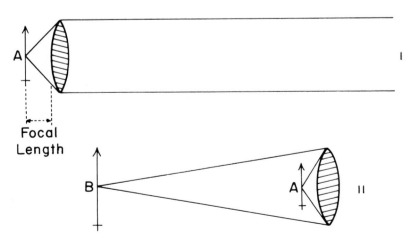

Fig. 3–10. Infinite and reflected focal points.

close that: (i) the image reaches infinity or (ii) the image is reflected rather than refracted (see Fig. 3–10 i, ii).

MAGNIFICATION

The magnification of a microscope is basically the product of the magnifying powers of the objective and the eyepiece. It further depends on: the focal length of the objective; the optical tube length; and the prism (when a binocular head is used, simply multiply the magnification by a further 1.5).

The focal length is the distance between the center of a lens and the point where a parallel beam of light is brought to a focus (see Fig. 3–10). This makes good sense if you realize that in a compound microscope we use a system of lenses. If an image is to be transmitted through a second lens in the system, the image should be projected evenly onto the next lens (see Fig. 3–11). Comparing Figs. 3–11 and 3–9, you will surmise that the magnification of a system of lenses, such as found in either the objective or the eyepiece, is limited and depends on the assigned focal length.

Some microscopes indicate only the focal length on their objectives; others may give their NA and magnifying power. When the magnifying power is indicated on both the objective and the eyepiece, simply multiply the two to obtain the total magnification of the microscope. When only the focal length is given, a slightly more involved calculation must be made:

$$\text{Eyepiece Magnification} \times \frac{\text{Optical tube length of the microscope}}{\text{Focal length of the objective}}$$

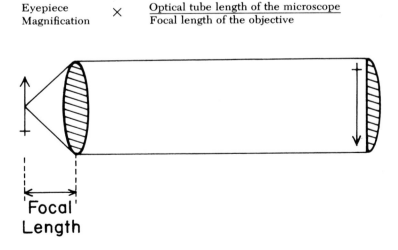

Fig. 3–11. The focal length in a system of lenses.

The optical tube length for most commonly used microscopes is 160 mm; it represents the distance from the image seen through the eyepiece to the object under study, when in focus (see Fig. 3–14). Hence, when the eyepiece gives a magnification of ten and the objective has a focal length of four, the total magnification will be

$$10 \times \frac{160}{4} = 10 \times 40 = 400.$$

Note that an increased focal length results in lesser magnification, which partly agrees with our explanation of Fig. 3–9. Partly? Yes, partly. By using a more or less convex lens, the light rays cause more or less refraction. In reality, therefore, it is a combination of the optical characteristics of the lens that influences the focal length, and hence the magnifying powers of the lens.

Clarity of Image. Is magnification all we want to achieve? Of course not. We also want clarity of image. Aside from resolution, as already discussed, the clarity of image is also affected by the quality of the lenses. Aberrations occur with less expensive lens systems. Two such aberrations are particularly important: chromatic and spherical aberration.

In the primary light spectrum, red light has the longest wavelength, 0.7 μm, blue, 0.45 μm, and violet, the shortest, 0.35 μm. The shorter the wavelength, the greater the effect a dense medium will have on the rate of travel. Therefore, white light passing through a prism or a convex lens will emerge at different points. Violet light will be refracted furthest by the slower speed (a) and red light refracted the least owing to its greater speed (c) (see Fig. 3–12).

This inability of a lens to converge white light at one central focal point is known as *chromatic aberration*; it may be noticed, when using inadequate or poorly adjusted microscopes, as the

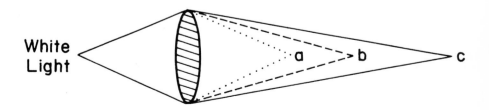

Fig. 3–12. Chromatic aberration.

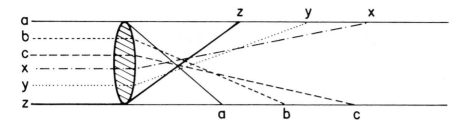

Fig. 3–13. Spherical aberration.

colored fringe surrounding the object under study. Chromatic aberration may be corrected by the use of achromatic lenses, which have been designed to compensate for the aberration.

Another phenomenon is due to the fact that when a beam of light is passed through a convex lens, most rays will enter and leave the lens at different points, and therefore are refracted to a variable degree (see Fig. 3–13). Hence, the rays do not converge at one single point. This shortcoming is known as *spherical aberration,* and it causes a fuzzy appearance at the rim of the microscope field. Spherical aberration may also be corrected by a system of compensating lenses. When shopping for a microscope, it is worth your while to remember the foregoing, because a better instrument saves money in the long run.

THE COMPOUND MICROSCOPE

Figure 3–14 portrays a simple diagram of the compound microscope. You should familiarize yourself with its various components and parts.

The base simply supports the instrument and should be placed on a level surface and left there. Students have the habit of pushing and pulling the microscope toward one another. This practice is not to be condoned, because the delicate mechanisms of gears and lenses are easily damaged by such rough treatment. If you must transport your instrument manually, use one hand on the arm and support the base with the other hand.

The light source is usually built in the base and can be adjusted so that the beam of light projects directly into the condenser. The condenser, too, can be adjusted and should be aligned with the light source and the objectives in a perfectly straight path. The most common fault in using the microscope is improper centering of the light source and condenser. The second most common mistake is

Optical and Mechanical Features of
THE MICROSCOPE

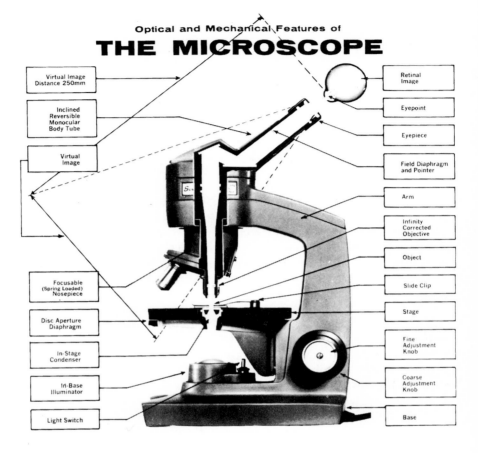

Fig. 3–14. The compound microscope, showing parts and the path of light through the instrument. (Courtesy of the American Optical Corp., Buffalo, N.Y.)

using too much light. Light intensity can usually be controlled by a transformer, which allows one to increase the voltage, and thus the light intensity.

The first thing a student is apt to do when the image is not immediately clear is to increase the light intensity. This is usually ineffective and, in the long run, damaging to the eyes and the lightbulb. When you have the urge to increase the light intensity, first ask yourself the following questions:

    a. Is the light source off center?
    b. Is the condenser off center?

c. Is the condenser incorrectly mounted?
d. Is the mirror misplaced?
e. Is the iris diaphragm opened far enough?
f. Is the objective lens dirty?
g. Is the oil dirty or mixed with air?
h. Is the eyepiece dirty?
i. Can I adjust the condenser higher?
j. Are any frosted filters inserted in the wrong places?

When all of these questions have been answered satisfactorily, more often than not you will reduce rather than increase the light intensity. Try it.

A few more hints may further improve your performance. The beam of light entering the objective may be regulated by the condenser. For most of your work, the condenser is best moved as close to the object as possible. For unstained wet preparations, a lower position will provide a better contrast because fewer light rays are required to obtain a clear image of the unstained objects. Lowering the condenser reduces the light intensity by throwing it out of focus.

The iris diaphragm is situated just beneath the condenser to guide the light beam effectively into the condenser. For most of your work, the best results are obtained with the iris diaphragm closed to 9/10 of its total capacity.

The coarse adjustment should be operated with both hands. The gears are usually fairly tight. Uneven strain will force them and may eventually jam the mechanism altogether.

The objectives are placed in a revolving nosepiece in a parfocal position. This means that when one of the objectives is in focus, all others are also in focus. Simply "zooming" in with different objectives saves much time and effort. Remember to zoom out again after using the high dry or oil immersion lens before you remove the slide, otherwise the slide may scratch these lenses.

The eyepieces of most modern microscopes can be set at different interpupillary distances. Use them to your best advantage.

Cover the microscope when not in use.

Remove all oil from the objective and the stage immediately after you remove the slide.

Do not tamper with eyepieces or objectives: they are factory aligned. Only clean the exposed (outer) lenses with lens paper.

Do not place a wet preparation on the stage without first wiping its bottom surface.

If the specimen appears blurred, switch over to another objective. If the image is then improved, the bottom-most lens of the previously used objective should be cleaned.

Blurred specks are usually caused by dust; if specks move when one eyepiece is rotated, clean the top-most lens of that eyepiece with a brush or lens paper. Never touch glass optics with your fingers—a fatty film will result on the surface. Instead, dust optics with a soft camel hair brush, or blow them free of dust with a syringe or a large rubber bulb, or wipe the lenses with clean lens paper. At best, moisten the lens paper with a little xylene.

MICROMETRY

Micrometry is the measurement of minute objects by means of a microscope and some measuring device. Micrometry may be performed with slide or eyepiece micrometers. The eyepiece micrometer is the most versatile device and thus, in the long run, the simplest method. Eyepiece micrometers may range from simple glass discs on which arbitrary linear scale divisions have been printed or engraved, to ocular micrometers with adjustable draw-tubes that contain similar discs and can be inserted into the ocular tube in their entirety. The simple disc type should be placed, scale side down, inside the ocular (eyepiece) on the top of the ocular diaphragm. Before accurate measurements can be made, an eyepiece micrometer must be calibrated for the particular micro-scope and lenses with which it is to be used. Calibration is the process of determining either the magnification factor or the value of a division of the eyepiece micrometer scale. A stage micrometer, which is a glass slide carrying a scale of precision-machined intervals, is required for this purpose. The actual process of calibration is relatively simple:

1. Put the slide micrometer onto the microscope stage with the scale uppermost.
2. Bring the scale into focus, using the objective and condenser as you intend to use them during your micrometry proper.
3. Insert the ocular micrometer or micrometer disc into its proper place.
4. Set the stage micrometer so that one line on its scale coincides with a line near the center of the scale on the eyepiece micrometer.
5. To the right of the coinciding lines, count the number of lines across the eyepice scale to the next point at which a line on the eyepiece scale again coincides with a line on the slide scale.

6. Determine the value of the eyepiece divisions with the
   following simple formula:

$$\frac{1 \text{ eyepiece}}{\text{division}} = \frac{\text{no. of slide divisions}}{\text{no. of eyepiece divisions}} \times \frac{\text{the value of each}}{\text{slide division}}$$

For example: If 10 slide divisions overlap 50 eyepiece
divisions, and the value of each slide division is 5 μm, then
the value of each eyepiece division will be

$$\frac{10}{50} \times 5 \ \mu m = \frac{1}{5} \times 5 = 1 \ \mu m$$

This must be done for each ocular-objective combination
you intend to use.

7. Remove the slide-micrometer and place the slide under
   study on the stage. Objects on any slide may now be
   measured using only the eyepiece micrometer and the
   factor determined in step 6. (If the same microscope-
   ocular-objective lenses are to be used repeatedly, it would
   be wise to keep the calibration values just derived for future
   use, by taping the record to the base of the microscope.)

DARKFIELD MICROSCOPY

In darkfield microscopy, oblique light, which ordinarily would
not enter the objective, is refracted by the object. Consequently,
the object appears as a self-luminous object against a dark background.

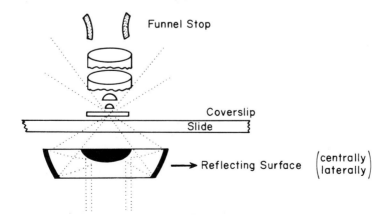

Fig. 3–15.   Darkfield condenser, and refraction of oblique light rays
by the object into the objective.

To better understand how this may be achieved, turn to Fig. 3–15 in which a darkfield condenser is represented. Comparing this darkfield condenser with that used for light microscopy, you will discover that the usual light path is blocked by a convex disc; the light is reflected so that it bypasses the objective lens. Only those light rays that are refracted by an object on the slide enter the objective.

Under optimal darkground conditions, even such delicate structures as the spirochetes, which measure only 0.1 μm in diameter, become clearly visible. However, wet preparations for examination must be as thin as possible in order to prevent the object from moving into different focal planes. Most modern microscopes can easily be converted into darkfield instruments by changing to a proper condenser and by increasing the light intensity.

PHASE CONTRAST MICROSCOPY

When you look at a living cell through the light microscope, the cell appears almost entirely transparent. Living cells are composed of minute structures, but these structures do not refract the light rays sufficiently to permit us to resolve them clearly; that is, they have only a slight difference in refractive index from the surrounding medium. However, besides being slightly refracted, the light rays passing through these structures have undergone another change: they have "slowed down" or, in optical terms, the phase of the light wave has changed.

Dr. F. Zernicke, a Dutch physicist, discovered these phase changes in 1940, and he received the Nobel prize in 1953 for further developing his discovery. In the phase microscope of today, the variations in phase changes are converted into visible changes of light intensity by a special optical system (see Fig. 3–16).

An ordinary light microscope can easily be converted into a phase contrast microscope. All that is required is:

    a. A special condenser with a built-in series of annular diaphragms. These diaphragms are really opaque discs of glass with a narrow clear ring. Each different objective requires a different size ring, depending on the NA of the objective.

    b. A special phase objective that has a phase-plate inserted in the back focal plane. The phase-plate is a glass disc with an etched circular trough. The light passing through the trough has a phase difference that is one quarter of the wavelength of the light passing through the rest of the plate. It is the contrast between these different light phases that allows us to distinguish the finer structures of the living cell.

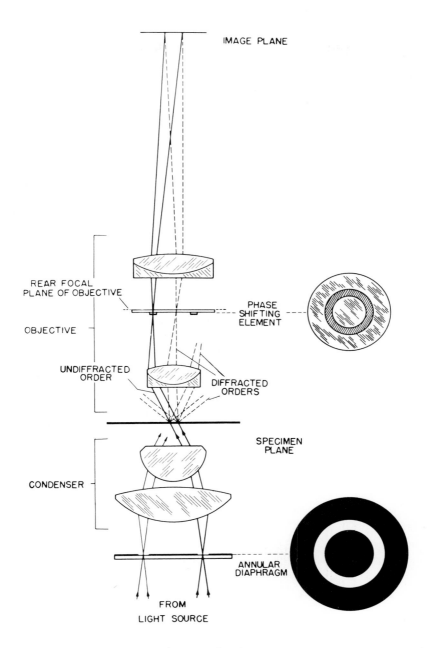

Fig. 3–16. Image formation by phase contrast microscopy.
(Courtesy of Bausch & Lomb, Rochester, N.Y.)

FLUORESCENCE MICROSCOPY

Certain dyes absorb light energy of one wavelength, such as ultraviolet, and emit light of another wavelength, such as yellow, green, or red. These dyes are known as fluorochrome or fluorescent dyes, because they fluoresce when subjected to ultraviolet light.

Since the wavelength of ultraviolet light is shorter than that of white light, we can improve the resolving power of the light microscope somewhat by making use of the foregoing principles. Some fluorescent dyes can be used to stain bacteria and other cells. When these cells are subjected to ultraviolet light, they appear as self-luminous objects against a dark background. Obviously, certain steps have to be taken to render a fluorescence microscope safe and effective. By following Fig. 3–17, some understanding of these safeguards will be gained.

A high mercury vapor lamp must be employed (HB 200) to supply an intense light source. The extreme heat given off by such a lamp must be blocked from the rest of the instrument by a system of heat-absorbing filters. It is also advisable to house the lamp in a protective shield, because these lamps often explode if used beyond 200 hours. A reflector should be placed within this shield to guide the light beam toward the focussing lens. Next to the focussing lens, a primary filter screens out the red to blue components of the light. A special condenser, the slide, and then the objective lens are next in line. Between the objective and the eyepiece, a secondary filter screens out the ultraviolet light, which is damaging to the eye. With a proper setup, only the altered ultraviolet light emitted by the dye is visible, usually in the yellow or green light spectrum.

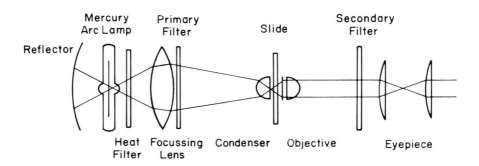

Fig. 3–17.   Diagram of the components of a fluorescence microscope.

ELECTRON MICROSCOPY

The electron microscope allows us to obtain useful magnification up to 1,000,000 times. A instrument that sensitive is obviously fairly sophisticated and expensive. By briefly comparing its main component parts with those of the light microscope, we will gain some knowledge of the principles underlying electron microscopy. Detailed descriptions of its mechansims and operational methods are beyond the scope of this text.

The image-forming radiation in the compound microscope is obtained from a light source; the electron microscope (E.M.) uses electrons as a source of radiation. The light beam travels mainly through air; the electrons must travel in a vacuum. Whereas the condensers we have studied so far are composed of glass lenses, the condenser of the E.M. has two electromagnets that narrow and concentrate an electromagnetic field. The specimen to be studied by E.M. needs careful attention. Ultra-thin sections of individual cells must be made and mounted on special grids to allow passage of the electrons. The image-forming mechanism of the E.M. is totally different from that of the compound microscope. Instead of absorption, refraction and projection of an image through an eyepiece directly onto the retina, in the E.M. the object scatters an electron beam. This scattering causes various degrees of excitement in a series of projectors, amplifiers, and coils until finally a fluorescent screen absorbs these different excitations and allows the operator to insert a photosensitive plate from which pictures can be taken.

FURTHER READING

1. Gray, P.: *The Use of the Microscope.* New York, McGraw-Hill Book Company, 1967.
2. Winstead, M.: *Instrument Check Systems.* Philadelphia, Lea & Febiger, 1971.

chapter 4

Sterilization and Disinfection

4-1 INTRODUCTION

In microbiology, sterilization implies the removal or destruction of all living organisms. A sterile object, therefore, is free from any viable (living) organisms. A microorganism is said to be alive when it is able to reproduce (see Chapter 5).

A point that is often forgotten is that destruction is not the same as removal. Particularly when sterilizing liquids, we should realize that some methods of sterilization leave dead organisms or other products behind. Even though the liquid may be sterile, these remaining products often interfere with whatever the liquid is designed to accomplish. We need only consider what would happen if we sterilized a heavily contaminated solution of glucose by heat and then used the sterile solution as intravenous food for a patient. The patient may benefit from the glucose but succumb from the toxic effect caused by the debris of dead organisms. It should be obvious, then, that in some instances, we have to do more than just sterilize an object or a liquid.

Several methods of sterilization are at our disposal. In general terms, these could be classified as:

a. *Chemical methods*, by which the destruction of organisms is effected by the application of a chemical.
b. *Physical methods*, by which destruction is accomplished by heat or radiation, or removal of organisms by filtration or centrifugation.
c. *Biologic methods*, by which destruction occurs through interference with life processes by biologic products.

Some methods of sterilization, of course, utilize combinations of these general methods. One could even argue whether some of the biologic methods are not really chemical, physical, or both.

Before entering into a discussion on any one particular method, a few general terms should be understood:

A state of infection is known as a *sepsis*, infectious material is said to be *septic*.

Asepsis or *aseptic* refers to a noninfective state or the absence of infectious material respectively.

An agent that interferes with the infectious potential of septic matter is called an *antiseptic;* one that neutralizes septic matter, a *disinfectant*. Note the subtle difference between an antiseptic and a disinfectant. In practice, an antiseptic may be seen as a weaker disinfectant that can be used to reduce the microbes on the skin or in the mouth. A disinfectant is useful in removing or destroying septic matter on instruments, floors or benchtops.

Microbiologists often use the terms *bacteriostatic*, which means preventing the growth and development of bacteria, and *bactericidal*, which means destroying or killing bacteria. Thus, antiseptics are generally bacteriostatic; disinfectants, generally bactericidal.

4-2 THE DYNAMICS OF DISINFECTION

The early Egyptians were the first to have used chemicals for the prevention of putrefaction. Their methods of preserving mummies, of course, were quite different from the antiseptic or disinfection methods in use today. However, they provided a start on the road to the development of more successful methods of sterilization.

The first medical applications of aseptic and antiseptic techniques were carried out simultaneously by Ignaz Semmelweis in Austria and Joseph Lister in Scotland during the latter part of the last century. However crude these early methods were, they were based on extensive studies of the various factors affecting disinfection. Many of these factors are still neglected by today's workers; such neglect often leads to improper disinfection, which really means no disinfection whatsoever.

What are some of the factors involved in the efficacy of disinfection? First of all, we should realize that the number of organisms present affects the rate of disinfection. If it takes 40 minutes to kill 1000 organisms of one type per milliliter, it may take twice that long, or longer, to kill a concentration of 100,000 organisms per milliliter of that same type (see Fig. 4–1).

We said "that type of organism," which implies that the rate of kill varies with different types of organisms, as it does. Each type of organism is affected to a different degree by the same disinfectant. We may go even further to state that some types of organisms vary in their susceptibility to the same disinfectant. Let us use a broth culture of a spore-forming bacillus for an example. If you subject

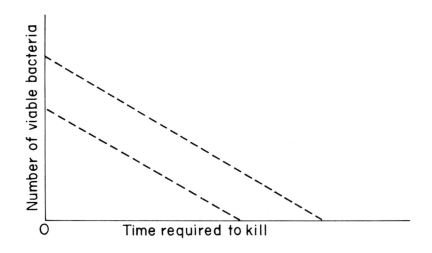

Fig. 4–1. Rate of kill related to the number of organisms per milliliter.

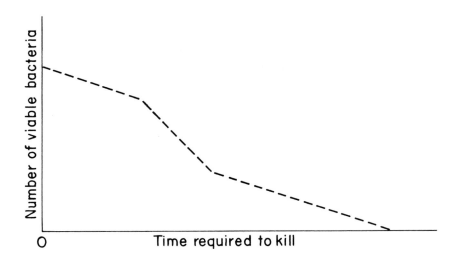

Fig. 4–2. Rate of kill of a broth culture of a spore-forming organism
by a disinfectant.

this culture to a particular disinfectant, you will find that only few
bacilli succumb at first, most of the remaining ones succumb in a
period shortly thereafter, and the last ones remain viable for a
rather long period (see Fig. 4–2).

Why the sigmoidal curve in Figure 4–2? A broth culture of a
spore-forming bacterium may contain three forms of that particular
type of bacterium. We may find: bacteria in the process of division
(these will be killed fairly easily); bacteria in the early vegetating
form (these will take somewhat longer to kill); and finally the spore
forms, which are the diehards.

The type of disinfectant used plays a further part in the
effectiveness of disinfection. Not all disinfectants are equally
powerful. Moreover, some disinfectants are designed to destroy
only certain types of organisms and are virtually ineffective when
used against other types.

The concentration of the disinfectant is another important
factor. It is often believed that the more concentrated the disinfectant, the more active it will be. This is true for some disinfectants,
but certainly not for all. Ethanol, for instance, is quite active at a
concentration of 70% but rather ineffective at either 60% or 80%.
Concentration and temperature are also critical with most of the

detergent compounds on the market today. These compounds act mainly by oxidizing bacterial proteins, a process that generally proceeds more rapidly when the temperature increases. Oxidizing compounds, such as iodine detergents, are generally more active at higher temperatures, provided they are properly diluted. Since many different products are marketed, no specific dilution factors can be referred to here. Some workers claim that increasing the temperature by 10°C doubles the rate of action of iodine compounds.

Temperature and pH are important factors in the use of some other disinfectants. For example, Zephiran at a concentration of 1:1000 is far more active at pH 8.0 than at pH 6.0.

Other factors to consider are the presence of extraneous materials, diluting agents, and physical barriers between the disinfectant and the bacteria to be killed. To elaborate on these factors:

a. When bacteria are coated with protein, mucus, or pus, they naturally are less accessible to a disinfectant.
b. To render some methods of disinfection even less effective, proteins and other materials sometimes neutralize the effect of certain disinfectants altogether. Quaternary compounds, such as Zephiran in particular, are often completely neutralized by proteins.
c. To decontaminate a broth culture by mixing it with disinfectant, the laboratory worker should know the dilution factor of the culture medium-disinfectant mixture.
d. Air bubbles in test tubes form natural barriers between disinfectant and culture. Even without air bubbles, the rate of diffusion of disinfectant into culture medium, and vice versa, greatly increases the time required to kill the culture.

The modes of action of disinfectants vary widely. Some disinfectants act primarily by coagulating or denaturing cellular proteins. Some may change the permeability of the cell wall or cell membrane, or otherwise damage these structures to cause lysis. Others still may alter the enzymatic activity, thereby interfering with the normal metabolic process, or upset the oxidation-reduction potential, thereby creating a lethal environment within the cell.

It should be clear by now that methods of disinfection are by no means the most reliable methods of sterilization. At best, they can be relied upon to reduce or kill vegetative bacteria. As such, they should render certain objects noninfectious, that is, free from pathogens; but the sterility of objects subjected to disinfectants only can never be guaranteed.

In summary, the ideal disinfectant should:

1. Have a high antimicrobial activity.
2. Be nontoxic, noncorrosive or nonirritative.
3. Be nonstaining and not damaging to fabrics.
4. Be odorless and free from undesirable vapors.
5. Be stable to heat and different pH levels.
6. Be highly soluble in water and in alcohol.
7. Have a low surface tension and good wetting properties.
8. Be unalterable by proteinaceous or other organic matter.
9. Leave no conductive or nonconductive film.
10. Act within a short period of time and not appreciably lose its activity during specified periods of storage.
11. Have a deodorizing effect and a dirt-carrying capacity.

4-3 GASEOUS STERILIZATION

Certain gases exert a lethal action on bacteria. They destroy various enzymes and biochemical structures essential to the survival of the organisms. The usefulness of some of these gases—chlorine, formaldehyde and sulfur dioxide—has long been recognized. More recently, ethylene oxide has been used in the sterilization of plastics and other thermolabile, disposable goods.

Gaseous sterilization methods are seldom used in today's hospital laboratory. Because we tend to use more and more disposable goods, however, it should be of interest to learn a little more about ethylene oxide sterilization. Ethylene oxide is a colorless liquid with an etherlike odor. It has a boiling point of only 10.7°C, and is highly inflammable in air. When mixed with 90% freon, carbon dioxide or nitrogen, it becomes safe to use. Ethylene oxide gas diffuses through porous materials and penetrates most plastics readily. It is most useful for sterilizing disposable goods and bulky instruments, such as heart-lung machines. At a temperature of about 50°C and a relative humidity of 33%, sterilization of most goods and instruments is accomplished within three hours. Because ethylene oxide gas is highly toxic, especially to tissues, products sterilized by this method should be used no sooner than 24 hours following sterilization.

4-4 STERILIZATION BY HEAT

Again, the early Egyptians provide the first recorded evidence of heat sterilization: they were the first to heat surgical instruments over an open fire. Only since Koch, in 1881, studied the properties of steam and hot air in their application to sterilization, however, can we speak of the development of scientifically sound methods of sterilization.

Before Koch's studies, Louis Pasteur had introduced "pasteurization" and had presented scientific evidence of its usefulness. Pasteurization is the heating of liquids, particularly milk, wines and beer, to about 63°C for 30 minutes or to 72°C for 20 to 30 seconds. However, pasteurization does not sterilize these liquids; it merely kills certain vegetative pathogens often found in these products and thereby renders the product safe for human consumption. By no means are they sterile.

Koch, together with his associates, demonstrated that dry heat at 100°C would destroy all vegetative bacteria within one and one-half hours. The spores of anthrax bacilli, however, could only be killed by dry heat at 140°C and, at that, it would take three hours. Not impressed by these results, Koch and his co-workers tried moist heat instead and found that its use greatly increased the efficiency of sterilization. We now know why this is so. In a dry atmosphere, heat kills only by oxidizing vital cell products. In a moist environment, heat causes coagulation of cell proteins. Much higher temperatures are required to cause detrimental oxidation than are required for destructive coagulation. The process of destructive coagulation is enhanced even further when steam under pressure is applied, and more so when saturated steam is applied.

Although methods of heat sterilization are among the best available, we must again realize that even by extreme heat, not all organisms will be killed at once. However, a more consistent pattern of destruction can be established when heat is applied than when disinfectants are used.

Bacteriologists had long accepted as fact the belief that when a suspension of bacteria is gradually heated, a point is reached at which all bacteria in that suspension will be killed instantly. They referred to this point by the term "thermal death point." The thermal death point was defined more precisely as the lowest temperature at which an aqueous suspension of a given type of bacterium was killed. This definition implies that a certain temperature would be instantly lethal to a certain bacterial population. If we remember from our discussion of disinfection that the rate of kill is also affected by exposure time and other factors, this definition seems deceptive. More recent studies have shown that the rate of destruction of bacteria subjected to certain temperatures follows an orderly, almost logarithmic, pattern of decline in numbers of viable organisms. Therefore, time of exposure is a factor of the rate of destruction equal in importance to the temperature applied.

The term *thermal death time* has gained prominence over the previously-used term of "thermal death point." Thermal death time is defined as the shortest period of time in which a known population of a particular bacterial culture is killed when suspended in a specific medium and exposed to a given temperature. Obviously, it would be impractical to determine the thermal death time for each object, culture or combination thereof imaginable. We do know, however, that the most resistant vegetative forms of microorganisms are killed within three minutes at 121°C. The most resistant spores require 12 minutes to be destroyed at this same temperature. We should use these figures in our assessment of the following methods of heat sterilization.

STERILIZATION BY DRY HEAT

As already discussed, dry heat kills mainly by oxidation of vital cell proteins. Relatively high temperatures are required to render dry heat sterilization effective.

Flaming. The red-hot flame of a Bunsen burner is particularly suited for sterilizing and decontaminating metal instruments such as inoculating loops, needles and forceps. For decontamination, it is best to employ a shielded flame, as the infectious material that may spatter will then remain within the "sleeve."

Incineration. Although recommended for disposal of contaminated dressings, paper goods, and animal carcasses, incineration should not be relied upon to decontaminate cultures and specimens. These should be autoclaved in the laboratories and then disposed of as ordinary garbage. To obtain the desired high temperatures, incinerators must be fitted with forced air jets.

Hot Air Ovens. Glassware and other bulky items that can withstand heat are best sterilized by dry heat as supplied by a hot air oven. Even the highly resistant spores of *Bacillus stearother-mophilus* will be destroyed at 160°C within one hour. This temperature and time period, therefore, are recommended as standards in the use of sterilization by hot air. Some other factors must also be taken into consideration:

    a. Warm-up time for oven and materials.
    b. Heat conductivity of materials, or air flow through the objects being sterilized.
    c. Air flow throughout the oven.

In Chapter 3 we already discussed some of these factors in regard to ovens and incubators. As a general guide, refer to Table

Table 4–1. Times required for sterilization by dry heat at 160°C

	Time in minutes	
	Heating up	Sterilizing
Syringe wrapped in cotton	60	60
Syringe placed in glass tube	90	60
Petroleum jelly, 16-oz jar	120	60
Flask—500 ml	60	60
Flask—volumetric, closed, 500 ml	90	60

4–1 to determine minimal times required to sterilize materials and objects in a hot air oven set at 160°C. To be safer still, many workers routinely set the hot air oven for four hours at 160°C from time of loading to completion of sterilization. At that temperature and for that period of time, even the most resistant spores will die. Most articles routinely sterilized in ovens withstand these conditions well.

STERILIZATION BY MOIST HEAT

Moist heat is the most efficient means of sterilization, since relatively low temperatures will ensure sterilization. To understand why this is so, we must review some elementary physics. You may remember that 80 kilo calories of heat are required to raise the temperature of 1 liter of water from 20°C to the boiling point, 100°C. Roughly seven times that amount of heat energy is required to convert the same liter of boiling water into steam. When this steam is allowed to condense onto cooler surfaces, this amount of heat energy is almost instantly released and passed onto the cooler surroundings.

As a result of this physical phenomenon, the temperature of articles heated by moist heat will be raised much more quickly than that of articles heated by dry heat. When bacteria are exposed to moist heat, this rapid increase in temperature is responsible for coagulation of vital cell proteins. Several methods of moist heat sterilization may be employed.

Boiling. This method is little more effective than dry heat at 100°C. However, it is easier to control the temperature of a boiling waterbath than that of a hot air oven. Furthermore, the waterbath is more efficient than the hot air oven because the warming-up period of objects to be sterilized is reduced. Finally, it is more practical, in that a pan of water may be brought to a boil almost anywhere. Realizing that boiling does not kill spore-forming bacteria, one can apply this method of sterilization with reasonable success wherever spore-formers do not play a role.

Tyndallization, or Flowing Steam. Many biological products such as culture media and other solutions may decompose when subjected to temperatures greater than 100°C for a lengthy period. Nevertheless, these products often contain a spore-forming bacteria that must be destroyed before the product can be used. If subjected to flowing steam for periods of 20 to 30 minutes on three successive days, these products are usually sterile.

We emphasize *usually* here, because the theory of this practice (advanced by Tyndall) is that spores will vegetate during the periods between heating and then be killed in their vegetating form during the next heating. This theory holds true for most spores. However, anaerobic spore-formers and some members of the genus *Bacillus* do not conform to this theory.

Steam under Pressure. Saturated steam under pressure (autoclaving) is the most dependable means of sterilization. We specify saturated steam here, because a mixture of air and steam greatly reduces the usefulness of the autoclave, no matter how great the pressure applied. We must again return to a physics lesson to appreciate this necessity for saturated steam. When water is boiled in a closed vessel, the resulting steam soon raises the pressure inside the vessel. The increased pressure raises the boiling point of the rest of the water, so that liberated steam gradually becomes hotter and hotter. The steam already formed does not necessarily heat up; only the newly liberated steam has a higher temperature, corresponding to the increased boiling point. Releasing the steam generated first (the relatively coolest) results in higher and higher temperatures of the newly generated steam, provided the pressure is allowed to increase gradually. Thus, to use an autoclave properly, it is most important to realize that mixtures of air and steam result in greatly reduced temperatures.

We have already discussed what happens to the heat absorbed by steam when that steam condenses onto cooler objects. The more heat absorbed by the steam, the greater the heat that is transferred to the cooler object. Hence, saturated steam under pressure has a greater effect than flowing steam.

Temperatures attainable by pressurized saturated steam are: 109°C at 5 lbs psi; 115°C at 10 lbs; 121°C at 15 lbs; and 126°C at 20 lbs. We could of course list many more data, but these are the ones most commonly used for sterilization.

The practical applications of sterilization by saturated steam can be better understood by taking a closer look at the apparatus most commonly employed for that purpose.

The Autoclave. Figure 4–3 illustrates a basic model of an autoclave. Surrounding the loading chamber on all sides except the front is a "jacket," in which we can build up a predetermined pressure by regulating the steam supply with a pressure valve at the intake. The front of the loading chamber has a door that is securely fitted to close off the chamber. When the required pressure in the jacket has been reached, the autoclave is ready for use.

Materials to be sterilized are placed in the chamber. The autoclave must be loaded properly to ensure a free flow of steam through the articles to be sterilized. Empty glass vessels should be tilted so that the air can be replaced easily by steam. Avoid overloading the chamber. After loading, the door must be closed securely. (The sealing gasket on the door should be checked

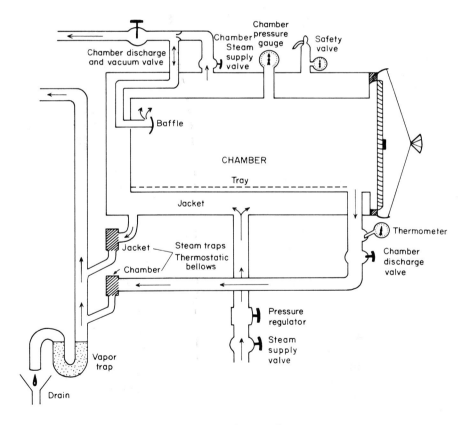

Fig. 4–3. The autoclave.

Table 4–2. Commonly used data in autoclaving

	Temperature	Time	Pressure psi
Culture media, broth	115°C	15	10
Culture media, agar	121°C	15	15
Infected material and cultures	126°C	15	20
Bottles, instruments	126°C	15	20

periodically. The gasket must be replaced when the least bit of leakage is observed, if not sooner.)

The chamber may now be filled with steam by opening the chamber steam valve. At this time, the chamber discharge valve remains open to allow proper evacuation of all the air. Only when the thermometer at the chamber discharge valve reads 100°C or higher should this valve be closed. Both temperature and pressure now increase rapidly. When the required temperature has been reached, the timing of the actual sterilization period begins. When this time has expired, the chamber steam valve is closed and the pressure within the chamber is released slowly by gradually opening the chamber discharge valve. The door should not be opened until the temperature gauge reads less than 100°C, unless the operator wishes to be met with a gush of steam and boiled-over vessels inside.

Modern autoclaves are equipped with timers, controls, thermostats, and alarms that allow us to preset the entire sterilizing cycle beforehand. Thus, sterilization methods are reduced in complexity to the mere press of a button. Completely automated sterilization methods still require supervision by a technologist capable of detecting and correcting operational flaws. Because models differ considerably, refer to the manufacturer's manual to learn more about the autoclave in use at your institution. Table 4–2 lists autoclave temperatures and pressures for sterilizing commonly used articles.

4-5 CONTROL OF HEAT STERILIZATION

There is only one way to sterilize and that is the perfect way. No in-betweens are possible. Sterile objects are like pregnant women: they either are or they aren't. How do we know whether an object is sterile?

The only sure way to determine whether or not an article is sterile is to test it thoroughly for microbiologic contents, and even that would not always be a perfect measure (see Chapters 6 and 24). The methods available for sterility control, therefore, are only checks on the procedures used in sterilization. When properly used, they give a reasonable assurance of safety; when improperly used, they constitute a major hazard to the maintenance of public health. Probably the best method of sterility control is the use of resistant, nonpathogenic spore-formers. The most commonly used spores are those of *Bacillus stearothermophilus*, a thermophilic bacillus that grows only at 56°C or above. Spore cultures are allowed to reach 10^6 organisms per milliliter. Filter paper strips are then soaked in the culture, dried at room temperature, and placed in small envelopes.* When the autoclave has been loaded, one of the envelopes is placed inside at a strategic location. Following sterilization, the strip is recovered and put in a tube of broth. If no growth occurs within a 48-hour incubation at 56°C, the articles autoclaved along with the strip can safely be assumed to be sterile.

Chemical indicators and reversible autoclave tape are also commonly used for quality control, but these are not as reliable as properly placed spore strips.

4-6 FILTRATION

Microorganisms may be removed from fluids and from air by a variety of methods. When all living organisms present in a medium are removed, that medium is sterile, be it fluid or air. Sera, antibiotic solutions and other liquids that would lose their usefulness if subjected to heat for any length of time are among the fluids most commonly sterilized by filtration.

FILTRATION OF FLUIDS

Several different filters may be employed. In general, the filter must be capable of holding back particles somewhat smaller than the smallest organisms present in the liquid to be sterilized. Hence, we have bacteria-proof and virus-proof filters. The British Pharmaceutical Code states that a filter must have average pores of 0.75 μm or less to qualify as a bacteria-proof filter. Virus-proof filters, of course, must have pores much smaller than that. No authoritative standard has yet been set, but to be virus-proof, the pores of the filter should be smaller than 10 nm. Some of the filters available today do even better than that!

---

*These envelopes and strips are commercially available (Baltimore Biological Laboratories, Cockeysville, Md.)

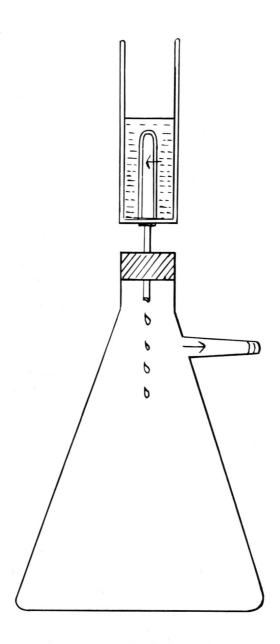

Fig. 4–4. A "candle" type filter.

Earthenware Filters. These may be made from kieselguhr, plaster of paris, kaolin, or a combination of these substances. The most common types are the German Berkefeld filter and the French Chamberland filter. Berkefeld filters are available in coarse (V = viel), normal (N) and fine (W = wenig) grades. The Chamberland filters are made in various porosities. Both are usually built in the shape of a hollow candle surrounded by a wider sleeve of metal (see Fig. 4–4).

The entire apparatus fits a rubber bung, which can be placed in a flask with a sidearm. The liquid to be sterilized is poured into the metal sleeve, and a suction pump is attached to the sidearm of the flask; the negative pressure inside the candle and flask forces the fluid through the pores and into the flask. Earthenware filters may be cleaned by brushing and subsequent boiling in distilled water. Their porosity should be checked after cleaning by checking the rate of flow of running distilled water. When clogged with organic matter to the point of inefficiency, the actual filter may be heated in a flame until red hot and cooled slowly. Wrapped in Kraft paper, the apparatus can be sterilized before use. Alternatively, the assembled filter and a fitting flask can be protected and sterilized together.

Seitz Filters. These consist of asbestos pads held in a funnel-like apparatus. The pads are supported by a wire screen and can be discarded after use. They come in various sizes and grades of porosity. The entire mechanism can be cleaned and reassembled easily. It is wise to moisten the pads slightly with distilled water before assembling the apparatus to allow a better "fit." The entire apparatus can be sterilized in a manner similar to the earthenware filters.

Cellulose Membrane Filters or Millipore Filters. These have largely replaced the more bulky Seitz filters. They offer some distinct advantages: smaller volumes may be sterilized, as the wastage of fluid remaining on the pads is almost negligible; porosity control is virtually unlimited; differentiation between particles of ± 10 nm by the use of graded filters is possible (which is a fairly rapid and reasonably accurate method to measure the size of a virus).

Various mechanisms are on the market to house different sizes and makes of membrane filters, ranging from the larger funnel type to the tiny Swinney type. Several manufacturers supply these filters.*

---

*Gelman Instruments Co., Ann Arbor, Mich.; Millipore Filter Corp., Bedford, Mass.; Sartorius, Göttingen, Germany.

FILTRATION OF AIR

The air filter most commonly used in the microbiology laboratory is the cotton plug. Various other fibers can be used to filter the air entering test tubes and "sterile" rooms or leaving contaminated environments such as fume hoods or inoculation chambers. In fact, cotton wool is one of the least satisfactory fibers because it packs tightly and absorbs moisture readily. Glass wool is much better suited for larger filters, as used in air conditioners. In the laboratory, however, a loosely-packed cotton plug is satisfactory in some instances.

For filtration of air in safety cabinets or air conditioners, the best filter to use is the HEPA filter.* These filters are made of a glass asbestos medium with aluminum separators mounted in a plywood frame on a rubber-based, self-adhesive gasket. The flow-rate of these filters should be monitored regularly to ensure maximum safety, as directed by the manufacturer.

CENTRIFUGATION

Centrifugation can be utilized as a method of sterilization. By spinning a liquid fast enough, any living matter will eventually be deposited at the bottom (see Chapter 3). When the supernatant is then aspirated aseptically, the fluid collected will be sterile.

A more effective method of sterilization is achieved by combining centrifugation with filtration. A Swinney type filter apparatus is available that allows two small vessels to be attached to either end of a filter (see Fig. 4–5). By filling one container with the fluid to be sterilized, attaching a sterilized filter and then a sterile vessel to the other end of the filter, the entire assembly can be placed in a centrifuge and the liquid forced through the filter into the sterile container.

4-7 STERILIZATION BY RADIATION

Various kinds of radiation can be used to destroy microorganisms. The more commonly used kinds are: ultraviolet light, infrared light, gamma rays, and high energy electron radiations.

Ultraviolet (UV) light is absorbed by the cellular proteins and acts by altering the chemical reactions of nucleoproteins. Ultraviolet light penetrates only slowly and must be applied directly

---

*Available from: Contamination Control Inc., Kulpsville, Penna.

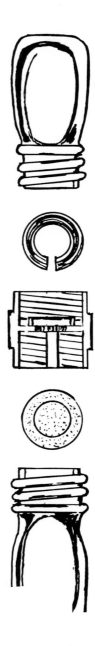

Fig. 4–5. A filter assembly that can be
centrifuged.

and for considerable periods of time. It is mainly useful as a sterilizing agent for benchtops and aerosols suspended in the air of operating rooms and inoculating cabinets. The operator should remember that ultraviolet light is particularly damaging to the eyes.

Infrared rays are employed mainly to reduce contamination of food during preparation. Infrared rays sterilize by imparting heat energy rapidly and thus oxidizing the organisms.

Gamma and high electron radiation is known as ionizing radiation because an electron is removed from certain atoms. The altered atoms are thus turned into reactive ions. Radiations such as these are highly effective as sterilization methods, but unless properly controlled, they constitute a major health hazard to the operator. It is possible to build operable and safe units, but high cost is a limiting factor.

FURTHER READING

1. Block, S. S. (ed.): *Disinfection, Sterilization and Preservation,* 2nd ed. Philadelphia, Lea & Febiger, 1977.
2. Borick, P. M. (ed.): *Chemical Sterilization.* Stroudsburg, Pa., Dowden, Hutchinson & Ross, Inc., 1973.
3. Perkins, J. J.: *Principles and Methods of Sterilization in the Health Sciences.* 3rd ed. Springfield, Illinois, Charles C Thomas, 1976.

chapter 5

Basic Structures and Functions of Bacteria

Microbes are far too diverse in nature to permit a general discussion of structure and function. Therefore, we shall limit ourselves here to the bacteria and study the features of other types of microbes in Chapters 21 to 23. In discussing compact living things such as bacteria, we shall combine our study of bacterial structures with the basic functions of those structures. The study of structure is known as morphology; that of function, as physiology. In Chapter 6, we combine the study of physiology with biochemistry. In fact, we should start out with the realization that any living organism is a highly complex unit. Whatever aspect we choose to study of that unit is interrelated with the unit as a whole, if not with the population of which the unit is a part.

5-1 COMPARING BACTERIA TO PLANTS AND ANIMALS

When first observed, bacteria appear to be more like plants than animals, but a closer analysis will reveal distinct differences.

We shall first compare the basic differences between animals and plants, and then compare bacteria; this process will clearly illustrate the distinct features of bacteria.

Animals may ingest their nutrients by engulfing (the amoeba), or by swallowing (the higher animals). All animals utilize rather complex substances for nutrition. Their cells have a flexible or elastic covering.

Plants ingest their nutrients by diffusion, utilize relatively simple substances, and have rigid coverings on their cells.

Cells, of course, are structural units of living matter enclosed within a membrane and consisting of a mass of cytoplasm that surrounds a controlling mechanism called the nucleus. Cytoplasm consists of a colloid, a substance of finely divided particles somewhat larger than molecules that fail to go into solution, yet too small to settle out by gravitational forces. It is a substance like eggwhite that is composed of carbohydrates, fats, proteins, salts and water.

Animal and plant cells are called eukaryotic cells because they have morphologically distinct nuclei. Bacteria are designated prokaryotic cells because they lack an organized nucleus and a mitotic apparatus (centrosome).

5-2 DEFINING BACTERIA

Bacteria are minute, prokaryotic unicellular organisms, without chloroplasts. They multiply by binary or transverse fission. They take in simple foods by diffusion and have a rather rigid cell wall. The individual cells are physiologically independent but are influenced by environmental changes brought about by neighboring cells or cellular products.

Let us examine this definition in greater detail. How small is minute? Bacteria are measured in micrometers. One micrometer (μm) is one millionth part of a meter, or one twenty-five thousandth of an inch. The average bacterium is less than 1½ μm wide and about 2 μm long. Each weighs only 10^{-12} g, or 1 g of bacteria will contain 1,000,000,000,000 organisms. If we realize that a newspaper page is usually between 20 and 30 μm thick, we should have some concept about the minuteness of bacteria.

What do we mean by binary fission? In a suitable environment, the bacterial cell eventually divides to form two identical bacteria by an asexual process. We use the term "asexual" advisedly, since certain bacteria are known to exchange some genetic material. This exchange of genetic material, known as a transduction, is not a prerequisite for reproduction, however.

The process of binary fission proceeds as follows:

a. The inner covering—cytoplasmic membrane—grows inward.
b. As this constriction continues, a new outer covering—cell wall—is produced. During this period also, the intracellular material (cytoplasm and nucleic material) divides equally within the two parts of the cell.
c. Following completion of the constriction, the two new cells break apart to form two daughter cells that are anatomically and physiologically identical.

This brings us to the consideration of *physiologic independence* and environmental changes. It is quite evident that the higher forms of life are composed of cell units that are organized into groups or organs. Each organ performs highly specific functions, thereby making all groups of cells, and all cells, interdependent on one another. The lower plants, if we may call the fungi so, also demonstrate some specialization and interdependence of cells. However, each bacterial cell carries on all the functions necessary

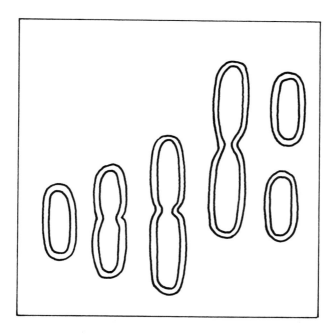

Fig. 5–1. Progressive binary fission.

to maintain its existence and to propagate. This does not imply that bacterial cells have no effect on one another whatsoever. They most certainly do. Some members of bacterial populations, for instance, may exert a beneficial effect on some of their "neighbors," whereas others may have an adverse effect on those same neighbors. Moreover, the same activity of one type of bacterium may benefit some types and yet harm others. To illustrate this, suppose we have three types of bacteria—A, B, and C—and A produces a substance, Y, that aids B but harms C. To some extent, the natural control of many infectious diseases is governed by these principles. The variety and numbers of the multitude of microorganisms living within our body are thus kept in delicate balance.

Antibiotics are some of the products produced by certain microorganisms that can kill or harm others. Unfortunately, we do not know precisely all the antibiotics produced by all organisms, nor the exact interaction that one or a combination of many antibiotics may have on mixed populations of bacteria. We do know, however, that if we use antibiotics indiscriminately, they may change the pattern of bacteria commonly found at various body sites, and that these body sites may then become more vulnerable to infections by other organisms that would have been warded off had the balance not been destroyed. This is discussed in more detail in Chapter 9.

5-3 GROSS MORPHOLOGY OF BACTERIA

Having defined bacteria, we may now return to the main topic of this chapter, morphology. Bacteria not only vary in size but also in shape. The more typical forms are:

   a. The cocci (singular, coccus), which are perfectly spherical when mature.
   b. The bacilli (singular, bacillus), which are straight or slightly curved rods.
   c. The vibrios, which are comma-shaped.

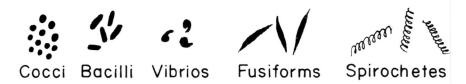

Cocci   Bacilli   Vibrios   Fusiforms   Spirochetes

Fig. 5–2.   Different forms of bacteria.

d. The fusiforms, which are spindle-shaped.
e. The spirochetes, which are shaped like a corkscrew (see Fig. 5–2).

5-4 EXTERNAL BACTERIAL STRUCTURES

Although bacteria may take different forms, all bacteria function in much the same way, and are composed of all, or most, of the following structures:

THE CELL WALL

This structure has been compared to a corset, because it is tough and rigid and allows the cell to maintain its distinct shape. The cell wall generally protects the cell. It prevents immediate lysis of the cell should the cell be placed in an environment with different osmotic pressures (review, if you wish, the principles of the process of osmosis). Because the cell wall is the chief means of protection for the bacterial cell, chemotherapy is often directed toward the wall in an effort to weaken it and permit other agents to effect the final destruction of the cell (see also Chapter 9).

The cell wall also permits the rapid differentiation of bacteria into two distinct groups: the gram-positive and the gram-negative bacteria. By following a simple procedure (see Gram's Staining Method, p. 416), use is made of a variance in the cell wall structure that results in a difference in permeability of the walls of the two groups of bacteria. Thus, after staining the bacteria with a crystal violet-iodine complex, the gram-positive bacteria will retain the dark purple stain when subsequently treated with alcohol; the gram-negative bacteria do not. Note that aging cells often lose their ability to retain the complex, so that older cultures of gram-positive bacteria may display gram-negative characteristics by this method.

THE CELL MEMBRANE

This is an elastic membrane situated directly underneath the cell wall. The cell membrane is semipermeable, allowing only certain substances to enter or leave the cell and barring others. Selective permeability is a highly complex process; we are only at the threshold of understanding it. A few general terms associated with this process should be understood:

a. *Endocytosis* is the term applied to any process by which the cell takes in any material from its environment.
b. *Phagocytosis* is the process by which a cell eats. The Greek "phago" means "to eat." Truly, phagocytosis is the process

by which the cell engulfs particles. These particles may
range from entire bacteria engulfed by certain white cells,
to portions of cells, small granules or macromolecules taken
in by some bacteria.

c. *Pinocytosis* is the process by which a cell engulfs tiny
droplets and substances dissolved therein. "Pinein" means
"to drink."

d. *Diffusion*—bacteria take in most of their nutritional requirements by simple diffusion. Membrane pores of about
7.5 Ångstroms (an Ångstrom is 0.1 nanometer) allow fluids,
basic elements and compounds smaller than that to enter
freely. Remember that simple diffusion continues until
both the intracellular and extracellular environments reach
an equilibrium in the concentration of whatever particles
are in solution. If particles are too large or are otherwise
barred from entry or departure, the cell will either take in
more water (when the concentration inside is greater), or
expel water (when the concentration outside is greater).
This may result in damage to the cell by either lysing
(bursting) or shrinkage. Because of the added protection of
the cell wall, the bacterial cell membrane is somewhat
restricted in its outward expansion.

Furthermore, simple diffusion is complemented by a
more complex process whereby certain enzymes produced
by the organism aid or inhibit the diffusion of many substances.

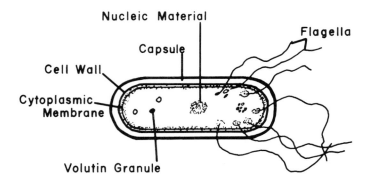

Fig. 5–3.   The bacterial cell.

e. *Expulsion or excretion*—most of the forementioned processes work both ways. Expulsion may be seen as reverse
pinocytosis, or any process by which the cell excretes
substances into its environment.

THE CAPSULE

Many bacteria are surrounded by a slime layer that is far less
rigid than the cell itself and is called a capsule. The thickness of
this capsule may range from undetectably narrow to several times
the diameter of the organism. The outer fringes of capsules are

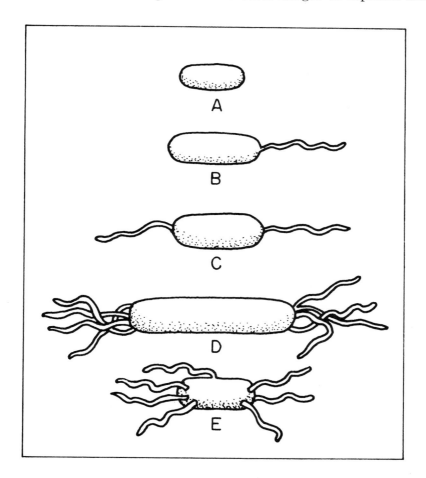

Fig. 5–4.   Different types of flagellation of bacteria. *A*, atrichous; *B*, monotrichous;
C, amphitrichous; *D*, lophotrichous; *E*, peritrichous.

difficult to determine unless aided by negative staining. Unstained, the capsule appears as a highly refractile halo surrounding the organism. Experience only will allow you eventually to distinguish between true capsules and the true halo produced by light diffraction under most light microscopes.

The capsule may act as a protective covering to combat phagocytosis or help to create an external storage depot of nutrients by adsorption.

THE FLAGELLA

These are threadlike processes that originate beneath the cell membrane. They are the organelles of locomotion and may be distributed indiscriminately over parts or over the entirety of the organism's surface. Organisms with only one flagellum at one pole are called monotrichous; those with one at each pole, amphitrichous; with a tuft of flagella at one or both poles, lophotrichous; and with flagella over the entire surface, peritrichous (see Fig. 5–4).

THE FIMBRIAE (Pila)

These hairlike structures are much shorter than flagella. They do not seem to take part in locomotion. The pila of some pathogens (such as gonococci) assist attachment to the host cells. They may also take part in genetic exchange between cells.

5-5 INTERNAL BACTERIAL STRUCTURES

Looking within the bacterial cell, which may be facilitated by staining, phase contrast microscopy, or electron microscopy, one may detect spores, granules or even smaller structures.

SPORES

These are refractile, poorly staining bodies. They are actually intermediary forms of the organism. Only a few types of bacteria are capable of forming into spores. When the going gets rough, when certain nutrients in the environment become exhausted, or when other environmental changes (temperature or pH) occur, the bacterium may build a protective core around its nucleic material. This core is able to survive changes in temperature and other harmful conditions that would kill the normal "vegetating" form. Upon entering a favorable environment, the spore "germinates" and develops into a normal vegetative bacterium.

When forming, spores may be located at certain areas of the bacterium. These locations, and the size of the spore in relation to

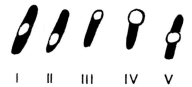

I   II   III   IV   V

Fig. 5–5.   Endospores, i, ii, iii, and exospores, iv, v. Figures i, v are central spores; iii and iv, terminal spores.

the width of the organism, are somewhat characteristic for certain species. Spores that extend beyond the width of the organism are called exospores, those that remain within the boundaries of the cell, endospores (see Fig. 5–5).

GRANULES

Large granules are evident in many bacterial cells. They may consist of phosphate complexes (volutin granules), or glycogen. They usually disappear when the organisms are transferred to a nutritionally poor medium and are therefore thought to serve as a food reserve. Many granules stain different colors with certain stains, and are thus called metachromatic granules.

MITOCHONDRIA

The chemical reactions that sustain life are many and varied. In the cells of plants and animals, certain areas are responsible for the completion of chemical reactions. These areas are particulate and known as mitochondria. Distinct mitochondria have not been demonstrated within the bacterial cell.

FURTHER READING

1. Brock, T. D.: *Biology of Microorganisms.* Englewood Cliffs, Prentice Hall, 1970.
2. Davis, B. D., *et al.: Microbiology,* 2nd ed. Hagerstown, Md., Harper & Row, 1973.

chapter 6
Culture, Growth and Development of Bacteria

The basic criteria to determine whether an organism is dead or alive are: Does it grow? Does it respire? Does it reproduce? Under favorable conditions, bacteria carry out all three of these functions.

In the previous chapters, we have briefly discussed the basic means of bacterial reproduction (see p. 58). In this chapter, we shall first discuss growth, then development, and finally, how both growth and development must be controlled or guided in order for us to cultivate bacteria in the laboratory.

We have already noted that bacterial physiology and biochemistry are closely interwoven disciplines. We shall not necessarily attempt to divorce one from the other here. The material covered in Section 6–1, however, is generally considered bacterial physiology; that of Section 6–2, biochemistry. Section 6–3 is an attempt to outline practical applications of both.

6-1 BACTERIAL GROWTH

Cells grow by absorbing nutrient materials, which they utilize as building blocks to produce new protoplasm. This aspect of growth is discussed more fully in Section 6–2.

When bacterial cells reach maturity—maximum size—they divide into two, and each daughter cell starts a new, independent "life."

We should point out that cell growth and division are cyclic processes and that when discussing bacterial growth, we usually refer to large populations rather than to individual organisms. In dealing with populations, then, we must realize that not all members of that population go through the same phase of the cycle at the same time. As some members divide, others may have reached only partial "maturity," whereas others still may find the going too rough and die. Being aware of these basic facts, we now consider how populations of bacteria generally behave.

THE BACTERIAL GROWTH CYCLE

The time lapse between the initial formation of a bacterium and its ultimate division into two daughter cells is referred to as *the generation time*. Generation time varies for different types of bacteria. It also varies for any one type of bacteria when the incubation temperature, the atmospheric conditions, or any other growth requirement is altered. Generation times of bacteria range from 20 minutes to several hours.

In the following discussion, let us assume that all possible variables remain relatively constant. Suppose then that we inoculate a certain number of a certain type of organism into a suitable medium in a flask. If we incubate this flask at a temperature and atmosphere optimally suitable for that organism, we will notice that during the first few hours, no cell division and consequently no increase in the number of viable organisms occur. (The estimation of viable numbers per 0.1 ml of broth culture is a relatively simple technique, discussed in Section 6–3.) During these first few hours, the cells are adjusting themselves to their new environment, increasing their metabolic rate, and building-up new protoplasm, all in readiness for a reproductive phase. This first period of adjustment and build up is known as *the lag phase*, because an expected increase in numbers seems to be lagging (see Fig. 6–1).

Assuming that optimal conditions prevail, the organisms multiply during the next phase, *the log phase*, at a rate governed by their minimum generation time. For most types of bacteria, this

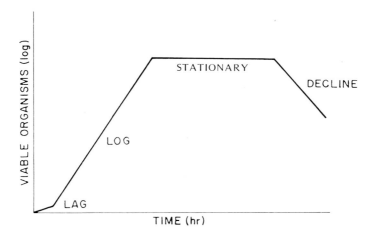

Fig. 6–1. The bacterial growth cycle.

means a doubling of the number of viable organisms every 20 minutes. This rate of growth is maintained as long as nutrients are abundantly available and the accumulation of toxic waste products is kept below a critical level. The log phase can be extended by adjusting the environment so that changes that would occur naturally are not allowed to develop. This may be effected by aeration of the medium, adjustment of the pH, aspiration and substitution of medium, or a combination of such means. When unchecked, the changing environment causes the culture to enter the next phase, *the stationary phase.*

During this third phase, the changing environment reaches a stage at which the number of organisms dying equals the number being reproduced. This phase is referred to as the stationary phase, because the number of viable organisms maintains an equilibrium.

The duration of this phase is determined by the rate of nutrient exhaustion and waste accumulation. It soon leads to the final phase, *the phase of decline.* During this fourth and final phase, the number of organisms dying exceeds that of the number being reproduced. This phase continues until all organisms in the culture have expired.*

___

*We did not speak of being killed, which is a different matter altogether (see Chapters 4 and 9).

THE BASIC GROWTH REQUIREMENTS OF BACTERIA

In the laboratory, we try to simulate as much as possible optimal growth requirements for any organism under study. These requirements vary tremendously from organism to organism. Generally, we may list the following requirements:

a. A suitable medium providing nutrients.
b. A suitable atmosphere.
c. A suitable osmotic pressure and pH.
d. A suitable temperature.
e. Moisture.

Specific media are discussed at length in Chapter 29 and in general terms in Sections 6–2 and 6–3. A *suitable atmosphere* may mean the presence or absence of oxygen, or the provision of other gaseous environments. In this respect, we must distinguish between:

a. *The obligate aerobes*, which cannot grow without oxygen.
b. *The obligate anaerobes*, which cannot grow in the presence of oxygen.
c. *The facultative anaerobes*, which can grow in either the presence or the absence of oxygen.

Some organisms also require other atmospheric conditions such as increased CO_2 or increased H_2S. Some rare bacteria, of no medical importance, require hydraulic pressures of up to 1000 inches of mercury in order to grow. These latter ones have been called barophilic.

A *suitable osmotic pressure* refers to the salt or sugar concentration of the media. Some bacteria are said to be *halophilic*, because they require a minimum of 10% of salt, NaCl, to grow. Staphylococci, on the other hand are said to be *haloduric;* they withstand, or endure, salt concentrations of up to 10%. Most other bacteria would die at these salt concentrations and prefer concentrations of 0.9% sodium chloride. The so-called *osmophilic* bacteria can grow only in the presence of at least 70% sugar, whereas most other bacteria, mainly those responsible for food spoilage, will not survive sugar concentrations of 50% or more.

A suitable pH refers to the hydrogen ion concentration, which must be regulated with appropriate buffers (see p. 18).

The most suitable temperature varies also from the *psychrophils*, organisms that grow only at temperatures lower than room temperatures, to the *mesophils*, which grow best at temperatures from 15°C to 45°C, and the *thermophils,* which grow only at temperatures above 45°C.

Moisture is one requirement all living things seem to have in common. Without water, no organism can develop. Some other peculiarities have been noted with respect to light requirements. Whereas most bacteria grow best in the dark, some can grow only in the presence of light; these are said to be *photogenic.* Some bacteria produce pigments only in the presence of light, the *photochromogens;* others produce pigments only in the dark, the *scotochromogens.*

6-2 BACTERIAL DEVELOPMENT

In the previous section, we concerned ourselves mainly with the general relationship of bacterial cells to their environment, and the influence a changing environment has on the increase, or decrease, of a viable bacterial population. In this section, we consider the chemical changes within the bacterial cell, and how some of these changes alter the environment.

METABOLISM AND ENERGY PRODUCTION

Numerous chemical activities take place within each bacterial cell. Basically, these chemical reactions are of two types:

a. *Catabolism*—the breakdown of products presented to the cell into simpler substances.
b. *Anabolism*—the formation of new products from these broken-down products.

Of course, both catabolism and anabolism occur simultaneously. The combined process is referred to as *metabolism.* The speed at which metabolism occurs is referred to as the *metabolic rate.* The metabolic rate is at its peak under optimal conditions, and it decreases when conditions deteriorate.

Catabolism usually releases energy and anabolism uses it. But what is energy, and how do you measure it? Energy is a capacity to do work. From the bacterium's point of view, energy is the capacity to drive biochemical reactants to produce the desired end products required to make more bacterial protein. There are two kinds of energy:

a. kinetic energy, which is energy in motion, or active energy;
b. potential energy, which is energy at rest, or stored energy.

Basically, energy is never lost. It may be stored in chemical compounds and released in the breakdown of such compounds. It may also be taken up again by the formation of new chemical compounds. Chemical reactions that release energy, as in catabolism, are said to be *exergonic*; those that store energy, as in anabolism, are called *endergonic*.

Energy is usually measured in *calories*. One calorie is the amount of energy required to increase the temperature of one gram of pure water by one degree centigrade. Plants, and some bacteria, can utilize the radiant energy from the sun to produce glucose and oxygen from carbon dioxide and water:

$$6 \ CO_2 + 6H_2O + 688,500 \ Cal \rightarrow C_6H_{12}O_6 + 6O_2$$

Bacteria that can utilize simple inorganic compounds and build these into carbohydrates and protein are called *autotrophs*. Unfortunately for us, most bacteria of medical importance are *heterotrophs*. They require more complex organic compounds as a source of carbon, and a more complex, biochemically that is, source of energy.

How is energy stored between catabolic and anabolic reactions? This mystery was solved when the process of cellular *phosphorylation* was unravelled. *Adenosine triphosphate* (ATP) is found in most living cells. It may be seen as a store of chemical energy, since the rupture of its anhydride linkage will release 8000 cal/mole:

$$ATP + H_2O \rightleftharpoons ADP + PH_2O_4 + 8000 \ calories.$$

From the equation, it can be seen that the reaction is reversible. In fact, both ATP and ADP *(adenosine diphosphate)* act as relay stations within the cell. ADP stores both phosphates and energy in the process of conversion to ATP, and ATP releases both energy and phosphates the other way around. You may also have noted that water is needed for the release of energy from ATP, which partially explains the requirement for moisture as earlier stated.

NUTRITIONAL REQUIREMENTS

Let us suppose that we have provided an optimal environment for a particular type of bacterium. What will happen to the nutrients within the medium?

The most important single point you should remember is that whatever happens to any medium depends as much on the composition of the medium as it does on the organisms we put into the medium. We must ensure that:

a. The medium contains all the ingredients called for.
b. The ingredients are not altered during preparation or storage of the medium.
c. The medium does not become contaminated by unspecified ingredients or organisms.

What are some of the ingredients we may incorporate in bacterial media? Chapter 29 outlines many different media, all of which serve some specific purpose. As we are now concerned only with the development of bacteria in general, we shall use as an example a nutrient medium that will allow most bacteria to grow. Such a medium should contain:

a. *Water*, which serves both as a solvent and as a transport medium for both nutrients and byproducts.
b. *Vitamins*. Bacteria have a definite need for vitamin B, which acts as an enzyme or coenzyme (a biochemical catalyst). Because of this catalytic activity, the supply of vitamins need be minimal.
c. *Carbohydrates*, which serve primarily as a source of carbon and secondarily as a source of energy, both through the process of glycolysis. There are three main groups of carbohydrates:
1. *Monosaccharides* $(C_6H_{12}O_6)$. These are the simple sugars such as glucose and fructose. They are water-soluble and can be utilized directly by most bacteria.
2. *Disaccharides* $(C_{12}H_{22}O_{11})$. These "double" sugars, such as sucrose and lactose, must be broken down to monosaccharides before bacteria can utilize them. Several bacteria produce enzymes that facilitate this breakdown, which is called hydrolysis.

$$C_{12}H_{22}O_{11} + H_2O \rightarrow 2C_6H_{12}O_6$$

3. *Polysaccharides* $(C_6H_{10}O_5)_x$. These are generally insoluble in water. Starch, glycogen, and cellulose are prime examples of polysaccharides. The molecules of many of these substances are so large that they cannot diffuse into the bacteria. Only bacteria that produce and excrete enzymes (*exoenzymes*) capable of facilitating partial external hydrolysis of these polysaccharides are able to utilize them at all.

d. *Amino acids,* which are built from amino (NH_2) and carboxyl (COOH) groups. By linking amino groups of one amino acid to carboxyl groups of others, peptides are formed. Several peptides linked together form polypeptides; several polypeptides form proteins. In order to build any protein at all, the heterotrophic bacteria must be supplied with ready-made amino acids, or with peptides, polypeptides, or proteins that can be degraded into the required amino acids.

Amino Acid Metabolism. The simplest amino acid is glycine:

$$NH_2\text{—}CH_2\text{—}COOH$$

Each amino acid has one amino group and one carboxyl group that are free; that is, by which they can enter into chemical reactions. Moreover, many amino acids have in addition another amino or carboxyl group that is free, or some other functional group free:

$$Lysine:\ NH_2\text{—}CH\text{—}COOH$$
$$|$$
$$CH_2\text{—}CH_2\text{—}CH_2\text{—}CH_2\text{—}NH_2$$

Glutamic acid:
$$NH_2\text{—}CH\text{—}COOH$$
$$|$$
$$CH_2\text{—}CH_2\text{—}COOH$$

The linkage of two or more amino acids to form peptides results in the release of water.

$$NH_2\text{—}CHR_1\text{—}COOH + NHH\text{—}CHR_2\text{—}COOH \longrightarrow$$
$$NH_2\text{—}CHR_1\text{—}CO\text{—}NH\text{—}CHR_2\text{—}COOH + H_2O$$

R_1 represents amino acid one, or its intermediate chain; R_2, amino acid two. On closer examination, we can see that the first amino acid has been *decarboxylated* and the second has been *deaminated* in the process.

Bacterial enzymes can build amino acids into peptides and these peptides further into bacterial proteins. As we said earlier, most bacteria must be presented with amino acids, peptides or proteins, in order to be able to build bacterial proteins. They do not necessarily have to be presented with the exact amino acids required to build their specific proteins. When presented with the "wrong kinds" of amino acids, bacteria can often convert them into the required kinds. Let us examine a few such conversions:

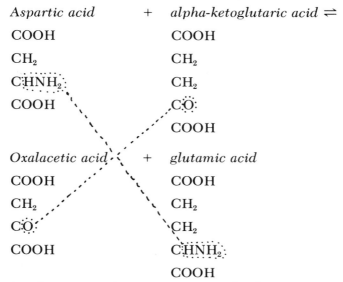

In the above example, an amino group has been removed from
aspartic acid and shifted to alpha-ketoglutaric acid, producing
oxalacetic acid and the "new" amino acid, glutamic acid. This
process is known as *transamination*. In transamination, one amino
acid loses an amino group (deamination), and another amino acid
gains an amino group (amination).

Many amino acids can be broken down by deamination, or by
decarboxylation (the removal of a carboxyl group), without the
formation of "new" or other amino acids:

Aspartic acid ⇌ Fumaric acid + Ammonia

$$\begin{array}{lll}
\text{COOH} & \text{COOH} & \\
\text{CHH} & \text{CH} & \\
\text{CHNH}_2 & \text{CH} & \text{NH}_3 \\
\text{COOH} & \text{COOH} &
\end{array}$$

Here, the aspartic acid is simply deaminated with the production of
fumaric acid and ammonia. Since this reaction is reversible, it is
obvious that amino acids can also be created from simpler substances.

Lysine ⟶ Cadaverine + Carbon dioxide

$$\begin{array}{lll}
\text{R} & \text{R} & \\
\text{CHNH}_2 & \text{CHNH}_2 & \\
\text{HOOC} & \text{H} & \text{CO}_2
\end{array}$$

Above, the amino acid *lysine* has been decarboxylated into
cadaverine and carbon dioxide.

Bacteria can utilize either simple deamination or simple decarboxylation reactions to stabilize their cellular pH or the pH of the medium. Many bacteria are capable of breaking down various amino acids into many different products. A technologist can often identify the organism under study by presenting the organism with a specific amino acid, knowing how the organism might change that amino acid, and then applying tests to detect the products of that expected change. For example, knowing the process of simple deamination of aspartic acid, one may present an organism with a medium containing only that amino acid. By checking the end result—ammonia production—we have a very simple means of estimating the organism's ability to deaminate this amino acid. Various other fairly simple tests have thus been developed (see Chapters 29 and 31).

Carbohydrate Metabolism. So far, we have discussed how bacteria can utilize amino acids to build proteins for the propagation of bacteria. We have also seen how we can utilize amino acids to effect changes in the medium, by which changes we can then characterize unknown bacteria. We have further discussed water, vitamin, and carbohydrate utilization by bacteria. We deferred our discussion on carbohydrate metabolism to the end of this section because it allows us to explain the origin of a number of cellular products hitherto unmentioned. Carbohydrate metabolism is a difficult subject, and this is only a brief synopsis of that process.

Carbohydrates are the principal, and often the only source of carbon from which bacterial carbohydrates, lipids, amino acids and all other organic substances are synthesized. In addition, carbohydrates are oxidized to supply the main source of energy for the cell.

We shall follow the use of glucose as an example, since most bacteria can utilize glucose directly. Glucose ingested by bacteria reacts with ATP (adenosine triphosphate) to form glucose-6-phosphate. From this point, three alternate pathways are possible (see Fig. 6–2):

a. Glucose-6-phosphate may be converted to glucose-1-phosphate, which is required for the production of polysaccharides such as glycogen and mucopolysaccharides found in capsules and the cell wall.

b. Glucose-6-phosphate may be oxidized to pyruvic acid by way of the fructose-6-phosphate path. From pyruvic acid, an array of different products may be produced, such as lactic acid, acetic acid, formic acid, propionic acid, ethanol, butanol, isopropanol, methanol, and many others.

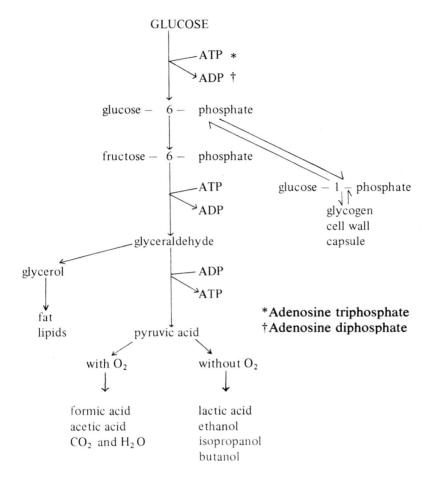

Fig. 6–2. Simplified pathways of glucose metabolism.

c. Glucose-6-phosphate is converted to glyceraldehyde (an intermediate product preceding formation of pyruvic acid). Glyceraldehyde is then converted into lipids (fats).

CELLULAR OXIDATION

Oxidation is the process by which energy is released through the transfer of electrons from one chemical reactant to another. While such chemical reactions primarily involve oxygen, elements other than oxygen may be the principal reactants. In strict chemical terms, oxidation may take at least three forms:

a. $X + O_2 \rightarrow XO_2$, in which case substance X is oxidized by combining with the oxygen.

b. $XH_2 \rightarrow X + H_2$, in which case substance X is oxidized by dehydrogenation, removal of the hydrogen.

c. $X^{++} + Y^{++} \rightarrow X^+ + Y^{+++}$, in which case substance X is oxidized by the loss of an electron.

In all of these cases, substance X lost electrons.

All living cells obtain their energy primarily through oxidation. This cellular process is often called respiration. However, in bacteriology, the term "respiration" has been given a narrower meaning—it simply refers to those energy-yielding reactions in which free oxygen is the ultimate acceptor of electrons. Therefore, it would always be an aerobic process. Thus, we will always refer to aerobic bacterial oxidation as *respiration*, and to anaerobic bacterial oxidation as *fermentation* (see Fig. 6–3). All you really need to remember is that if oxygen does not take part in oxidation, we speak of fermentation.

If you further remember that vitamins, carbohydrates, amino acids and other assortments of ingredients may all be found in a single bacteriological medium, and that any or all of the reactions mentioned, plus several others, may all go on simultaneously within a flask or test tube, you will be well-prepared to meet some of the difficulties you will undoubtedly experience in the laboratory.

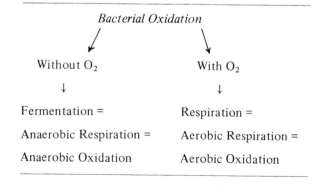

Fig. 6–3. Terminology applied to bacterial oxidation.

6-3 THE CULTURE OF BACTERIA

So far, we have discussed how bacteria grow and what they need to develop. In this section, we are concerned with how we can provide the required conditions to allow a culture to grow. A culture is a growth or cultivation of any organism. A pure culture contains only one type of bacterium; a mixed culture contains two or more different types of organisms.

Most specimens sent to laboratories for analysis contain mixtures of different organisms. A prime function is to isolate these different organisms in pure cultures. Only then can reliable assays of microorganisms be made.

METHODS TO OBTAIN PURE CULTURES

The Dilution Method. By diluting mixed cultures in broth, a final dilution will ultimately be reached that will contain only one type of organism. This method of separating organisms is useful only when the sought-after organism is present in greater numbers than all other types of organisms combined. To visualize the difficulties and limitations of this method, consider this example: A bag contains 200 red marbles, 100 blue ones, 50 green ones and 10 yellow ones. A total of 360 right? Now, without looking into the bag, try to pick out first 180, then 90, 45, 22, 6, 3 and finally the last two marbles, one by one. How often will this exercise result in a final red marble being pulled from the bag? How often a yellow one?

The Plating Method. We have already briefly mentioned the pure culture technique developed by Koch (see Chapter 2). By incorporating a solidifying agent such as agar into a liquid medium, a solid gel will form after the medium is poured into a Petri dish while still warm (above 45°C) and allowing it to cool. By spreading a tiny portion of a specimen, or a tiny drop of a mixed broth culture over the surface of this plate, distinct colonies will develop on the surface of the plate. Colonies, you remember, are the descendants of a single bacterium grouped together in a visible "heap."

Different spreading methods or patterns are in vogue. An easy and effective method may be carried out as follows:

    a. Use a thin platinum wire, or loop, to transfer specimen or culture. This wire or loop may be conveniently sterilized between manipulations by holding it in a Bunsen flame until red hot.

    b. Spread the inoculum, culture or specimen thinly over a small area of the plate.

Fig. 6–4.   Plating technique for isolating colonies.

c. From this area, dilute the inoculum by running a series of streaks from that area over the remaining area of the plate in a predetermined pattern (see Fig. 6–4).

Since the idea is to dilute the inoculum, run the streaks only one way, and prevent touching any streaks already laid down as you go along. If the inoculum contains relatively few bacteria, isolated colonies will appear along the first streaks.

The experienced bacteriologist can differentiate between many bacteria just by looking at the colonies. Some of the colonial characteristics he would recognize are illustrated in Figures 6–5 and 6–6. Others are:

a. *Consistency:* the colony may be butyrous, mucoid, slimy or friable (crumble).
b. *Transparency:* the colony may be transparent, translucent or opaque.
c. *Pigmentation:* all shades of colors may be produced by different cultures.

Selective Inhibition Methods. In medical bacteriology, we can often be fairly selective in our approach when trying to isolate pathogens from certain specimens (see Chapters 24 and 25). When we know which bacteria we do not wish to isolate, we can create conditions that will prevent these undesirable bacteria from growing. (Unfortunately, those methods that prevent the unwanted organisms from growing may inhibit the ones we are after as well.) Furthermore, technologists often forget that, although many inhibitory conditions prevent the growth of several bacteria they wish to eliminate, few conditions actually destroy these bacteria. Consequently, they often regard as "pure" cultures many mixtures consisting of apparently pure colonies that are growing over other types of viable bacteria. When transferring the "colony" plus the underlying contaminants to another medium for further assay of the "colony," the results will naturally be unreliable.

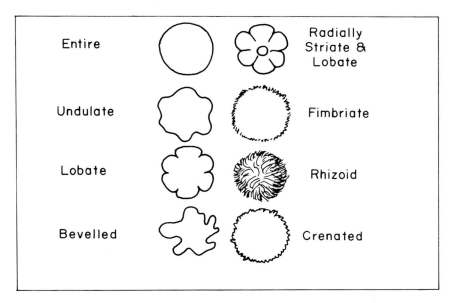

Fig. 6–5. Periphery differences of bacterial colonies.

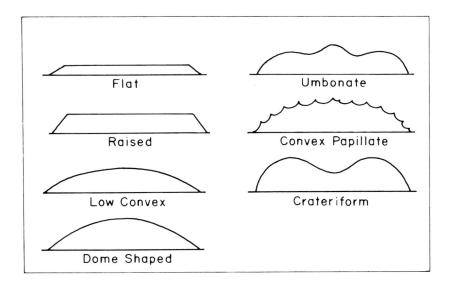

Fig. 6–6. Elevation differences of bacterial colonies.

Regardless of these disadvantages, several selective inhibition methods give excellent results when carefully used. Some selective inhibition methods commonly employed are:

   a. Growth at high or low temperatures for isolation of thermophils and psychrophils respectively.
   b. Anaerobic or aerobic incubation to exclude aerobes and anaerobes respectively.
   c. Variation of pH.
   d. Incorporation of specific inhibitors such as antibiotics, antisera, and various chemicals. For example, bile salts inhibit many gram-positive bacteria.

ANAEROBIC CULTURE

A number of different methods have been employed in the anaerobic culture of bacteria. The following are some of the more popular.

Liquid media, such as thioglycolate broth, cooked meat broth and others, may serve to culture most anaerobes, but are practical only when relatively fresh (see Chapter 29).

Spray's dish is a specially designed two-compartment jar on which the bottom of a Petri dish fits snugly. The two compartments are separated by a low ridge on the bottom of the jar.

One gram of pyrogallic acid is placed in one of the compartments, and 10 ml of 2.5 M NaOH in the other. The Petri dish bottom containing the seeded agar medium is inverted over the jar, and the jar is tilted gently to mix the NaOH with the acid. The resulting chemical reaction produces enough hydrogen to consume all the oxygen in the jar. This method allows a rapid set-up of one culture plate at a time. It is of some advantage in the busy lab when a specimen arriving late could otherwise necessitate the disturbance of cultures previously set up in larger batches (see Gaspak jars).

*Gaspak jars** have quickly replaced the more conventional Torbal jars. With the Torbal jars, oxygen is replaced by hydrogen with the aid of a vacuum pump, a hydrogen source, and an internal catalyst. The Gaspak jar follows a principle similar to that employed in Spray's technique, with the added benefit of disposable reagent packages and a large jar to accommodate up to ten plates at a time.

To a disposable Gaspak, 10 ml of water are carefully added. The Gaspak and an indicator are placed with the cultures in the jar,

_____

*Registered trademark, Baltimore Biological Laboratories, Cockeysville, Md.

and the lid is closed. A catalyst that works at room temperature activates a chemical reaction between the water and the magnesium and zinc chloride contained in the Gaspak envelope, thereby consuming all the oxygen within the jar in approximately 30 minutes. Detailed literature is available from the manufacturer on request.

In anaerobic culture, it is mandatory that culture media be reduced (kept free of oxygen) as much as possible. Plated media are particularly difficult to maintain in the reduced state; they may require re-reducing before setting up an anaerobic culture. A simple, though relatively costly, method of reducing plated media is to place them in an activated Gaspak jar for a few hours prior to inoculation. Special reducible plated media are available commercially, along with a simple apparatus that allows the reduction of large numbers of plates in a more economic fashion.†

VIABLE COUNT CULTURE

A fairly simple technique may be followed to estimate the number of viable bacteria in a fluid specimen or culture.

Dilutions of the sample may be made in sterile broth in 1-ml doubling or tenfold dilutions. Each 1 ml of diluted specimen may then be mixed with melted agar medium at 45°C, and the mixture poured into a sterile Petri dish. Upon suitable incubation, viable bacteria will develop into detectable colonies that will be embedded in the medium. By counting the number of colonies produced, and by multiplying these with the dilution factor, exact counts of the number of viable bacteria present in 1 ml of the original specimen may be ascertained.

FURTHER READING

1. Davis, B. D. *et al.: Microbiology*, 2nd ed. Chapters 3–5, Hagerstown, Harper & Row, 1973.
2. Holdeman, L. V., and Moore, W. E. C. (eds.): *Anaerobe Laboratory Manual*. 4th ed. Blacksburg, Va., Virginia Polytechnic Institute, 1977.

†Robbin Reducible Media Plates, Scott Laboratories, Inc., New York, N.Y., 10036.

chapter 7
Classification of Microbes

7-1 EARLY ATTEMPTS IN CLASSIFYING LIVING THINGS

A brief review of early attempts at classifying living things may help us to understand more clearly some of the difficulties that still plague us today.

Little attention was paid to biologic classification until the sixteenth century. In 1583, Cesalpino produced his "De Plantis," which established botany as an independent science. During the next two centuries, classifying living things became fashionable, and a variety of systems and an even greater variety of names came into being.

In the mid-eighteenth century, Carl von Linne, a Swedish count, set out to shape order among the various systems. He made popular the binary Latin naming of all living things, as first proposed by J. Bauhin in the late 1500s. In 1758, Linnaeus published his *Systema Natura* which was an attempt to classify all living things. When Linnaeus came upon the "wee little beasties," however, he gave up in despair and simply said: "They are too small, too confused, no one will ever know anything exact about them, we will simply put them in the class of *Chaos*." If he put a curse on the subject, it has certainly been most effective, as the classification of microbes is still a subject of much debate.

7-2 CLASSIFICATION SYSTEMS

The study of systems by which living organisms are placed in a distinct rank or group is called taxonomy. A rank or group is referred to as a *taxon* (plural *taxa*). The scientific naming of living things is called *nomenclature*. Basically, there are three systems by which living things may be classified: natural, artificial, and phylogenetic classifications.

NATURAL CLASSIFICATIONS

These are based on the order believed to occur in nature. Obviously, it is difficult to state objectively what the natural order of microorganisms should be. Until we know far more about the various microorganisms than we do at present, we shall not be able to classify them on purely natural grounds.

ARTIFICIAL CLASSIFICATIONS

These are based on any convenient characteristics that may differentiate one organism, or for that matter any one item, from another. Artificial classifications, therefore, are subjective. An example of extreme subjectivity in classifying items is the index of this book, in which the only criteria for differentiation are the letters of the alphabet.

PHYLOGENETIC CLASSIFICATIONS

These are based on the evolutionary history of groups of organisms, and should convey their evolutionary relationships to other groups. Phylogeny, at best, is presumptive. Furthermore, microorganisms were around long before mankind, but failed to leave any fossilized relics. Classifying microorganisms by phylogeny is therefore not only impractical but simply impossible.

It should be obvious by now that classifying living things, particularly microorganisms, is not a simple matter, and that microbes can only be classified according to a highly artificial system.

7-3 CLASSIFYING MICROBES

The classifications of many microorganisms leave much to be desired. The main reasons for our present difficulties may be stated as follows:

    a. Microbiologists have usually been far more interested in what microorganisms can do and what they look like than in what taxon they should belong or by what name they should be called.
    b. Microbiology has never gone through a definite descriptive phase.
    c. Names, where applied, were often chosen for convenience only and were seldom based on rules of classification or nomenclature. Hence, a variety of names have been given to many identical organisms.
    d. Many microorganisms lack the criteria used to classify the higher forms of life.

You have by now surmised that we will run into some difficulties in our attempts to classify microorganisms. These difficulties are compounded by the fact that microbes may belong to either one of Linnaeus' main taxa, the plant and animal kingdoms, main differences of which were discussed in Section 5-1. It is presently commonly accepted that a third main taxon be established, the Protista, composed of organisms of relatively simple organization. The Kingdom Protista would contain the protozoa, fungi, algae, yeasts, bacteria and rickettsias. This would still leave the viruses as a distinct entity. A further division of the Protista would create the Subkingdom Eucaryotae, composed of the truly nucleated, higher protists such as the protozoa, the fungi, and most algae; and the Subkingdom Procaryotae, containing the blue-green algae, most yeasts and the bacteria (including the rickettsias).

Mainly for convenience, we shall continue to refer to protozoa as animals and defer their treatment to Chapter 23. From a medical diagnostic point of view, fungi and yeast may also best be lumped together, and they are discussed in Chapter 22. The viruses are covered in Chapter 21. The algae are of no medical interest and therefore are not further mentioned. The classification of bacteria warrants a more careful analysis and is dealt with in the next section, where we will also further elaborate on the general principles of nomenclature and taxonomy.

7-4 CLASSIFYING BACTERIA

The classification and naming of the bacteria is governed by a Committee of the International Association of Microbiological Societies. The Committee meets at least once every four years to consider changes that may have been proposed, in the interim period, to the International Code of Nomenclature of Bacteria.

The first general consideration of the latest International Code of Nomenclature of Bacteria reads:

> Progress of bacteriology can be furthered by a precise system of nomenclature which is properly integrated with the systems used by botanists, zoologists and virologists, and accepted by the majority of bacteriologists in all nations. The Code applies to bacteria and related organisms. Botanical and zoological codes now provide, and a virological code when approved will provide, for the nomenclature of certain other microbial groups such as fungi, algae, protozoa and viruses.

The Code is based on twelve firmly stated principles that become workable by adhering to the accompanying rules.

The main principles that are applicable to diagnostic medical microbiology are stated as follows:

a. To aim at fixity of names.
b. To avoid or to reject the use of names that may cause error or ambiguity or throw science into confusion.
c. Scientific names of all taxa are usually taken from Latin or Greek. The classical Latin rules for latinization of Greek and other non-Latin words should be followed.
d. Every individual is treated as belonging to a number of categories of consecutive rank and consecutively subordinate; of these the species is the basic one. The principal categories in ascending sequence are species, genus, family, order, class, division (see Table 7–1).
e. Each category or rank is called a taxon. The word group should be used sparingly, preferably only to designate related serotypes.
f. The primary purpose of giving a name to a taxon is simply to supply a name to refer to it and not to describe the characteristics or the history of its members.

These and several other principles have led to the following applications: 1. each distinct kind of bacterium is called a

Table 7-1. A presentation of the various taxa designated by the International Committee on Nomenclature of Bacteria

I*	II	III	IV	V
Division				
	Subdivision			
Class				
	Subclass			
Order				
	Suborder			
Family				
	Subfamily			
		Tribe		
			Subtribe	
Genus				
	Subgenus			
			Section	
				Series
Species				
	Subspecies			
		Variety		

*Only those taxa listed in columns I and III are commonly used in the classification of bacteria encountered in the diagnosis of infectious diseases of man.

species; 2. each species is given a name that consists of two words, e.g., *Bacillus subtilis*. The first word, *Bacillus*, is the generic title, and it is always written with a capital letter. It is the name of the genus to which the species belongs. It is a Latin or latinized noun, and regardless of its derivation, it must be treated as a Latin name.

The generic title usually describes the morphology of the organism, though this is not a necessity; for example: *Bacillus*—small rod; *Sarcina*—packet or bundle; *Micrococcus*—small grain; *Clostridium*—small spindle. Other generic titles have been given in honor of persons or places (*Borrelia, Pasteurella*), but all have been latinized. The genus name is a noun in the singular. It is not a collective noun and should never be used in the plural.

The second word is the species epithet and should never be capitalized. It is usually, but not necessarily, an adjective modifying the generic title; for example: *Staphylococcus albus*—the white *Staphylococcus; Clostridum welchii*—Welch's *Clostridium.*

GENERAL TERMINOLOGY

At this stage, the general terminology applied to the taxa used in the classification of bacteria and other organisms is defined further.

Species: The basic unit of classification. A species consists of a group of individuals with certain dominant characteristics in common.

> a. A *variety* is sometimes called subspecies. Some members of species, although their dominant characteristics are the same, differ enough to warrant further subdivision, e.g., *Corynebacterium diphtheriae*, variety *gravis*, etc.
> b. A *strain* is a pure culture of bacteria derived from a single isolation. Each pure culture that has a different source or time of origin constitutes a separate strain; for example, no two isolates are alike—all constitute different strains.
> c. A *clone* is a culture composed of the descendants of a single cell.
> d. When a new species is first described, the original culture is termed the *type culture*.

Genus (plural, genera). A group of closely related species. Genera that include only one species are said to be monotypic genera. *Type species* is chosen to represent a genus; in other words, it has all the characteristics considered typical of that particular genus.

Family. A group of closely related genera. A family name usually consists of the stem of the name of its earliest known genus plus the suffix *aceae*.

> a. *Type genus* is chosen to represent the typical characteristics of a family.
> b. *Tribe*—some genera of families vary enough to warrant further division between the family and genus ranks. Thus, tribes are groups of closely related genera. The name of a tribe is usually derived from the stem of the name of its earliest known genus plus the suffix *-eae*.

Order. A group of closely related families. The name of an order is also derived from the stem of the name of its earliest known genus and the suffix *-ales*.*

---

*The suffix for suborder is *-ineae*; for subfamily, *-oideae*; and for subtribe, *-inae*.

Class. A group of related orders. In one classification system, all bacteria and related forms are considered to belong to one class, the Schizomycetes.

CLASSIFICATION

Although the principles of taxonomy and nomenclature are objective in nature, the actual classification of bacteria remains a relatively subjective procedure. The principal guide in bacterial classification is *Bergey's Manual of Determinative Bacteriology.* The Introduction to the eighth edition of this Manual reads in part: "The Manual is meant to assist in the identification of bacteria. No attempt has been made to provide a complete hierarchy, ... because a complete and meaningful hierarchy is impossible. Instead the Manual is presented in 19 parts based on a few readily determined criteria."

The main criteria as far as medical bacteriology is concerned are:

    a. Physical growth requirements
    b. Main morphologic differences
    c. Fundamental staining reactions
    d. Ability to produce spores
    e. Biochemical and metabolic activities
    f. Antigenic structure and reactivity

As a general overview of bacteriology, Table 7–2 lists all the genera within their respective taxa; those genera of medical importance are printed in boldface. In the ensuing chapters, we shall endeavor to present the medically significant bacteria as orderly as possible, and within the general framework of the eighth edition of *Bergey's Manual of Determinative Bacteriology.*

Table 7–2. The bacteria

Part 1. Phototrophic Bacteria	Genus IX. *Amoebobacter*
Order I. Rhodospirillales	Genus X. *Ectothiorhodospira*
Family I. Rhodospirillaceae	Family III. Chlorobiaceae
Genus I. *Rhodospirillum*	Genus I. *Chlorobium*
Genus II. *Rhodopseudomonas*	Genus II. *Prosthecochloris*
Genus III. *Rhodomicrobium*	Genus III. *Chloropseudomonas*
Family II. Chromatiaceae	Genus IV. *Pelodictyon*
Genus I. *Chromatium*	Genus V. *Clathrochloris*
Genus II. *Thiocystis*	
Genus III. *Thiosarcina*	Part 2. Gliding Bacteria
Genus IV. *Thiospirillum*	Order I. Myxobacterales
Genus V. *Thiocapsa*	Family I. Myxococcaceae
Genus VI. *Lamprocystis*	Genus I. **Myxococcus**
Genus VII. *Thiodictyon*	Family II. Archangiaceae
Genus VIII. *Thiopedia*	Genus II. *Archangium*

Table 7–2. *(cont.)*

Family III. Cystobacteraceae
    Genus I.   *Cystobacter*
    Genus II.   *Melittangium*
    Genus III.   *Stigmatella*
Family IV. Polyangiaceae
    Genus I.   *Polyangium*
    Genus II.   *Nannocystis*
    Genus III.   *Chondromyces*
Order II. Cytophagales
  Family I. Cytophagaceae
    Genus I.   *Cytophaga*
    Genus II.   *Flexibacter*
    Genus III.   *Herpetosiphon*
    Genus IV.   *Flexithrix*
    Genus V.   *Saprospira*
    Genus VI.   *Sporocytophaga*
  Family II. Beggiatoaceae
    Genus I.   *Beggiatoa*
    Genus II.   *Vitreoscilla*
    Genus III.   *Thioploca*
  Family III. Simonsiellaceae
    Genus I.   *Simonsiella*
    Genus II.   *Alysiella*
  Family IV. Leucotrichaceae
    Genus I.   *Leucothrix*
    Genus II.   *Thiothrix*
Families and Genera of Uncertain
Affiliation:
    Genus   *Toxothrix*
  Family Achromatiaceae
    Genus   *Achromatium*
  Family Pelonemataceae
    Genus   *Pelonema*
    Genus   *Achroonema*
    Genus   *Peloploca*
    Genus   *Desmanthos*
Part 3. Sheathed Bacteria
    Genus   *Sphaerotilus*
    Genus   *Leptothrix*
    Genus   *Streptothrix*
    Genus   *Lieskeella*
    Genus   *Phragmidiothrix*
    Genus   *Crenothrix*
    Genus   *Clonothrix*
Part 4. Budding and Appendaged
Bacteria
    Genus   *Hyphomicrobium*
    Genus   *Hyphomonas*
    Genus   *Pedomicrobium*
    Genus   *Caulobacter*
    Genus   *Asticcacaulis*
    Genus   *Ancalomicrobium*
    Genus   *Prosthecomicrobium*
    Genus   *Thiodendron*
    Genus   *Pasteuria*

    Genus   *Blastobacter*
    Genus   *Seliberia*
    Genus   *Gallionella*
    Genus   *Nevskia*
    Genus   *Planctomyces*
    Genus   *Metallogenium*
    Genus   *Caulococcus*
    Genus   *Kusnezovia*

Part 5. Spirochetes
  Order I. Spirochaetales
    Family I. Spirochaetaceae
    Genus I.   *Spirochaeta*
    Genus II.   *Cristispira*
    Genus III.   ***Treponema***
    Genus IV.   ***Borrelia***
    Genus V.   ***Leptospira***
Part 6. Spiral and Curved Bacteria
  Family I. Spirillaceae
    Genus I.   *Spirillum*
    Genus II.   *Campylobacter*
Genera of Uncertain Affiliation
    Genus   *Bdellovibrio*
    Genus   *Microcyclus*
    Genus   *Pelosigma*
    Genus   *Brachyarcus*

**Part 7. Gram-Negative Aerobic Rods and
Cocci**
  Family I. Pseudomonadaceae
    Genus I.   ***Pseudomonas***
    Genus II.   *Xanthomonas*
    Genus III.   *Zoogloea*
    Genus IV.   *Gluconobacter*
  Family II. Azotobacteraceae
    Genus I.   *Azotobacter*
    Genus II.   *Azomonas*
    Genus III.   *Beijerinckia*
    Genus IV.   *Derxia*
  Family III. Rhizobiaceae
    Genus I.   *Rhizobium*
    Genus II.   *Agrobacterium*
  Family IV. Methylomonadaceae
    Genus I.   *Methylomonas*
    Genus II.   *Methylococcus*
  Family V. Halobacteriaceae
    Genus I.   *Halobacterium*
    Genus II.   *Halococcus*
Genera of Uncertain Affiliation
    Genus   *Alcaligenes*
    Genus   *Acetobacter*
    Genus   ***Brucella***
    Genus   ***Bordetella***
    Genus   ***Francisella***
    Genus   *Thermus*

Table 7–2. *(cont.)*

Part 8. Gram-Negative
Facultatively Anaerobic Rods
    Family I. Enterobacteriaceae
        Genus I.   *Escherichia*
        Genus II.   *Edwardsiella*
        Genus III.   *Citrobacter*
        Genus IV.   *Salmonella*
        Genus V.   *Shigella*
        Genus VI.   *Klebsiella*
        Genus VII.   *Enterobacter*
        Genus VIII. *Hafnia*
        Genus IX.   *Serratia*
        Genus X.   *Proteus*
        Genus XI.   *Yersinia*
        Genus XII. *Erwinia*
    Family II. Vibrionaceae
        Genus I.   *Vibrio*
        Genus II.   *Aeromonas*
        Genus III.   *Plesiomonas*
        Genus IV.   *Photobacterium*
        Genus V.   *Lucibacterium*
  Genera of Uncertain Affiliation
        Genus   *Zymomonas*
        Genus   *Chromobacterium*
        Genus   *Flavobacterium*
        Genus   *Haemophilus*
        Genus   *Pasteurella*
        Genus   *Actinobacillus*
        Genus   *Cardiobacterium*
        Genus   *Streptobacillus*
        Genus   *Calymmatobacterium*
    Parasites of *Paramecium*
Part 9. Gram-Negative Anaerobic
Bacteria
    Family I. Bacteroidaceae
        Genus I.   *Bacteroides*
        Genus II.   *Fusobacterium*
        Genus III.   *Leptotrichia*
  Genera of Uncertain Affiliation
        Genus   *Desulfovibrio*
        Genus   *Butyrivibrio*
        Genus   *Succinivibrio*
        Genus   *Succinimonas*
        Genus   *Lachnospira*
        Genus   *Selenomonas*
Part 10. Gram-Negative Cocci and
Coccobacilli (Aerobes)
    Family I. Neisseriaceae
        Genus I.   *Neisseria*
        Genus II.   *Branhamella*
        Genus III.   *Moraxella*
        Genus IV.   *Acinetobacter*
  Genera of Uncertain Affiliation
        Genus   *Paracoccus*
        Genus   *Lampropedia*

Part 11. Gram-Negative Cocci
  (Anaerobes)
    Family I. Veillonellaceae
        Genus I.   *Veillonella*
        Genus II.   *Acidaminococcus*
        Genus III.   *Megasphaera*
Part 12. Gram-Negative,
Chemolithotrophic Bacteria
  a. Organisms oxidizing ammonia or
    nitrite
    Family I. Nitrobacteraceae
        Genus I.   *Nitrobacter*
        Genus II.   *Nitrospina*
        Genus III.   *Nitrococcus*
        Genus IV.   *Nitrosomonas*
        Genus V.   *Nitrosospira*
        Genus VI.   *Nitrosococcus*
        Genus VII.   *Nitrosolobus*
  b. Organisms metabolizing sulfur
        Genus   *Thiobacillus*
        Genus   *Sulfolubus*
        Genus   *Thiobacterium*
        Genus   *Macromonas*
        Genus   *Thiovulum*
        Genus   *Thiospira*
  c. Organisms depositing iron or man-
    ganese oxides
    Family I. Siderocapsaceae
        Genus I.   *Siderocapsa*
        Genus II.   *Naumanniella*
        Genus III.   *Ochrobium*
        Genus IV.   *Siderococcus*
Part 13. Methane-Producing Bacteria
    Family I. Methanobacteriaceae
        Genus I.   *Methanobacterium*
        Genus II.   *Methanosarcina*
        Genus III.   *Methanococcus*

Part 14. Gram-Positive Cocci
  a. Aerobic and/or facultatively
    anaerobic
    Family I. Micrococcaceae
        Genus I.   *Micrococcus*
        Genus II.   *Staphylococcus*
        Genus III.   *Planococcus*
    Family II. Streptococcaceae
        Genus I.   *Streptococcus*
        Genus II.   *Leuconostoc*
        Genus III.   *Pediococcus*
        Genus IV.   *Aerococcus*
        Genus V.   *Gemella*
  b. Anaerobic
    Family III. Peptococcaceae
        Genus I.   *Peptococcus*
        Genus II.   *Peptostreptococcus*

Table 7–2. *(cont.)*

After *Bergey's Manual of Determinative Bacteriology*, 8th ed., 1974, with permission of the Williams & Wilkins Co.

FURTHER READING

1. Buchanan, R. E., and Gibbons, N. E. (eds.): *Bergey's Manual of Determinative Bacteriology*. 8th ed. Baltimore, Williams & Wilkins Co., 1974.
2. International Code of Nomenclature of Bacteria.* Washington, D.C., American Society of Microbiologists, 1975.

*This code is available from International Microbiological Fund, 221 Science Hall, Iowa State University, Ames, Iowa for one dollar.

chapter 8

Infectious Diseases

8-1 INTRODUCTION

The practice of modern medicine is a blend of the arts and the sciences. This blend has not always existed, and it is far from being a stable mixture today. The common senses of smell, taste, sight and touch were the only tools of medicine for a long time. Little logic prevailed in early days, and medicine was almost a totally subjective or even mystical art. Hippocrates, about 500 B.C., was the first to relate signs and symptoms with specific disease syndromes and to try to correlate these findings in order to arrive at some logical diagnosis.

Today, signs and symptoms are still the primary facts that guide the physician in his diagnosis. More and more, however, the physician relies on other purely scientific data in order to arrive at a diagnosis. In fact, one might say that this reliance on scientific data

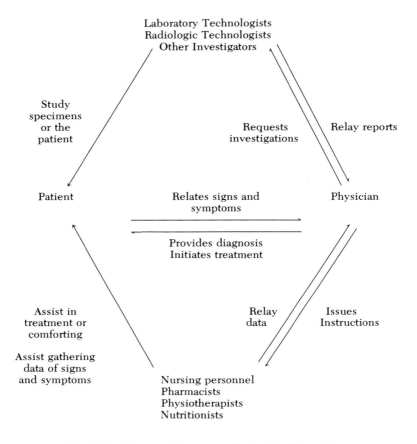

Fig. 8–1. The varied functions of allied health workers.

is overdone, and that certain patients might receive better treatment more promptly if the physician carefully analyzed the signs
and symptoms and logically applied them in determining the
diagnosis. Be that as it may, there is a great need for scientific
data-gathering in medicine. Indeed, it is difficult to imagine a
modern hospital without its x-ray or laboratory departments. Utilization of these and other allied health departments has increased
greatly over the last few decades and has altered the practice of
medicine tremendously. Where 50 years ago a patient would be
visited by his doctor and perhaps treated by a nurse, today's
hospital patient is served directly or indirectly by an array of
personnel that would astonish him if they were all lined up in front
of his bed. Figure 8–1 illustrates some functions of the various

allied health workers and their relationship to the patient. It should be evident from the illustration that even though the physician remains the key figure in the practice of medicine, he would be severely handicapped without the assistance of the other allied health workers.

In this chapter we shall consider the various causes and effects of infectious disease and their relationship to the diagnosis and treatment of the disease. Chapter 9 considers the factors that control or prevent these diseases.

8-2 BASIC PRINCIPLES OF DISEASE

All diseases are produced by changes in either structure or function or both in one or more organs. These changes must be of such a magnitude that the normal function of a significant part of the body is impaired. Impaired function of the body is usually manifested by outward signs or symptoms, such as fever, headache, cough, sore throat, malaise, rash, paralysis, vomiting, diarrhea, photophobia, hydrophobia, and delirium. Some signs may not be evident unless more in depth investigations are undertaken, such as spots on internal organs as revealed by x-ray studies, increased or decreased sugar or ion levels as determined by biochemical analysis, irregular heart beat as detected by electrocardiography, irregular brain impulses as detected by electroencephalography, and abnormal behavior patterns as determined by psychoanalysis. The study of signs and symptoms often leads to a specific diagnosis. A correct diagnosis will guide the physician to elect the proper therapeutic, remedial, or comforting procedures. Incorrect diagnoses may further impair the patient by improper treatment.

Some impairments may be acute, manifest themselves at short notice, and be short in duration; others may be chronic, manifest themselves over a period of time, and be relatively long in duration. If the disease can be cured completely, the impairment is said to be reversible. If permanent damage is suspected or evident, the impairment is irreversible. When the symptoms subside without treatment, the disease is said to be self-limiting. Given time, many infectious diseases are self-limiting (see Basic Immunology, Chapter 9). Prompt diagnosis and correct treatment, however, reduce much hardship.

8-3 INFLAMMATIONS

An inflammation is the sum total of all the responses of the host in its encounter with an irritant. Such irritants may be organic (microbial), chemical (toxins), physical (injuries and burns), or a combination of these. The inflammatory responses are basically the same in all instances, regardless whether relatively minor or major damage results. Let us therefore examine, in a much simplified way, what happens when a minor injury to the skin, such as a sliver cut, results in the development of a boil. In the first instance, the defense mechanism will concentrate on removing the extraneous material by physical means—bleeding and contraction. Secondly, the phagocytes and other leukocytes will increase near the sites of injury. The phagocytes and leukocytes will attempt to destroy any foreign invaders, such as bacteria, that may have also entered. Some of these invaders are specially protected. Bacteria that produce capsules, for example, are particularly resistant to phagocytosis. Other bacteria produce enzymes or toxins that will destroy the phagocytes or leukocytes or will invade underlying tissue to cause necrosis. Some bacteria produce potent toxins that may cause more generalized effects or even death.

The degree of damage, or the severity of discomfort caused by invading bacteria, relates to the pathogenicity or virulence of the organisms. Bacteria that cause no apparent damage are referred to as nonpathogenic (not able to produce disease); those that cause damage or have the ability to cause damage are called pathogens (capable of causing disease). Some pathogens may temporarily lose the ability to produce a certain harmful toxin or enzyme, or may require special conditions in order to produce the harmful substance. Pathogens that have lost their ability to produce disease are said to be avirulent (harmless), but could become virulent (harmful) in the appropriate environment. The ability of certain bacteria to change from virulent to avirulent is utilized in the production of some vaccines used for immunization (see Chapter 9). One simple method is to grow the bacteria on basic media and subculture them time and again on the basic medium. The process of reducing the virulence of bacteria by repeated passage to basic media is known as attenuation. The reverse—repeated passage to enriched media or live animals to increase virulence—is also possible and is known as exaltation.

If the invading organisms or materials are removed by bleeding or contraction, the remaining clean cut will usually heal by itself without much discomfort. If the invaders must be attacked by leukocytes or phagocytes, a local swelling (edema) and some redness is usually noticeable. In pronounced attacks by leukocytes and phagocytes, the swelling results in a boil. Gradually, the leukocytes, phagocytes and dead local tissue degenerate into pus, the boil breaks, and the pus is released. Boil rupture and subsequent healing often lead to scar formation. Other complications may lead to organisms entering the bloodstream, causing generalized discomfort or localized infections at distant sites (see Section 8–4).

8-4 INFECTION AND INFECTIOUS DISEASES

DEFINITIONS

An infection is any process whereby a microorganism enters into a relationship with a host. This relationship need not necessarily be harmful to the host. In fact, most infections result in a symbiotic relationship between the invader and the host which is of mutual benefit.

An infectious disease results when the invader is antagonistic to the host. The antagonism may be direct or indirect. Direct antagonism occurs when the invader itself harms the host. An example of direct antagonism would be the biting of a flea, or the tissue damage caused by migrating roundworms. Indirect antagonism may be caused by deprivation, when the invader utilizes nutrients intended for the metabolism of the host, or by intoxication, when the host is poisoned by products produced by the invader. Examples of different types of indirect antagonism are the infestation by tapeworms and the paralytic effect of diphtheria toxins.

In some instances, different types of microbes work together to effect changes that neither could effect by itself. Such "cooperation" is referred to as *synergism*. The relationship of *Fusobacterium fusiforme* and *Borrelia vincentii* in cases of Vincent's angina is a prime example of synergism.

As already stated, the mutually beneficial relationships predominate. Of these, the association between man and the many microorganisms found in the lower alimentary tract is probably the most important to us. We often forget the delicate balance of flora that prevails in our intestines and frequently we upset this balance by taking antibiotics and other drugs. It is not unlikely that, nowadays, we more often induce disease by interfering with natural infections than we reduce disease by interfering with infectious disease agents. In other words, antibiotics, so often administered without real need, may do more harm than good.

A "natural infection" may result in an infectious disease in more ways than one. A more complete understanding of the normal flora of the body is necessary to appreciate some of these ways.

Besides the mutualists—the organisms living in mutual benefit with ourselves—the body also contains a large number of so-called commensals. *Commensals* are organisms that live off or on a host without causing any apparent harm. However, many of these commensals may cause disease when conditions change. Consider what might happen when some of the bacteria that inhabit the skin enter an inflicted wound. On the skin the bacteria may live an apparently harmless existence. Once entering the tissue or the bloodstream, many of these "harmless" bacteria might cause severe infectious diseases.

INFECTIOUS DISEASE REQUIREMENTS

To be successful in causing an infectious disease, then, an organism must meet certain basic requirements. Let us concentrate on the microbes, and for a moment forget about those that bite or cause harm by migration, such as the roundworms.

First, the organism itself must be able to invade those areas of the body where it can do some harm. To cause harm, it must be able to produce a toxin or other virulent product, or otherwise interfere with the life processes of the host. Secondly, the host must be susceptible to whatever virulent or toxic products the organism may produce, or vulnerable to interference with its life processes by the invaders. Both these factors center around the ability of the host to ward off infectious diseases, or the host's resistance to the infectious agent.

Resistance may be twofold: innate or acquired. *Acquired resistance* refers to specific immunity through antibodies produced by the host or its mother, a topic discussed more fully in Chapter 9.

Innate resistance refers to the normal nonspecific defense mechanisms. Some of these nonspecific defense mechanisms are of a genetic nature. This is why certain groups of individuals, or certain races of people, are more resistant to some types of infectious diseases than others. The mechanical barriers of the body offer protection against foreign invaders. The horny layers of the skin are difficult to penetrate. The moist mucous membranes will entrap many microorganisms before they can reach more suitable locations. Tears, sweat and other secretions will remove microbes and, more importantly, will destroy many of them through a component substance called lysozyme. The gastric juices kill most of the organisms we ingest. When entering the bloodstream, lymphatics, bone marrow or lungs, the microbes meet the phagocytes; these cells engulf most foreign particles and then proceed to digest or remove them. And finally, antibiotics produced by many members of the normal flora further help to control infectious diseases by reducing or eliminating a wide range of foreign invaders.

To be successful, the pathogens must overcome many barriers, and they may do this in many different ways. For example, they may invade in large numbers, turning the odds in their favor, or they may bypass or overcome some or all of the hazards.

TYPES OF INFECTIOUS DISEASES

The more important infectious diseases are described in Part II. Many infectious diseases manifest themselves in some general pattern, or produce similar signs and symptoms. Here we describe the more general disease patterns.

Abscess. This is a severe localized collection of pus in a tissue, organ, or confined space, caused by an infection with pyogenic (pus-forming) bacteria. An abscess may be deep-seated and may burrow to the skin surface and rupture to discharge its contents. Internal rupture of an abscess can disseminate the infection rapidly, often causing death unless treated promptly.

Necrosis. When cells degenerate to the point where tissues are damaged irreparably, we speak of necrosis. There are four major types of necrosis:

Coagulation necrosis. The arterial blood supply to a tissue is cut off and the tissue slowly "suffocates," or specific toxins actually cause coagulation of cellular proteins. In both cases, the degeneration is relatively slow.

Liquefaction necrosis. This is a fairly rapid and complete dissolution of cells, such as that caused by some bacterial toxins or cellular enzymes. This type of necrosis is usually associated with pus formation or abscess.

Caseous necrosis. This is the destruction of cells with the formation of granular or friable masses of amorphous fat and protein. Tubercles are specific examples of caseous necrosis.

Gangrenous necrosis. This is a combination of coagulation necrosis and further degeneration by actively growing bacteria at the necrotic site. This type of necrosis is associated with putrid odors and blackening of the tissue, as occurs in gangrene.

Toxicity. Various microorganisms produce different toxins that may affect the body in a variety of ways. Some effects have already been discussed under necrosis. Other, more generalized effects may occur when a toxin permeates the vascular or lymphatic systems and is thus disseminated throughout the body. Basically, there are two types of bacterial toxins—exotoxins and endotoxins. Exotoxins are excreted by the organisms and are generally disseminated quickly. They are sensitive to heat (60°C for 30 minutes), highly antigenic (stimulate the production of antibodies), and usually potent. The toxins produced in tetanus and diphtheria are prime examples of exotoxins. Endotoxins are released by a microorganism when its cell wall breaks down. Endotoxins are generally less potent than exotoxins, but they are potentially dangerous when the rapid destruction of bacterial cells by antibiotics causes the release of vast amounts of endotoxin. Endotoxins are heat-stable (60°C for 30 minutes) and are poor antigens.

Respiratory Diseases. Some infections are particularly detrimental to the respiratory system. Specific diseases caused by organisms may be found in Part II; the following are some of the more common disorders that may be caused by more than one type of organism:

Bronchitis often follows a cold, influenza or some other ailment. When the bronchial tree has been irritated by a relatively mild virus or by such irritants as dust or smoke, it becomes particularly susceptible to infection by purulent bacteria that would otherwise be warded off. In a normally healthy individual, bronchitis is usually self-limiting, but when associated with inhalation of industrial dust or heavy smoking, it may become chronic. In elderly or debilitated persons or infants, bronchitis often leads to pneumonia.

Pneumonia is a diffuse inflammation of the lungs that may occur from an infection with *Streptococcus, Staphylococcus, Klebsiella* or *Haemophilus* species or a viral agent. It may also be a complication of congestive heart failure and bronchial obstructions due to tumors, or it may follow aspiration (inhalation) of foods, gastric contents, or other foreign bodies in the lungs. Bacterial infection is usually the cause of lobar pneumonia, which is described in Chapter 11.

Emphysema refers to an increase in the size of the air spaces distal to the terminal bronchioles, and the consequent destruction of the bronchial walls. Emphysema is believed to be a delayed result of chronic infections or irritations. As a result of emphysema, the lungs are impaired by overstretching and a reduced capacity to exchange oxygen for carbon dioxide. These impairments put a strain on the heart, which must compensate for the deficiency in respiration by pumping more and more blood. Therefore, heart failure is a frequent end-result of emphysema.

Gastrointestinal Diseases. Obviously, these diseases are caused most frequently by organisms or toxins that are ingested. (Again, specific common diseases are described in more detail in Part II.)

Appendicitis is a common ailment that affects all age groups. It is less common in the very young and the aged, and most common in older children and young adults. It is the most common disease requiring intra-abdominal surgery. The chief cause of acute appendicitis is infection, which may be caused by a number of different bacteria and sometimes parasites. Initial symptoms are usually abdominal pain in the right lower region, followed by nausea, vomiting or anorexia. Pain may be diffuse or located in the epigastric or periumbilical region. A characteristic is an increase in white blood cells with a predominance of polymorphonuclear leukocytes. X-ray studies may reveal calcified fecaliths in the appendix. If the appendix is removed promptly, the prognosis is good, and the patient will probably be up and about in days. Delay in surgery often leads to rupture of the appendix, with a subsequent peritonitis that could be fatal.

Peritonitis is an infection of the peritoneal membrane. Symptoms are acute pains throughout the abdomen and high fever. Prompt treatment with massive doses of antibiotics is indicated.

Cholecystitis is an infection of the gallbladder. It affects mainly persons in their fifties and sixties, particularly obese females. The disease is usually caused by stones obstructing the bile duct. The infection is usually secondary to the damage to the duct or gallbladder. Symptoms are not clearcut. Complications such as perforation causing peritonitis or abscess of adjacent organs are not uncommon. Diagnosis is usually made by x-ray studies, which reveal malfunction or stones. Surgery or prolonged treatment is often indicated.

Enteritis is an inflammation of the small intestine. It is fairly common, more frequent in males, and peaks at middle age. The true causes are not known. The symptoms are irregular but often associated with pain, diarrhea, loss of appetite, nausea, and vomiting. Complications are bleeding, perforation, and peritonitis.

Ulcerative colitis is an inflamed condition of the rectum and colon. Its true causes are unknown, but numerous organisms have been incriminated. It is one of the most frequent and serious disorders of the colon and has a long and protracted course. It may be complicated by obstruction, pericolic abscess, and perforation leading to peritonitis.

Genitourinary Diseases. *Glomerulonephritis* is an inflammation or degeneration of the glomeruli of the kidneys. It may be caused by bacteria, embolism, or hypersensitivity, and it may be acute, subacute, or chronic. Initial symptoms of acute glomerulonephritis are fever, weakness, chills, malaise, and loss of appetite. Hematuria (blood in the urine) is a classic sign, often accompanied by pyuria (pus), albuminuria, and also casts, which are found by microscopic analysis of the urine. Nitrogenous products are retained as measurable by blood urea nitrogen. Anuresis may develop, and lead to fatal results, which are not frequent. Acute forms may clear up in a few weeks, progress to more severe symptoms, or lead to subacute or chronic forms.

Pyelonephritis is an interstitial inflammation of the parenchyma of the kidney and the renal pelvis. It may be caused by a range of different bacteria, but it is most frequently caused by *Escherichia coli.* Acute pyelonephritis manifests itself by a sudden pain in the back, radiating to a region over the gallbladder, the lower abdomen, and into the loin. Chills, fever, nausea and vomiting may also be present. Urination is painful and gives a burning sensation. The urine is highly colored, infrequent, and scanty. Pyelonephritis is often associated with renal obstruction and may lead to uremia and bacteremia, and it is frequently fatal.

Circulatory Diseases. These often result from more localized infections that have gone unnoticed or untreated.

Pericarditis is an infection of the membrane that surrounds the heart, the pericardium. It may result from rheumatic inflammation, as a part of pancarditis, or from a variety of infections as caused by bacteria, fungi, viruses or parasites. Pericarditis is usually a complication of other infections such as pneumonia, influenza, tuberculosis, and tonsillitis. The organisms reach the pericardium by way of the lymphatics, the blood, or as an extension of a neighboring infection. The inflammation produces a serous exudate within the pericardial sac. The exudate may become so voluminous that it compresses the heart, the great blood vessels, or the lungs. In healing, a dense constricting scar may form around the heart, which permanently impairs proper filling of the heart (constrictive pericarditis).

Rheumatic fever often results in damage to the heart. This disease is difficult to recognize because it mimics many other diseases. It is preceded by infections with hemolytic streptococci, and occurs most commonly in persons between the ages of five and fifteen years. Repeated attacks of rheumatic fever may occur, causing some damage to the heart during each attack. The pumping action of the heart may be impaired for a short time, or the damage may be permanent.

Joint and bone diseases include *arthritis*, a disease of unknown origin, which may follow a sprain, an infection or joint injury. Some believe it to be caused by bacterial or viral infections; others suspect it to be an allergy. It takes many different forms, and may affect both sexes, the young and the old.

Osteomyelitis is an infection of bone. It is caused most commonly by staphylococci, except in infants, in whom streptococci are more frequently involved. The infection may be localized or diffuse, and may affect the periosteum, the cortex, or the marrow. The organisms may invade the bone by way of the bloodstream or directly from a neighboring abscess in soft tissue. The infection may spread and cause pronounced necrosis of the bone. Treatment tends to be difficult.

8-5 HYPERSENSITIVITY

Hypersensitivity is an acquired capacity of the body to react in an intensified fashion to a foreign body or substance that is introduced into the body. The introduction to the body may occur by way of the parenteral (injection), respiratory, oral, or other route. Hypersensitivity is useful when it protects the body from the harmful effects caused by microorganisms or their byproducts (immunity). It is harmful when it causes violent tissue reactions, such as allergic responses. The protective characteristics of hypersensitivity appear in Chapter 9 (Basic Immunology); here we shall briefly consider the harmful aspects of hypersensitivity.

Hypersensitivity diseases form a complex group of disorders that basically relate to the immune response (see Section 9–2). They range in severity from relatively mild hay fever, to debilitating asthma or systemic lupus erythematosus, to fatal anaphylactic shock. An antibody-antigen reaction is believed to be responsible in all hypersensitivity reactions. Two major types of hypersensitivity are known: immediate and delayed. In both types, a person exposed to the foreign substance for the first time does not necessarily demonstrate any ill effects. What does happen, however, is that antibodies to the foreign substance are produced. These antibodies may be bound to certain cells, and when the person is exposed to the same substance a second time, a reaction occurs between the substance and the cells containing the antibody.

In immediate types of hypersensitivity, the reaction may occur within a few minutes to a few hours from the time of contact with the foreign agent. The most dramatic reaction is "anaphylactic shock," which may be characterized by collapse, cyanosis, choking, unconsciousness, and even sudden death. Anaphylactic shock is known to have followed such seemingly harmless processes as repeated horse-serum injections (serum sickness), repeated bee or wasp stings, and repeated injections of penicillin or some other drug.

Delayed hypersensitivity usually occurs only 12 to 24 hours after the contact. The most typical delayed type hypersensitivity is that displayed by the tuberculin test (see p. 245). Other examples are contact dermatitis, reactions to poison ivy, and various drug reactions.

FURTHER READING

1. Boyd, W., and Sheldon, H.: An Introduction to the Study of Disease. 7th ed. Philadelphia, Lea & Febiger, 1977.

chapter 9

Control of Infectious Diseases

9-1 INTRODUCTION

In Section 8–3, we briefly discussed how microorganisms spread from a localized infection to other body sites. In this section, we shall discuss how microorganisms spread from person to person, and some of the factors involved in the control of such spreading.

The branch of medicine concerned with the various factors and conditions that determine the frequency and distribution of diseases is known as epidemiology; the practitioner, as an epidemiologist. The epidemiologist collects data on diseases in population groups and interprets the data to determine the state of health of the group. When a certain disease occurs that is abnormal for the group, or abnormal at a specific time period for a particular group, or is found more frequently than is known to be normal for a group, the epidemiologist may declare that an epidemic exists. Epidemics are not restricted to infectious diseases. In fact, an epidemiologist studies all factors affecting the physiologic state of a population, such as malnutrition, occupational hazards, genetic constitution, neoplasm, and the process of aging. An epidemic, then, is any unusually large outbreak or incidence of any type of disease in any one population group at a given time and place. An epidemic that is worldwide may be referred to as a pandemic. In this chapter we must limit ourselves to those aspects of epidemiology that apply to infectious diseases. We should not lose sight, however, of the many factors that play a role in the total disease process. In discussing the spread and control of infectious diseases, several factors must be considered:

    a. the sources of infection
    b. the modes of spread
    c. the means of prevention

The most common source of infection is the patient. As we have already seen in Section 8–4, not every infected person is infectious. Similarly, one need not be sick in order to be infectious—many apparently healthy individuals carry one or more types of infectious agents. These individuals are referred to as *carriers*, many of whom have recuperated from an infectious disease but have not been successful in eliminating the infectious organisms from their systems. The classic example of such cases is the typhoid carrier. Typhoid bacilli may be found in some individuals long after they have recovered from the disease. Indeed, typhoid bacilli can only be eliminated from some carriers by surgical removal of the gallbladder.

Other carriers of typhoid and other agents may be contact carriers. *Contact carriers* are individuals who pick up bacilli or other infectious agents from the sick but do not demonstrate any clinical symptoms themselves.

Infections derived from animals and animal products are generally known as *zoonoses*. In North America, many infectious diseases have been all but eliminated from domestic animals. Pasteurization of dairy and other produce has further reduced the most common hazards. The danger that relaxed attitudes may foster major hazards, however, looms larger than is generally realized, especially with the more widespread use of factory-prepared foods.

With increased urbanization, wild animals also play less important roles in the spread of infectious disease. However, they remain a major source of infection which is why many infectious agents will never be eradicated.

The soil is the final major source of infectious organisms. Again, with the widespread use of chemical fertilizers and the elimination of animals as beasts of burden in many countries, the soil has become less and less important as a source of infection.

Whatever the source, control measures must be geared to the organisms most commonly expected to be a hazard. Consequently, a wildlife worker should be vaccinated against rabies because many wild rodents carry this virus; a meat-cutter should be vaccinated against brucellosis; and a correspondent off to India, against cholera.

This chapter deals with the general principles underlying the control of infectious diseases. Part II considers more specific details of spread and control as they apply to the various diseases caused by specific organisms.

9-2 BASIC IMMUNOLOGY

It has long been known that many patients who recover from an infectious disease are resistant to future attacks of the same disease. This resistance is known as immunity, and the protected individual is said to be immune. Immunity has been found to be specific; that is, an individual may build up resistance to one type of disease, but this resistance does not usually protect him against other types of diseases. The study of these variable resistances to different types of infectious diseases is known as immunology. In fact, immunology includes all responses to foreign agents, regardless whether the agent is infectious or not. Immunology has revealed that much of the resistance may be attributed to a substance called antibody.

ANTIBODIES, ANTIGENS AND IMMUNITY

Antibodies are *globulins*, carried by the serum, which are produced by the body upon stimulation by another substance called *antigen*. Antibodies react with their respective antigens in some observable way. More precisely, the antibodies are *immunoglobulins*, of which there are five groups: IgG, IgA, IgM, IgD and IgE. Each group of globulins has specific physical and biochemical characteristics. The IgG is the largest group—most bacterial and viral antibodies belong to the IgG group. The second largest group is composed of IgA immunoglobulins, which contain antibodies against insulin, the thyroid, and apparently other autoantibodies.

IgG has a molecular weight of 150,000 and IgA has a molecular weight ranging from 170,000 to 500,000; both have sedimentation rates of about seven. The relatively small size of IgG allows it to pass across the placenta. Antibodies of the IgM group, on the other hand, are known as the macroglobulins, and these have a molecular weight of 900,000 and a sedimentation rate of 19. IgD has been associated with activity against penicillin, diphtheria toxoid, insulin, and a variety of other substances. IgE is a heat-labile antibody related to allergies and hypersensitivities (see also Section 8–5).

Modern immunologists use the term "immunoglobulin" almost exclusively when referring to "antibodies." We shall use both terms interchangeably in this text.

In our definition of antibody, we referred to the term antigen. An *antigen* is any substance which, when introduced into the body, will stimulate the production of another substance, antibody, and will react with *that antibody* in some observable way. Are we going around in circles? Not really. Consider this analogy: an antigen is like a hand, and an antibody is like a glove. General definitions of either object would be similar, as are our definitions of antibody and antigen. Furthermore, as no two hands are exactly alike, so the antibody is an exact-fitting glove, custom-made specifically to fit only one antigen.

In analyzing these definitions, you may have pondered the question of whether antibodies can also function as antigens. They can and often are, which brings us to another important aspect of immunology: not all antibodies are beneficial. The body learns very early in life how to distinguish between antigens that are foreign to it and those that are not. In normal individuals, this results in the body producing antibodies to foreign antigens only. The *autoantibodies*, which are produced upon stimulation by our own antigens, may react and destroy these same antigens in our body. When this happens, we speak of an autoimmune disease. Some autoimmune diseases are eventually fatal.

When the body produces antibody upon stimulation by an antigen, the immunity is referred to as *active immunity*. Active immunity may be incurred by an infection, in which case we speak of *natural active immunity*, or by immunization or vaccination which would result in *artificial active immunity*. Active immunity, then, results whenever the individual who carries the antibodies was actively engaged in the production of the antibodies. Active immunity is not always a blessing, as a short review of unsuccessful organ and tissue transplants will bear out. In order to benefit a person in time of need, antibodies need not be produced by the individual himself. Most of us were endowed with a number of different antibodies at birth. As already mentioned, these antibodies of the IgG group cross the placenta from mother to fetus. They may then be referred to as maternal antibodies.

Maternal antibodies help to protect the newborn during the early stages of life, when the newborn is unable to produce antibodies. The immune mechanism, the ability to produce antibody, does not mature until about the sixth month of life. It is believed that until that time the body "learns" to distinguish between foreign antigens and those carried by the body. If antibodies would be produced during that time, antibody production would be indiscriminate and could react with body tissues, to the detriment of the individual.

Immunity obtained without actual production of antibodies by the carrier is referred to as *passive immunity*. Besides maternal antibodies, we can also acquire other antibodies. Many antibodies can be produced on a large scale in animals, or may be obtained from blood products from immune individuals. Administration of such antibodies, either in animal sera or in concentrated gamma globulin from human sources, will also result in passive immunity. The acquisition of maternal antibodies, of course, would result in *natural passive immunity*; that of other antibodies, in *artificial passive immunity*.

A discussion of immunology, a clinical problem, must of necessity be too brief in a text such as this. It is, however, an extremely interesting and timely topic of study.

9-3 IMMUNIZATION

Immunization (vaccination) had its origin in the late 18th century. Edward Jenner, in 1796, observed that milkmaids rarely came down with smallpox. He attributed this to their frequent contact with cowpox and introduced the practice of vaccination (Latin *vacca* = cow) by injecting healthy individuals with the exudate of pustules on the udders of infected cows. Since then, the practice of immunization has been expanded to routinely confer protection against a number of infectious diseases. Immunization schedules should be initiated at the age of three months. They should first be directed against those diseases that are most prevalent in the community in which the baby resides, or against those diseases that would be most debilitating should they be contracted. In North America the initial vaccination is generally directed against diphtheria, pertussis (whooping cough), tetanus (lockjaw) and poliomyelitis (infantile paralysis). A combined vaccine containing antigens to all agents responsible for the above diseases (DPT-polio vaccine) is readily available and is most effective when used in three successive doses during the first year of life. The first dose should be administered at the age of three months or when the baby reaches a weight of twelve pounds, whichever is the later. A second dose should be given one month after the first, and a third one month later. A booster dose should be given one year following completion of the initial vaccination schedule, and again at the time of primary school entry (age six). High-risk groups should be given single doses of tetanus-diphtheria vaccine (Td) every ten years, or single doses of polio vaccine every five years.

Other vaccinations may be directed against measles, mumps, smallpox, rubella, yellow fever, tuberculosis, cholera, typhoid, and a range of other diseases. The practice and schedules vary among states if not among areas. Local conditions should be studied before entering the health professions or before planning a foreign visit. Certain vaccinations are mandatory in order to be allowed to enter or return from certain territories or countries.

In addition to vaccination, antitoxins are also widely used. Antitoxins are antibodies that have already been formed to neutralize specific toxins. Whenever a person sustains a potentially dangerous wound and has not been immunized or is not known to have been immunized, a dose of tetanus antitoxin is usually prescribed as a prophylactic measure. Antitoxins to other specific agents (such as diphtheria), or gamma globulin (which potentially contains an array of antibodies) may be indicated under various conditions or circumstances.

9-4 ANTIMICROBIAL AGENTS

Undoubtedly, antimicrobial agents provide the most effective treatment for infectious diseases. Because of their importance in therapy and disease control, we shall discuss these agents in some detail. First, we attempt to define and classify them. Then we consider their origin, their activity, and finally their usefulness in treatment. In Chapter 27 we shall also discuss the laboratory aspects of bacterial susceptibility and resistance to antimicrobial agents.

DEFINITIONS AND CLASSIFICATIONS

An antimicrobial agent is any substance that acts against microorganisms. An antibiotic is a substance derived from living organisms that is capable of inhibiting some of the life processes of some microorganisms. Antibiotics may be obtained from bacteria, fungi, molds, algae, lichens and higher plants. The antibiotics may be classified by one or more of the following criteria:

a. their chemical composition
b. their source
c. their activity range on different types of microorganisms in vitro
d. their therapeutic value

From a diagnostic point of view, the third criterion would be the most useful, and we shall use that criterion for our classification. Antibiotics may be divided into four large groups:

a. Those acting primarily against gram-positive bacteria: bacitracin, most penicillins, erythromycin, lincomycin, oleandomycin, vancomycin, and others.
b. Those acting primarily against gram-negative bacteria: few penicillins, colistin, gentamicin, novobiocin, polymyxin B.
c. Those acting against both gram-positive and gram-negative bacteria: some penicillins, streptomycin, chloramphenicol, tetracycline, cephalosporin, kanamycin, neomycin. (Although streptomycin acts mainly on gram-negative bacteria, it does act against some gram-positive bacteria. The other agents listed here are popularly known as the broad-spectrum antibiotics because they interfere with a wide variety of microorganisms.)
d. Those acting especially against fungi: amphotericin, nystatin, griseofulvin.

If we were to include all antimicrobial agents in this classification, the sulfonamides would come under group C. We could then also conclude the series with a fifth group, comprised of isoniazid (INH) and para-aminosalicyclic acid (PAS), the agents primarily active against tubercle bacilli.

SOURCES OF ANTIBIOTICS

Most antibiotics are derived from microorganisms that inhabit the soil. Various *Bacillus* species and the common molds supply the largest number of different antibiotics.

Sir Alexander Fleming, in 1928, was the first to discover the antagonistic effect of some *Penicillium* molds on the growth of certain bacteria. The value of his discovery was not fully realized until ten years later, and five years more were required to exploit this phenomenon on a scale large enough to benefit the sick. Today, penicillin is produced commercially from *P. chrysogenum, P. notatum* and some other species. The penicillin radical may be altered in several ways to produce an array of different, yet similar, antibiotics (such as ampicillin, methicillin, oxacillin). During the late thirties and early forties, a number of other microorganisms were found to yield satisfactory antibiotics: *Bacillus brevis*–tyrothricin; *Bacillus polymyxa*–polymyxin; *Bacillus subtilis*–bacitracin; *Streptomyces griseus*–streptomycin.

Many others have since been discovered, and the "hunt" is still going on. To discover a suitable antibiotic is not a simple task. Announcements of newly discovered "super drugs" appear in the news at intervals. These announcements are usually followed by fizzles and blushed cheeks, when further studies may bring to light that the "drug" is even more potent in killing higher animals than it is in killing microorganisms.

As long as microorganisms continue to change their anti-microbial susceptibility patterns (and they probably always will), the search for different and better antibiotics undoubtedly will continue.

ANTIMICROBIAL ACTIVITY

Antimicrobial agents may affect microbes in one of two general ways:

   a. They may destroy microorganisms outright; that is, have a bactericidal effect.
   b. They may prevent the organisms from multiplying or grow-ing; that is, have a bacteriostatic effect.

Some more specific modes of action are competitive inhibition, interference with protein synthesis, and interference by surface action. Specific modes of action of the more common antibiotics are listed in Table 9–1.

Competitive Inhibition. Para-aminobenzoic acid (PABA) is an essential growth requirement for most living things. The basic chemical structure of PABA (NH_2 ⬡ COOH) is very similar to that of sulfonamides (NH_2 ⬡ SO_2NH—). Sulfonamides, there-fore, can compete with the reactive sites on the coenzymes affect-ing PABA utilization. When sulfonamide is present in large concen-trations, PABA utilization will be disrupted to the point at which the invading microorganisms can no longer replicate.

Interference with Protein Synthesis. Tetracyclines, streptomy-cins, erythromycins and chloramphenicol are capable of inhibiting

Table 9–1. Summary of data on common antimicrobial agents

Common Name of Agent	Primary Spectrum	Common Serum Level	Mode of Action
Ampicillin	Gram-positive and negative bacteria	2–5 μg/ml	Inhibition of cell wall synthesis
Amphotericin	Fungi	1–3 μg/ml	Interference with membrane function
Bacitracin	Gram-positive bacteria	Insignificant	Deterioration of cell membrane
Carbenicillin	Gram-negative bacteria	Up to 400 μg/ml	Inhibition of cell wall synthesis
Cephalosporin	Gram-positive and negative bacteria	5–40 μg/ml	Inhibition of cell wall synthesis
Chlortetracycline	Gram-positive and negative bacteria	1–5 μg/ml	Interference with ribosome synthesis
Cloxacillin	Gram-positive bacteria	14–20 μg/ml	Inhibition of cell wall synthesis
Colistin	Gram-negative bacteria	7.6 μg/ml	Deterioration of cell membrane
Erythromycin	Gram-positive bacteria	0.4–1.3 μg/ml	Interference with ribosome synthesis
Gentamicin	Gram-negative bacteria	2.3–5.4 μg/ml	Induces abnormal protein synthesis
Isoniazid (INH)	*Mycobacterium tuberculosis*	0.8–20 μg/ml	Uncertain
Kanamycin	Gram-positive and negative bacteria	14–35 μg/ml	Induces abnormal protein synthesis
Lincomycin	Gram-positive bacteria	0.6–2.5 μg/ml	Inhibition of protein synthesis
Methicillin	Gram-positive bacteria	50–80 μg/ml	Inhibition of cell wall synthesis
Neomycin	Gram-positive and negative bacteria	1–2 μg/ml	Induces abnormal protein synthesis
Nitrofurantoin	Gram-positive and negative bacteria	Insignificant	Inhibition of enzyme activity
Novobiocin	Gram-negative bacteria	100 μg/ml	Inhibition of DNA polymerization
Oleandomycin	Gram-positive bacteria	0.8 μg/ml	Uncertain
Para-aminosalicylic acid (PAS)	*Mycobacterium tuberculosis*	10–1000 μg/ml	Uncertain
Penicillin G	Gram-positive bacteria	1.2–400 μg/ml	Inhibition of cell wall synthesis
Polymyxin B	Gram-negative bacteria	0.4–8 μg/ml	Deterioration of cell membrane
Streptomycin	Gram-positive and negative bacteria	40–60 μg/ml	Induces abnormal protein synthesis
Sulfonamides	Gram-positive and negative bacteria	Vary widely	Competitive inhibition of PABA uptake
Tetracycline	Gram-positive and negative bacteria	1–5 μg/ml	Interference with ribosome synthesis
Vancomycin	Gram-positive bacteria	6–40 μg/ml	Inhibition of cell wall synthesis

(Modified after Poupard, J. A., et al., Lab. Med., 2:26–27, 1971.)

the protein synthesis of different bacteria. The exact reasons why one antibiotic interferes with protein synthesis of some but not other bacteria is still under study.

Interference by Surface Action. Various antimicrobial activities may affect the outer surfaces of bacterial cells:

    a. The *cell wall may be destroyed,* or prevented from forming. Many penicillins and bacitracin are primarily surface-acting agents. When the cell wall is destroyed, the organism is more vulnerable to attack by natural nonspecific agents.

    b. The *selective permeability* of the cell wall may be altered. Polymyxins, tyrocidin and other agents often demonstrate such activity. These effects may lead to an inability to take in vital nutrients, the loss of vital proteins, or the accumulation of harmful byproducts within the cell.

ANTIMICROBIAL TREATMENT

In vitro studies of antimicrobial agents do not always represent the effects that will occur in vivo. To be effective as a therapeutic drug, an antimicrobial agent must:

    a. Destroy, or cause the destruction of, all the organisms responsible for the disease in question.

    b. Be harmless to the patient.

In many instances, these ideals cannot be attained and certain risks must be taken in treatment. When these risks become paramount to the treatment, other forms of treatment should be substituted. Of course, the choice of treatment is the responsibility of the physician in charge. The allied health professional may be responsible for delivering the treatment (the nurse), or may provide the physician with data to guide his selection of the most appropriate drug (the laboratorian). Therefore, our discussion of antimicrobial therapy must be limited to general topics.

In the treatment of infectious diseases, the physician may take a number of different approaches:

    a. He may resort to the so-called shotgun therapy, and choose any of a number of broad-spectrum antibiotics. This course of action is sometimes necessary, particularly when the symptoms demand immediate attention.

    b. He may investigate the infection further, and upon receipt of the first laboratory report, confirmation of the isolation of a certain type of organism, choose an antibiotic to which that type of organism is usually susceptible.

    c. He may await further laboratory studies that will tell him more specifically to which antibiotics the pathogen in question is susceptible.

The course of action outlined under b usually requires a waiting period of 24 hours; that under c, at least 48 hours. Unfortunately, such waiting periods are not often permitted. Far too often patients arrive at a clinic to complain about ailments that have bothered them for months and, presto, they are subjected to immediate antibiotic therapy. Such indiscriminate use of antimicrobial agents must aid the development of resistant strains. The more often antibiotics are administered, especially when they are not specifically inhibitory to particular pathogens, the more frequent the appearance of resistant strains will be.

The entire subject of antimicrobial agents covers drug resistance, susceptibility, and dependence, as well as drug-induced alterations of microbes and effects of drugs on the heart. The subject is interesting and one from which the student can learn much about microbial behavior.

9-5 CONTROL OF NOSOCOMIAL INFECTIONS

Hospital-associated or nosocomial infections are not a new problem. They occurred long before microorganisms were known to be the cause of disease; they will continue to occur as long as the sick are gathered together in one area for treatment or care. During the past two decades, several factors have led to an increased awareness and interest in hospital-acquired infections. Some of these relate to antimicrobial therapy and the emergence of drug-resistant bacteria; others include the technologic advances of medicine in diagnosis and therapy. All these factors have resulted in an increased number of "compromised" hosts. A compromised host is a person who, for one reason or another, is more susceptible to infection than the average person. Examples of compromised hosts include patients who are immature, aged, immobile, receiving steroids, recuperating from surgery, or severely burned. The main task of medical personnel is to minimize the occurrence of nosocomial infections as much as possible. This task poses a number of simple questions: What should be done? When should it be done? Why should it be done? Who should do it? Owing to the scope of this subject, we shall be limited to discussing only the main principles and practices involved in the control of nosocomial infections. The student should consult the reading list for additional information.

SOURCES OF INFECTION

The first item to consider in the control of any infection is the source. The most common source of a nosocomial infection is the patient. Infection may occur when the patient himself contaminates diseased or exposed areas of his own body; when hospital personnel contaminate exposed areas with patient soils while treating the patient; when the patient contaminates other patients directly (for example, by coughing) or indirectly (by sharing common utilities or through the careless practices of hospital personnel). Other common sources of infection are foods, either made in the hospital or brought in; unsterile equipment or dressings; contaminated intravenous fluids; hospital personnel. The number of less common sources of infection could be virtually endless.

WHAT CONSTITUTES AN INFECTION?

A nosocomial or hospital-acquired infection may be defined as an infection that is not indicated or incubating at the time of the patient's admission, and does not manifest itself within the first 72 hours of hospitalization. (Some obviously hospital-acquired infections, such as postoperative wound infection, do occur within the first 72 hours.)

The foregoing definition of hospital-acquired infections is limited by the definition of infection itself, and this definition will vary from hospital to hospital if not from physician to physician. Some basic criteria must be set that are neither too narrow nor too broad. Table 9–2 lists some criteria that may serve as a basic guide. It should be the task of the Infectious Diseases (ID) Committee to determine what constitutes a nosocomial infection in a particular hospital or hospital ward.

Table 9–2. Some basic criteria for determination of nosocomial infection

Infective Site	Criteria
Blood	Isolation of organisms
Burns	New pus or an inflammation not present on admission
Respiratory tract	Isolation of pathogen or symptoms not present on admission
Intestinal tract	As above
Wounds	Presence of pus

WHO COMPRISE AN ID COMMITTEE?

An Infectious Diseases Committee is any group of individuals who have the knowledge and authority to determine what constitutes a nosocomial infection and what must be done to control such infections. In the smaller hospital, such a committee could be composed of the chief medical officer, the administrator, the senior laboratorian, the senior nurse, and a specific individual assigned the role of infectious control officer or epidemiologist. In the larger hospital, it could be a group of similar professionals and a full-time epidemiologist.

WHAT DOES THE ID COMMITTEE DO?

In general, the I.D. Committee monitors or surveys the incidence of infectious diseases and issues instructions on how to control or prevent them. More specifically, they should:

1. Review patient charts for clues that would detect new infections.
2. Follow-up the course of actual infections.
3. Monitor the use of antibiotic therapy.
4. Monitor staff sickness reports.
5. Review necropsy reports.
6. Prepare reports on the incidence of infections and review these monthly, quarterly and annually in order to study trends and detect shortcomings.
7. Meet frequently with appropriate staff members to discuss current problems in various areas.
8. Prepare a hospital ID Control Manual.
9. Review laboratory reports.
10. Initiate specific surveys when warranted.

In most hospitals, the majority of these tasks can best be carried out by two specific officers: a survey officer who screens all pertinent data for detection of infections, and an epidemiologist who follows up on the course of detected infections. In the smaller hospitals, the first task may be assigned as part of the duties of a nursing supervisor. The epidemiologist should be a medical officer. Both officers should be responsible to the Infectious Diseases Committee and should be given sufficient authority to allow them to carry out their tasks.

CONTROL OF HOSPITAL PERSONNEL

All personnel recruited to the hospital environment should undergo some degree of health screening. They should be required to present a general certificate of health. They should also have a chest x-ray study, and their immunization records should be reviewed. Immunization is advocated to protect against tuberculosis, polio, tetanus, diphtheria, rubella and smallpox. Laboratory personnel should be informed of the benefits of typhoid vaccination and encouraged to receive that vaccine. Immunization records should be maintained and schedules updated as required. Follow-up chest x-ray studies should be routinely conducted at least every two years. Personnel required to handle foods should be screened for febrile antibody levels. If antibody studies prove positive or doubtful, a fecal culture and analysis should be performed. When problems occur, special screening of specific personnel groups may be undertaken.

Hospital personnel should be encouraged not to report for work when they have symptoms of infectious diseases. Obviously sufficient arrangements must be made to replace sick employees as required.

CONTROL OF PATIENTS AND VISITORS

Visitations should be restricted everywhere in the hospital. No visitors with communicable diseases should be allowed to enter patient wards. Special restrictions should limit visitors to patients with burns, those in obstetrics, gynecology, or neonatology, and, of course, those who have infectious diseases.

Isolation techniques and protocols must be outlined and strictly practiced. The following are brief guidelines that should be expanded upon and made more specific in each hospital Infectious Disease Control Manual.

Strict Isolation. All visitors must report to the nursing station before entering the patient's room. The patient must be provided with a private room and the door must be kept closed. All persons entering the room must wear gowns, masks and gloves. All articles removed from the room must be wrapped and either disposed of by incineration or autoclaved before reuse.

The following diseases require strict isolation: pulmonary anthrax, extensive burns infected with *Staphylococcus aureus* or *S. pyogenes*, diphtheria, eczema vaccinatum, pulmonary or extrapulmonary melioidosis with draining sinuses, herpes simplex of neonates, plague, rabies, rubella, smallpox, staphylococcal pneumonia or enterocolitis, streptococcal pneumonia, and generalized or progressive vaccinia.

Respiratory Isolation. All visitors must report to the nursing station before entering the patient's room. The patient must be provided with a private room and the door must be kept closed.

Masks must be worn by all persons entering the room. Hands must be washed before entry and upon leaving the room. All articles contaminated with secretions must be incinerated or disinfected.

The following diseases require respiratory isolation: chickenpox, herpes zoster, measles, meningococcal meningitis, mumps, whooping cough, rubella, tuberculosis and Venezuelian equine encephalitis.

Enteric Isolation. Only children require a private room; adults should be instructed in proper toilet practices. All persons coming in direct contact with the patient must wear gloves and gowns. Hands must be washed before entry and upon leaving the room. Articles contaminated with urine or feces must be incinerated or disinfected, and should be removed only by persons wearing gloves.

The following diseases require enteric isolation: cholera, gastroenteritis caused by *Escherichia coli,* viral hepatitis, salmonellosis, and shigellosis.

Protective Isolation. All visitors must report to the nursing station before entering the patient's room. The patient must be provided with a private room and the door must be kept closed. Gowns and masks must be worn by all persons entering the room. Hands must be washed before entry and upon leaving the room. All persons having direct contact with the patient must wear gloves. Articles that could be hazardous to the patient must be excluded from the room or specially treated before entry.

Conditions requiring protective care are agranulocytosis, severe and extensive dermatitis, certain patients receiving immunosuppressive drugs or suffering from lymphomas or leukemia.

Wound and Skin Isolation. All visitors must report to the nursing station before entering the patient's room. A private room would be desirable. Masks must be worn when dressings are being changed, and gloves must be worn by anyone having direct contact with the patient. Hands must be washed before entry and upon leaving the room. Articles such as dressings, soiled linens and instruments must be decontaminated or incinerated.

Conditions requiring wound and skin isolation are extensive burns, gas gangrene, impetigo, staphylococcal skin and wound infections, streptococcal skin infections, and any other extensive wound infection.

ROUTINE PRECAUTIONS

All hospital garbage must be packed in closed containers and disposed of with care. All laundry must be sacked and labelled "contaminated" if at all suspicious. All instruments and furnishings must be kept spotless and must be disinfected whenever contaminated or between their use by different patients. Disposable items, such as needles, lancets, syringes, masks, gowns, gloves, cups, and specimen containers, must be discarded in a safe manner. They should preferably be placed in a container that cannot be pierced by sharp objects and can be incinerated easily.

Housekeeping and maintenance personnel must receive proper instruction to minimize the possible risk of their causing the spread of infection from one area to another, and, in general, they must be made aware of the differences between housekeeping practices performed in hospitals and those performed in hotels and other institutions that do not cater to the infirm. Sterilization and disinfection procedures must be monitored continually throughout the hospital to ensure their efficacy.

ENVIRONMENTAL CONTROL

Indiscriminate sampling of the hospital environment for microbial contents is not a positive approach to infectious disease control. No meaningful standards have been established to determine acceptable or unacceptable levels of microbial contents of air, floors, walls, doorknobs or other objects. Routine sampling of these objects only provides data that are difficult to interpret. Therefore, environmental sampling should be limited to the investigation of specific problems; e.g., as when a particular article or area is suspected to be the source of infection. When it is necessary to investigate a specific problem, the laboratory should be consulted to guide the selection and collection of specimens that would provide the best test material.

In some instances it may be desirable to spot-check certain equipment, especially when cleaning or operating procedures have been recently changed. Equipment that should be checked under these circumstances includes reusable face masks, endotracheal tubes, antiseptic solutions, ice, instruments sterilized by cold sterilization, humidifiers, nebulizers, and anesthesia apparatus. The checking and sampling procedures should always be coordinated with the service laboratory and its staff.

FURTHER READING

1. Boyd, W., and Sheldon, H.: *An Introduction to the Study of Disease.* 7th ed. Philadelphia, Lea & Febiger, 1977.
2. Lowbury, E. J. L. et al.: *Control of Hospital Infection: a practical handbook.* London: Chapman and Hall, 1975.
3. Gibson, G. L. (ed.): *Infection in Hospitals: A code of practice,* 2nd ed. Edinburgh: E. & S. Livingstone, 1974.
4. *Isolation techniques for use in hospitals.* Washington, D.C., Dept. H.E.W., Publication No. (H.S.M.) 71–8043, 1970.

Part II
SYSTEMATIC MEDICAL
MICROBIOLOGY

Gram-Positive Cocci

10-1 CLASSIFICATION

Bergey's Manual, Part 14
Gram-positive cocci
Group a, aerobic or facultatively anaerobic
  Family I. Micrococcaceae
    Genus   I. *Micrococcus*   Species: *luteus*
                                                  roseus
                                                  varians

                II. *Staphylococcus*   *aureus*
                                                  epidermidis
                                                  saprophyticus

                III. *Planococcus*   *citreus*

Family II. Streptococcaceae
   Genus   I. *Streptococcus*   Species: *pyogenes*
                                                    pneumoniae
                                                    faecalis
                                                    bovis
                                                    mitis
                                                    16 others
                  II. *Leuconostoc*   6 species
                  III. *Pediococcus*   5 species
                  IV. *Aerococcus*   *viridans*
                  V. *Gemella*   *haemolysans*
Group b, anaerobic
   Family III. Peptococcaceae
      Genus   I. *Peptococcus*   6 species
                   II. *Peptostreptococcus*   5 species
                  III. *Ruminococcus*   2 species
                   IV. *Sarcina*   2 species

DEFINITIONS

Micrococcaceae. Gram-positive cocci that occur in groups or pairs and divide on more than one plane. Nonsporogenous; may be motile or nonmotile. They are catalase-positive, attack carbohydrates fermentatively, and grow well on ordinary media either aerobically or anaerobically.

Micrococcus. Similar to *Staphylococcus* but do not ferment glucose.

Staphylococcus. Appear typically in clusters, are nonmotile, and ferment glucose and several other carbohydrates.

Planococcus. Appear typically in tetrads, are motile, and do not ferment glucose.

Streptococcaceae. Gram-positive cocci or ovoid cells, arranged in pairs, short chains, or in tetrads; nonsporogenous and usually nonmotile. They are catalase-variable, ferment carbohydrates, and have more complex nutrient requirements than members of Family I.

Streptococcus. Appear in pairs or chains in liquid media; all except some strains of Group D are nonmotile. Catalase-negative; glucose fermented by the hexose diphosphate pathway.

Leuconostoc. Divide in one plane, resulting in pairs or chains. Catalase-negative; glucose fermented by the hexose monophosphate pathway.

Pediococcus. Divide in two planes, resulting in pairs and

tetrads. Catalase variable. Yield inactive lactic acid from glucose fermentation.

Aerococcus. Like *Pediococcus,* but yields dextrorotatory lactic acid from fermentation.

Gemella. Gram-reaction is indeterminable, but cell wall structure resembles that of gram-positive bacteria. Catalase is negative and glucose is fermented.

Peptococcaceae. Gram-positive cocci that grow only anaerobically. Generic characteristics are summarized in Table 10–5.

10-2 STAPHYLOCOCCUS

Species of the genus *Staphylococcus* are among the bacteria most frequently isolated from human specimens. They are normally present on our skin, where most of them live as commensals. Most strains behave as opportunists, invading tissues when a person acquires minor or major injuries. Their invasive powers are related to their ability to produce the enzyme coagulase. Coagulase production is also the major characteristic by which the species are differentiated.

MORPHOLOGY

Staphylococcus microorganisms are gram-positive cocci arranged in irregular, grapelike clusters (Fig. 10–1). Their average diameter is 1 μm, depending on the age of the culture and the type of culture medium used. Older cultures display more single, enlarged forms, and are often gram-negative. In broth cultures, singles, pairs, and the odd short chain are apparent. Longer chains are rarely seen.

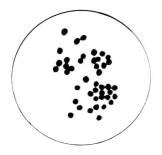
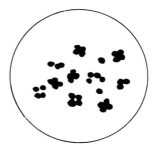

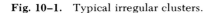

Fig. 10–1.   Typical irregular clusters.   **Fig. 10–2.**   Typical tetrads.

CULTURAL CHARACTERISTICS

Staphylococcus are aerobic and facultatively anaerobic. They grow well on simple media, at temperatures ranging from 10° to 42°C. Optimal growth temperature is 36°C and optimal pH is 7.4. Staphylococci grow well in media containing up to 10% sodium chloride; thus, salt mannitol agar (see p. 395) can be used for species differentiation. Only few strains produce scanty growth on Mac-Conkey agar. On blood agar after 24 hours at 37°C, the colonies will be circular, low convex, entire, opaque, shiny and butyrous. Some strains produce hemolysis. They all produce pigmentation, ranging from creamy white to deep golden. Pigmentation is no longer a dependable criterion for classification.

BIOCHEMICAL CHARACTERISTICS

Different species and even strains ferment a variety of car-bohydrates without producing gas. The most useful sugar to be used in differentiation of the species is mannitol.

Members of the species S. *aureus* produce the enzyme coagulase. Coagulase is an enzyme or coenzyme associated with the coagulation of blood plasma. It can be detected easily by a rapid slide or tube test (see Coagulase test, p. 427).

RESISTANCE

Staphylococcus are among the most resistant of the nonsporogenous bacteria. Nutrient agar cultures may remain viable for years. Many strains are resistant to drying and have been isolated from books and clothing up to 14 weeks following contamination. They are destroyed by heat at 60°C in 30 minutes, provided they are in suspension. In the absence of serum, pus or albumin, they are killed by 2% phenol in 15 minutes, by 3% hydrogen peroxide in three minutes, and by 70% ethanol in one hour.

Crystal violet at 1:500,000 and brilliant green at 1:10,000,000 are inhibitory and may be incorporated in certain selective media to eliminate *Staphylococcus* species.

Most strains of *Staphylococcus* are sensitive to a wide range of antibiotics. Several strains, however, have developed a high resis-tance to many of the commonly used antibiotics. Antibiotic resis-tancy patterns of *Staphylococcus* are constantly changing, resistant strains being found more readily in hospital personnel than in the population at large.

ANTIGENICITY

Staphylococcus species have been demonstrated to carry a number of agglutinating antigens. Since most antigens are carried by different species, no clear distinction can be made between the species on the basis of antigenic analysis.

PATHOGENICITY

The pathogenicity of *Staphylococcus* is associated with the ability of the organism to produce a number of different toxins. Of these, the enterotoxin is responsible for a common type of food poisoning. Ingestion of relatively small amounts of enterotoxin results in vomiting and diarrhea within about four to six hours. On the other hand, the exotoxin causes necrosis of the skin and lyses red blood cells during the development of boils or other local abscesses. From these local inflammations, the organisms frequently spread by way of the lymphatics and the blood. Hence, staphylococcal infections often develop into more serious diseases such as pneumonia, meningitis, endocarditis, osteomyelitis and many others.

TREATMENT

Toxoid treatment has been used but does not seem to be of much value. Antibiotics are useful in the treatment of many staphylococcal infections. The development of resistance and the ease of reinfection, however, are serious factors limiting effective treatment. The inability of antibiotics to act on organisms located in the central necrotic part of many lesions further complicates the picture. It is often necessary to drain closed lesions as part of the treatment.

TRANSMISSION

Staphylococcus are carried on most normal skins. *S. aureus* is frequently found in the nasopharynx of healthy individuals, more commonly in hospital personnel.

Invasive infections arise most frequently as complications of trauma, burns, or other skin lesions. They also occur more frequently with debilitating diseases such as cancer, diabetes, and cirrhosis of the liver. During puberty, recurrent superficial infections often occur in persons with hyperactive sebaceous glands, and in individuals subjected to oil, grease, and similar skin irritants.

The most common spread is from contaminated gauze, fomites and other materials directly associated with infected sites.

PREVENTION

Vaccines have been prepared to help protect individuals against staphylococcal infections. Their effectiveness in rendering protection is dubious indeed. The only preventive measure that meets with moderate success in reducing the number of staphylococcal infections is the exercise of scrupulous hygienic practice.

LABORATORY DIAGNOSIS

Specimens. Depending on the localization of the infection, the more common types of specimens from which *S. aureus* is isolated are pus, nasal swabs, wound swabs, ear swabs, blood, sputum, and even spinal fluid. The organisms are not very susceptible to environmental changes, so that no special precautions need be taken to preserve the specimens.

Direct Examination. Clinical material from staphylococcal infections usually reveals a large number of characteristic gram-positive cocci in clusters. The blood is an exception to this rule.

Isolation. Specimens planted on blood agar plates give rise to numerous, typical colonies when incubated at 37°C overnight. Specimens such as sputa, nasal swabs, and others which may contain a number of bacterial types other than *Staphylococcus* may be planted on salt mannitol agar. This medium is selective for *Staphylococcus* and further differentiates between mannitol fermenters and nonmannitol fermenters.

Identification. In the past, much emphasis has been placed on characteristics such as pigment production, hyaluronidase production, mannitol fermentation and so forth.

Presently, all coagulase producers are called *Staphylococcus aureus*, regardless of other characteristics the isolates may further exhibit.

S. aureus can be further typed on the basis of lysogenic characteristics when subjected to specific bacteriophages. A number of different bacteriophages—bacterial viruses—have been isolated, which demonstrate a predilection for some types of *S. aureus* and an indifference to others. By subjecting *S. aureus* to a number of different phages, all labelled with a specific number, a pattern of phage sensitivity may thus be ascertained.

10-3 STREPTOCOCCI

During the preantibiotic era, streptococcal infections, together with tuberculosis, resulted in more deaths than did any other infectious disease.

MORPHOLOGY

Individual organisms are spherical, gram-positive cells, measuring 0.5 to 1.0 μm in diameter. In liquid media, they frequently develop in long chains of eight or more. The cells may be somewhat elongated along the axis of the chain (see Fig. 10–3). They are nonsporogenous.

Older cultures tend to lose their gram-positivity. Several virulent strains produce capsules. Only a few saprophytic strains are motile.

CULTURAL CHARACTERISTICS

Streptococcus grow on ordinary media but much better on media containing serum or blood. Several pathogenic strains require enriched media.

The optimal temperature for most streptococci is 37°C; notable reduction in growth occurs above 40°C or below 30°C. The absolute growth range lies between 22° and 42°C. The pH growth range is narrow, 7.4 to 7.6. Additional glucose, at 0.5%, enhances the growth of most species but will alter the hemolytic activity.

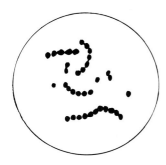

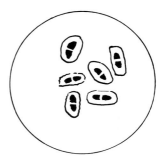

Fig. 10–3. Typical streptococci.   **Fig. 10–4.** Typical pneumococci.

Characteristically, hemolysis may be demonstrated as:

a. *Alpha hemolysis,* a partial or incomplete hemolysis, in which a greenish, somewhat slimy-appearing discolorization is produced in a narrow zone surrounding the colony *(S. viridans* and some *S. faecalis).*

b. *Beta, or complete hemolysis,* appears as a clearly transparent zone, usually extending several times beyond the diameter of the colony (most *S. pyogenes,* some *S. faecalis* and all *S. hemolyticus).*

c. *No hemolysis* (most *S. faecalis,* and almost all non-pathogenic *Streptococcus).*

To obtain clearly characteristic hemolysis, horse or rabbit blood should be employed. Sheep blood is reasonably satisfactory, but human blood is definitely unsatisfactory.

BIOCHEMICAL CHARACTERISTICS

Fermentation studies have been carried out extensively in the past in efforts to differentiate between various types, groups and species. Presently, serologic methods are gradually replacing fermentation and other biochemical methods. Much biochemical information has been obtained about streptococcal cell products. Evidence exists that relates some of these products with a variety of disease syndromes associated with streptococcal pathogenicity.

RESISTANCE

All except *S. faecalis* are sensitive to 60°C for 30 minutes (pasteurization). Most of the pathogenic species are sensitive to sulfonamides and a range of different antibiotics. Group A hemolytic streptococci are generally sensitive to penicillin and erythromycin.

In sputum, exudates and excreta, *Streptococcus* have been found to survive for weeks. Disinfectants are useful in eliminating them from instruments, furniture and general objects.

VARIABILITY

In general, mucoid and matt colonies contain large amounts of so-called M protein and are virulent. Glossy colonies contain little or no M protein and are usually avirulent. L forms (bacteria with deficient cell walls) of both alpha- and beta-hemolytic strains have been isolated.

ANTIGENICITY

Streptococcus species can be divided into serologic groups on the basis of 15 group-specific carbohydrates (mucopolysaccharides). Further subdivision of groups into types is also possible. The polysaccharide antigens were first discovered by Lancefield in 1933, hence the designation "Lancefield grouping." The 15 group-specific antigens are labelled from A to O. Most streptococcal infections in man are caused by members of Groups A, B, C, D or G. Infections by members of other groups are rare indeed. Certain streptococcal toxins are also antigenic, particularly streptolysin O and "Dick's toxin" (see below).

PATHOGENICITY

Streptococcal infections may occur in every organ or tissue of the body, in a pattern generally analogous to staphylococcal infections. The more common streptococcal infections include the following.

Epidemic Sore Throat. *S. pyogenes,* Group A, causes this disease.

Scarlet Fever. An erythrogenic toxin produced by certain strains of Group A causes this disease. Patients exposed to this toxin, also referred to as "Dick's toxin," usually develop antibodies in their serum. The Dick test makes use of this erythrogenic toxin. When small doses of "Dick's toxin" are injected intradermally, a typical rash will occur in the injected area within 24 hours unless the individual carries sufficient antibodies to neutralize the toxin.

Another skin test, the Schultz-Charlton test, uses an injection of homologous antitoxin at the height of the scarlet fever outbreak. The antitoxin will neutralize the toxic effect, resulting in a localized blanching of the rash. Consequently, the Dick test is useful in establishing the immune status of an individual; the Schultz-Charlton test, in diagnosing scarlet fever.

Subacute Bacterial Endocarditis (S.B.E.). This disease may be caused by any type of organism that enters the circulation and subsequently establishes itself on the heart valves. Most frequently, however, *S. viridans* is the cause of this condition, usually from bacteremia following tooth extraction.

Rheumatic Fever. This is probably the most serious condition resulting from streptococcal infections, caused mainly by *S. pyogenes,* group A.

Various skin diseases. Impetigo, erysipela, and carbuncles are among the conditions that may result from a variety of streptococcal infections.

Puerperal Fever. Also known as childbed fever, this infection may develop when streptococci enter the uterus after delivery. Fortunately rare today, puerperal fever claimed the lives of thousands of women only a hundred years ago.

Other streptococcal infections may result in sinusitis, tonsillitis, pharyngitis, laryngitis, mastoiditis, pneumonia, glomerulonephritis and even meningitis.

TREATMENT

Most streptococcal diseases respond well to antibiotic treatment. Some, particularly rheumatic fever, are frequently recurrent unless prolonged antibiotic treatment is administered in small doses.

TRANSMISSION AND PREVENTION

S. pyogenes seems more or less confined to man and is almost always acquired from another individual. Control of carriers greatly reduces the number of infections. Other *Streptococcus* species are very widely distributed. They are found in man, most domestic animals, rodents and also the lower animals.

Pasteurization of milk and other produce, as well as generally improved hygienic standards, have drastically reduced most of the once dreaded streptococcal diseases.

LABORATORY DIAGNOSIS

Specimens. Depending on the site of infection, different specimens may yield streptococcal isolates. Throat swabs constitute the type of specimen from which *Streptococcus* species are most frequently isolated. To increase the chances of isolation, serum-coated swabs have been advocated.

Direct Examination. Most areas of the body from which swabs may be taken normally harbor *Streptococcus* of one type or another. Therefore, examination of clinical material for the presence of streptococcal-like bacteria has little value. In the case of burns, wounds and other areas that should be sterile, the finding of bacteria would, of course, be more significant.

Isolation. This presents few problems in the laboratory. All *Streptococcus* grow reasonably well on blood agar and other routine media. Specimens that may contain a large number of "contaminants" can be planted on blood agar containing 1:500,000 of crystal violet, which renders the medium relatively selective for *Streptococcus*. *S. faecalis* also grows on MacConkey medium, on media containing 40% bile, or in broth containing 6.5% sodium chloride.

Identification. Table 10–4 outlines the patterns for differentiation of isolated pathogenic Streptococcacea. Differentiation from

Micrococcaceae and *Neisseriaceae* can readily be made by the catalase and oxidase tests respectively.

S. viridans can easily be differentiated from *S. faecalis* by its inability to withstand heat (60°C for 30 minutes) and its failure to grow in broth containing 6.5% sodium chloride.

Streptococcus isolates may be further typed on the basis of their antigenic composition (see Antigenicity).

Serology. Patients suffering from rheumatic fever usually develop antibodies against streptolysin O in their serum. Even though this antibody does not seem to render the patient immune, its detection offers a means of diagnosing cases of rheumatic fever. For antistreptolysin O titration, see Chapter 28.

10-4 PNEUMOCOCCI

This gram-positive coccus is a frequent cause of pneumonia in man. This organism was formerly classified as *Micrococcus pneumoniae* and as *Diplococcus pneumoniae*. Its similarity to *Streptococcus* has long been recognized, and it has now been placed in that genus in the eighth edition of *Bergey's Manual*. Because of its medical importance, we will consider it separately from the other streptococci.

MORPHOLOGY

Pneumococci appear in pairs and resemble two lancets with the opposite sides flattened, surrounded by a definite capsule (Fig. 10–4). They may form short chains in broth cultures. Swollen and irregular forms are frequently observed in cultures older than 24 hours, at which time they may also lose their gram-positivity.

CULTURAL CHARACTERISTICS

Streptococcus pneumoniae is rather sensitive to pH changes. For optimal growth, the pH should be between 7.6 and 7.8. It grows at a temperature range from 25° to 41°C, but only well at 37°C, ± 1. The organisms lyse rapidly in the presence of surface active agents such as bile, and spontaneously in culture (autolysis). The colonial morphology is characterized by this autolytic effect. Individual colonies appear as small craters (crateriform), surrounded by a greenish halo on blood agar owing to alpha-hemolysis.

Glucose and glycerine added to the culture aid the rate of growth, but also speed up autolysis by causing production of acid end-products. The chances for successfully isolating organisms in culture are improved under 10% carbon dioxide.

RESISTANCE

S. pneumoniae has been recovered from dried sputum after several months. On ordinary culture media it seldom survives more than a few days. Heat, 52°C for 10 minutes, and routine disinfectants rapidly destroy these organisms, which are sensitive to many antibiotics, particularly to penicillins.

The fact that S. pneumoniae is sensitive to optochin (1:4000 ethyl hydrocupreine hydrochloride) and to bile salts (2% sodium deoxycholate or 10% ox bile) has great diagnostic significance (see Laboratory Diagnosis).

ANTIGENICITY

All strains of S. pneumoniae carry a group-specific somatic antigen by which they can readily be classified. Further classification of some 85 different serotypes is possible, on the basis of specific capsular polysaccharides, by the "capsular swelling test" or the "Quellung reaction." In this reaction, a certain type of S. pneumoniae is mixed with a type-specific antiserum. The antibodies form a precipitate at the outer fringe of the capsules of individual cells when they react with their corresponding antigen on the capsule. The capsule is then more clearly delineated, and appears as though it had swollen.

PATHOGENICITY AND TREATMENT

The most characteristic human infection by S. pneumoniae is lobar pneumonia. The onset is usually sudden with the appearance of fever, chills and sharp pains in the chest. The sputum is a characteristic "rusty" color owing to an outpouring of bloody exudate. Bacteremia is common during the early stage (25%) and may develop into sinusitis, mastoiditis, and not infrequently, meningitis. With the advent of antibiotic therapy, the incidence of pneumococcal meningitis and other complications is rare. The administration of pneumococcal antisera, once a common treatment, is no longer used.

TRANSMISSION AND PREVENTION

In some areas, about 50% of the population carry virulent types of S. pneumoniae in their nasopharynx. However, certain predisposing factors must be present before these organisms manifest themselves clinically:

a. Injuries to the respiratory tract. These may be caused by virus infections, excessive smoking, or environmental factors such as silicoses of miners.

b. Circulatory or respiratory defects resulting in obstruction or congestion.

c. Malnutrition, fatigue, or general debility.

LABORATORY DIAGNOSIS

The most common specimen, of course, is sputum. The technologist should examine the mucopurulent portion (flecks) rather than the saliva. Blood cultures and, in the event of a pneumococcal meningitis, spinal fluid, may also yield pneumococci. Pneumococcal meningitis may occasionally be diagnosed by testing the spinal fluid with specific antisera in a capillary tube precipitation test.

Isolation of the organisms under increased CO_2 presents few problems. Identification may be aided by comparing cultural characteristics and consulting Table 10-4 and Chart 10-1. Optochin sensitivity is the most reliable means of identifying S. pneumoniae. Optochin discs placed on blood agar inhibit growth of S. pneumoniae in zones up to 30 mm in diameter. Other commonly isolated alpha-hemolytic colonies are not affected by the optochin.

10-5 DIFFERENTIATION

The medical bacteriologist should determine which characteristics of the organisms in question would yield the fastest, most reliable, and most clinically significant test results. When dealing with gram-positive cocci, the primary differentiation is based on cellular arrangements (Figs. 10–1 to 10–4) and on colonial characteristics. Since the emphasis is on clinically significant pathogens, the recognition of these among possible mixtures of other bacteria (see Chapter 25) is important. With a little experience, spotting staphylococcal- or streptococcal-like colonies becomes relatively simple. A quick gram-stain yields the morphology and gram-reaction, and a catalase test further differentiates between Staphylococcus (+) and Streptococcus (−). A coagulase test then differentiates S. aureus from other Staphylococcus species, and phage-typing may be performed if necessary.

Differentiation of Streptococcus species is more involved. Of primary importance is the identification of Group A beta-hemolytic Streptococcus and S. pneumoniae. These may be detected by the relatively simple bacitracin and optochin susceptibility tests.

Beta-hemolytic streptococci susceptible to bacitracin may be label-led *Streptococcus pyogenes* Group A; optochin-susceptible gram-positive cocci are *S. pneumoniae*.

In most diagnostic laboratories, only the foregoing procedures are done routinely. If gram-positive cocci other than *Staphylococcus aureus, Streptococcus pyogenes* Group A, or *Streptococcus pneumoniae* need to be identified, the primary characteristics listed in Chart 25–1 should be determined and that table utilized as a guide to initial differentiation. Secondary identification within the respective families should then proceed as follows.

Micrococcaceae. Isolates belonging to this family can be placed in their respective genera on the basis of morphology, motility, pigmentation, and glucose fermentation (see Table 10–1).

Micrococcus species may be identified by pigmentation and glucose oxidation (Table 10–2). For clinical purposes, however, this is hardly necessary. *Staphylococcus* species are differentiated by coagulase production, mannitol fermentation, and novobiocin susceptibility (Table 10–3).

Planococcus is a monotypic genus and requires no further testing.

Table 10–1. Differentiation of Micrococcaceae

	Micrococcus	*Staphylococcus*	*Planococcus*
Irregular clusters	+	+	−
Tetrads	∓	−	+
Ferment glucose	−	+	−
Motility	−	−	+
Yellow-brown pigment	−	−	+

Table 10–2. Differentiation of *Micrococcus*

	M. luteus	*M. roseus*	*M. varians*
Yellow pigment	+	−	+
Red pigment	−	+	−
Oxidize glucose	−	±	+

Table 10–3. Differentiation of *Staphylococcus*

	S. aureus	*S. epidermidis*	*S. saprophyticus*
Produce coagulase	+	−	−
Ferment mannitol	+	−	+
Sensitive to novobiocin	Yes	Yes	No

Table 10–4. Differentiaion of Streptococcaceae

	Hemolyse sheep blood agar	*Grow at 45°C*	*Survive 60°C for 30 min.*	*Grow at pH 9.6*
Streptococcus	+ (β, α); −	∓	∓	∓
Leuconostoc	−	−	−	−
Pediococcus	−	+	−	−
Aerococcus	α	−	+	+
Gemella	−	−	−	−

Streptococcaceae. Isolates of this family can be grouped in genera by following Table 10–4.

Streptococcus species may be differentiated on the basis of their hemolytic activity, after which Charts 10–1, 10–2 or 10–3 may be consulted. Serologic differentiation of streptococci may also be done.* It is advisable to corroborate serologic results with the biochemical analysis.

Leuconostoc species are seldom encountered in the clinical laboratory. They are important only in the brewing and food-canning industries.

Pediococcus and *Aerococcus* divide in two planes and produce some tetrads in broth. *Aerococcus* survive 60°C for 30 minutes and grow at pH 9.6; *Pediococcus* species do not. There is no need to further differentiate *Pediococcus* species isolated in the clinical laboratory.

Gemella can be identified by following Chart 10–3.

---

*Antisera for streptococcal identification are available from Difco Laboratories, Detroit, Mich., or Baltimore Biological Laboratories, Cockeysville, Md.

Chart 10–1. Identification of beta-hemolytic streptococci.

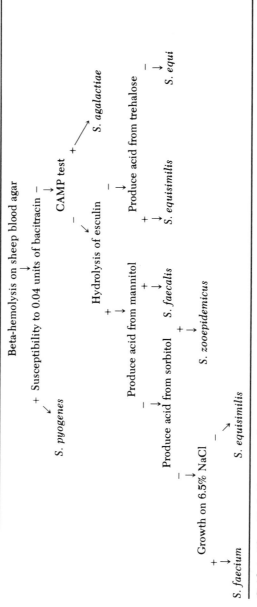

Guide to Chart 10–1: Determine bacitracin susceptibility, perform CAMP test, determine hydrolysis of esculin, acid production from mannitol, trehalose, and sorbitol, and growth in 6.5% NaCl. Record results and follow chart.

Chart 10–2. Identification of alpha-hemolytic streptococci.

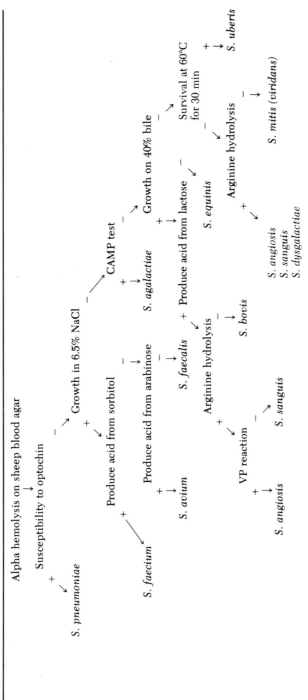

Guide to Chart 10–2: Determine optochin susceptibility, growth in 6.5% NaCl, CAMP reaction, acid production from sorbitol, acid production from arabinose, growth on 40% bile, acid production from lactose, survival following exposure to 60°C for 30 minutes, and hydrolysis of arginine. Record your results and follow the chart.

144

Chart 10–3. Identification of nonhemolytic streptococci and Gemella.

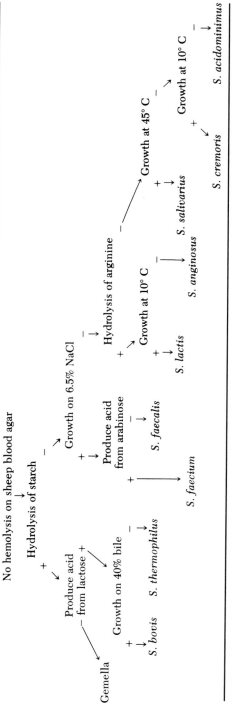

Guide to Chart 10–3: Determine hydrolysis of starch, growth on 40% bile, growth on 6.5% NaCl, acid production from arabinose, hydrolysis of arginine, growth at 10° C and at 45° C. Record your results and follow the chart.

Table 10–5. Differentiation of Peptostreptococcaceae

	Appear in long chains	Appear in cubic packets	Digest cellulose
Peptococcus	−	−	−
Peptostreptococcus	+	−	−
Ruminococcus	±	−	+
Sarcina	−	+	−

Peptostreptococcaceae. These anaerobic gram-positive cocci are frequently isolated from clinical materials; however, their clinical significance has not been clearly established. They are generally saprophytic in nature and play a part as opportunistic invaders when other bacteria are primary infectious agents.

The genera can be differentiated (see Table 10–5). Differentiation is difficult, however, and requires the services of a competent reference laboratory.

FURTHER READING

1. WHO Expert Committee on the Prevention of Rheumatic Fever. Technical Report No. 342, World Health Organization, Geneva, 1966.
2. Deibel, R. H.: The Group D streptococci. Bact. Rev., 28:330–366, 1964.
3. Dowling, H. F.: The rise and fall of pneumonia control programs. J. Infect. Dis., 127:201–206, 1972.
4. Kimler, A.: Some clinical laboratory briefs on staphylococci. J. Bact., 83: 207–208, 1962.
5. Symposium on staphylococci and micrococci. J. Appl. Bact., 25:309–455, 1962.
6. Wentworth, B. B.: Bacteriophage typing of the staphylococci. Bact. Rev., 27:253–272, 1963.

chapter 11

Endospore-Forming Bacteria

11-1 Classification
11-2 *Bacillus*
11-3 *Clostridium*
11-4 Differentiation

11-1 CLASSIFICATION

Bergey's Manual, Part 15
Endospore-forming rods and cocci
    Family I. Bacillaceae
        Genus   I. *Bacillus*   Species: *anthracis*
                                              cereus
                                              subtilis
                                              45 others
                II. *Sporolactobacillus*   *inulinus*
              III. *Clostridium*   *botulinum*
                                                perfringens
                                              sporogenes
                                                tetani
                                              57 others
                IV. *Desulfotomaculum*   3
                 V. *Sporosarcina*   *ureae*
      Uncertain genus: Oscillospira   *guilliermondi*

DEFINITIONS

Bacillaceae. Gram-positive spore-forming bacteria.

Bacillus. Aerobic or facultatively anaerobic rods, catalase-positive and gelatin-liquefying. *Bacillus* may occur in long thread-like forms, particularly in rhizoid colonies; usually motile.

Sporolactobacillus. Aerobic to microaerophilic rods that are catalase negative.

Clostridium. Obligate anaerobic rods that do not reduce sulfate.

Desulfotomaculum. Obligate anaerobic rods that reduce sulfate to sulfide.

Sporosarcina. Aerobic coccus that grows only in complex media.

Oscillospira. Gram-negative, spore-forming rods that reproduce by transverse fission, are motile, anaerobic, and appear to be very fastidious.

11-2 BACILLUS

Nonpathogenic *Bacillus* species are among the most frequently isolated bacteria in any laboratory, largely because they are highly resistant and almost ubiquitous, occurring as saprophytes in the soil, water, plants and animals.

Most *Bacillus* organisms are fairly large, 0.4 by 3.0 μm wide to 2.0 by 9.0 μm long. They are usually straight rods with parallel sides and may be arranged in varying configurations. In older cultures, long disjointed filaments are often seen. Round or oval spores develop and may be located centrally, terminally or subterminally. Spores of *Bacillus* species are endospores; they do not extend beyond the width of the vegetating organism.

All routine media readily support the growth of bacilli, which is another reason for their frequent occurrence. They display a number of different colonial characteristics (finely granular, moist, membranous with or without obvious folds or wrinkles, butyrous, and even-spreading). Most species display rather large, opaque, dull, flat, and pigmented colonies that frequently hemolyze blood agar.

In the spore form, *Bacillus* are highly resistant to heat and to most disinfectants. They are killed by dry heat at 160°C in one hour and by moist heat at 120°C in about 20 minutes. The vegetating forms are no more resistant than are *Staphylococcus* species.

In the medical laboratory, aerobic gram-positive spore-formers that bear no resemblance to *Bacillus anthracis* are simply reported as "*Bacillus* species." Further identification serves no real purpose, although some outbreaks of food poisoning have been attributed to *B. cereus*, and *B. subtilis* occasionally causes human eye infections. The latter species is also of interest because it produces the antibiotic bacitracin (see p. 115).

BACILLUS ANTHRACIS

This organism, the only pathogenic species of the genus *Bacillus*, primarily infects cattle and sheep, less frequently horses, goats, and dogs, and occasionally man. First discovered by Pasteur in 1881, the once common anthrax bacillus is a rarity in the North American medical world of today.

Morphology. *B. anthracis* microorganisms are straight or slightly curved rods that measure 1.0 to 1.2 μm by 3.0 to 8.0 μm. Their ends are usually truncated, and smears from cultures on solid media demonstrate the characteristic bamboostick appearance of bacilli in chains (Fig. 11–1). Oval endospores are located at the center (Fig. 11–2). In exudates and serum-enriched media, capsules surrounding entire chains are prominent. Anthrax bacilli are nonmotile.

Cultural Characteristics. *B. anthracis* grows well on routine media at 37°C, with a growth range between 12°C and 45°. The colonial morphology varies with the type of medium employed. On nutrient agar, irregular, round, raised, dull, opaque, grayish-white, slightly undulate colonies, about 3 mm in diameter, appear in about 24 hours. In gelatin stabs, a rather characteristic "inverted fir tree" type of growth is displayed at first, with progressive liquefaction. Blood agar is not hemolyzed, and the colonies appear larger than those cultured on nutrient agar.

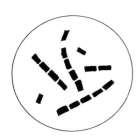

Fig. 11–1. Anthrax bacilli.

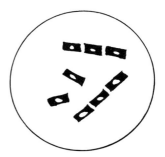

Fig. 11–2. Anthrax spores.

Biochemical Characteristics. Acid but no gas is produced from dextrose, sucrose and maltose. Litmus milk is decolorized and coagulated. The lecithinase reaction is feebly positive (see L.E.Y. medium, p. 410).

Pathogenicity. The disease anthrax may take one of three forms:

  a. *Cutaneous anthrax* manifests itself as a malignant pustule, usually on the forearms of persons who work in tanneries or with hides.
  b. *Pulmonary anthrax,* or "wool sorters" disease, is the more classic form of anthrax. Primary pneumonia results from the inhalation of anthrax spores from animal hides, hair, or wool.
  c. *Intestinal anthrax* is rare but severe and therefore worthy of note.

Treatment and Prevention. Specific antisera were used extensively in the past for treatment. More recently, antibiotics, particularly tetracyclines, have been used effectively against anthrax. Detection and control of anthrax-laden animals and vaccination of cattle and sheep in endemic areas have reduced the incidence of anthrax to fewer than ten human cases per year in North America.

Evidence of anthrax in carcasses or hides can be obtained by the Ascoli test. In this test, a small piece of spleen or hide is boiled for 15 minutes in about 10 ml of saline. Cooled and filtered, this preparation serves as an antigen. Placed with an equal portion of anthrax antiserum in a capillary tube so that the two will slowly diffuse into one another, a ring of precipitate will form at the interface within 20 minutes when anthrax antigens are present.

Laboratory Diagnosis. The typical microscopic structure of anthrax bacilli and the relative ease of their isolation when associated with one of the previously mentioned clinical pictures allows early identification. Results obtained from direct examination should be corroborated by isolation or by animal pathogenicity tests. Guinea pigs and mice develop generalized septicemia two days following subcutaneous injection. Many organisms can be seen in specimens from the spleen and in heart blood from carcasses. The spleen is also enlarged.

11-3 CLOSTRIDIUM

Pasteur, in 1861, originated studies of organisms belonging to this genus in his work on butyric acid and *Clostridium butyricum,* the type species of the genus. Until World War I, little further had become known about these anaerobic spore-formers. The frequency of gas gangrene infections among soldiers suffering bullet wounds prompted much research and the discovery of several *Clostridium* species.

MORPHOLOGY

Among *Clostridium* species, pleomorphism is common. The morphology has been found to vary from one subculture to another, even on the same type of medium. This variability causes difficulties when one attempts to differentiate between *Clostridium* species solely on the basis of microscopic morphology.

Generally, individual organisms belonging to species of this genus range from 0.4 to 1.2 μm in width and from 3 to 8 μm in length. Most individuals appear as straight rods; some may be

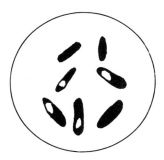

Fig. 11–3. *Clostridium perfringens* spores.

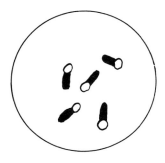

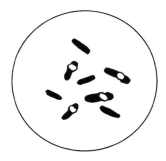

Fig. 11–4. *Clostridium tetani* spores.   **Fig. 11–5.** *Clostridium botulinum* spores.

curved. Their sides are usually parallel, and their ends may be rounded or truncated. They may be arranged singly, or in pairs, or in small groups in parallel bundles or short chains. Long filaments, as described under *Bacillus*, are also common.

All members of this genus are able to form spores; however, some do so more readily than others. The shape and location of the spore are aids in diagnosis. *C. perfringens* seldom forms spores unless it is grown in media containing magnesium sulfate. Then, oval, subterminal spores may be seen (Fig. 11–3). *C. tetani* sporulates readily, producing spores that extend two to three times the width of the bacterium itself. They are terminally located, and give this species its characteristic "drumstick" appearance (see Fig. 11–4). *C. botulinum* sporulates more readily when grown at 25°C than when grown at 37°C. Its spores are subterminal but slightly larger than the diameter of the organism (Fig. 11–5).

All *Clostridium* species are gram-positive, but oxidation of older cultures may cause changes in this reaction. *C. perfringens* is the only nonmotile species of the genus. *C. septicum* and *C. perfringens* are encapsulated when grown in media containing serum; *C. perfringens* is also encapsulated in serous exudates.

CULTURAL CHARACTERISTICS

All *Clostridium* species grow on blood agar, peptone water or meat infusions. Media must be freshly prepared, since they will absorb oxygen readily and thus become toxic to the obligate anaerobes. Liquid media can conveniently be boiled just prior to use in order to drive off absorbed oxygen. The number of boilings should be kept down to a maximum of two, however, because boiling destroys or alters some of the essential nutrients.

C. perfringens and *C. histolyticum* are microaerophilic; all other species are strict anaerobes. On solid media, most strains grow relatively slowly, sometimes producing only a thin, effuse, often spreading film on primary isolation. This film is easily missed unless the examiner is observant or experienced. For most species, the optimal pH range is 7.0 to 7.4, and the optimal temperature is 37°C. Some species are thermophilic, preferring temperatures between 50° and 60°C. The colonial morphology, as the microscopic morphology, is not constant and may vary from the same strain when subcultured on the same type of medium. On blood agar:

1. *C. perfringens* is generally round, smooth, opaque and butyrous. Characteristically the microorganisms show a double zone of partial and more complete hemolysis (the so-called target zone hemolysis).

2. *C. tetani* often spreads over large areas or over the entire surface of the plate. It is translucent and has a moist appearance.

3. *C. botulinum* is glistening, translucent, effuse, smooth or granular, with butyrous, somewhat filamentous colonies. It usually produces a narrow zone of beta hemolysis.

BIOCHEMICAL CHARACTERISTICS

A variety of sugars are readily fermented by *Clostridium* species. Species differentiation on this basis, however, is not as simple as it may seem. Some species decolorize indicators irreversibly, and other indicators are affected by anaerobic culture. To determine fermentation of carbohydrates by anaerobes, a special medium is recommended (see p. 401). *C. perfringens* produces acid and gas abundantly when inoculated in litmus milk. Associated with coagulation of proteins, this produces the so-called stormy clot. Other species demonstrate different reactions on litmus milk.

Some *Clostridium* species have the ability to produce the enzyme lecithinase. On L.E.Y. agar (see p. 410), lecithinase will precipitate lecithin, as demonstrated by a zone of opalescence surrounding a growth streak. Specific antitoxins inhibit lecithinase and hence opalescence on the medium.

RESISTANCE

Stock cultures of *Clostridium* may be kept on cooked meat broth at room temperature for several months and sometimes years. Most species are sensitive to sulfonamides, penicillins, and tetracyclines. For heat and disinfectant resistancy, see *Bacillus.*

PATHOGENICITY

Clostridium species causing disease in man have been divided into three groups:
  a. The gas gangrene group—*C. perfringens, C. novyi, C. septicum,* and others.
  b. The tetanus group—*C. tetani,* several types.
  c. The botulinum group—*C. botulinum,* A, B, C, D, E, and F.
Botulinus and tetanus toxins are among the most lethal toxins known. It has been estimated that 1 mg of botulinus toxin could kill 20 million mice and probably one thousand men.

Gas Gangrene. This disease is most commonly caused by *C. perfringens.* Other organisms that cause gangrene do not produce the abundant gas in tissues that characterizes infection with *C. perfringens.* Gangrene is a result of the activity of several enzymes and toxins produced by invading organisms. Collagenase digests collagen of subcutaneous tissue and muscle, thereby permitting the spread of the infection. Actual necrosis is mainly caused by lecithinase and theta-toxin.

The organisms are usually introduced through a deep wound, such as a bullet or stab wound. *Clostridium* grows slowly at first, but as the bacterial byproducts "pave the road," invasion becomes more and more rapid. Until the advent of antitoxin therapy, the only cure for this grotesque disease was amputation. Antibiotic therapy has further reduced the hazards of gas gangrene.

Tetanus Bacilli. These organisms are not invasive, but their potent toxin causes a more generalized disease. Following infection of a wound, burn or other injury, an incubation period of four to seven days or sometimes a month may elapse. A severe headache followed by difficulty in swallowing and in opening the mouth (lockjaw) are the earliest symptoms. The toxin is a neurotoxin that increases reflex excitability and often causes muscle spasm. Antitoxin should be administered promptly to neutralize the toxin before it becomes cell-bound. Untreated, tetanus is usually fatal.

Botulism. This is a food poisoning resulting from the ingestion of botulinus toxin. Seldom do *C. botulinum* invade wounds or tissues. The disease syndrome is characterized by difficulty in speech, inability to swallow, and diplopia (double vision) beginning twelve hours to four days following toxin ingestion. Even when specific antitoxins are administered quickly, the patient's chances for recovery are limited.

TRANSMISSION AND PREVENTION

C. perfringens and many other *Clostridium* species belong to the normal intestinal flora of animals and man. Unless they enter injured tissues, they have no invasive powers. Proper care of wounds, particularly those inflicted by farm implements and other articles that may be contaminated with manure and prophylactic antibiotic treatment are recommended.

C. tetani are commonly found in the feces of horses and other related animals. Tetanus toxoid is particularly antigenic to man. Early and repeated vaccinations have greatly reduced the incidence of tetanus. Because of the relatively long incubation period preceding tetanus, a "booster dose" of vaccine is routinely given to persons previously immunized when they accidentally injure themselves with articles thought to harbor tetanus bacilli. Patients suffering such wounds who have not been previously immunized may receive tetanus antitoxin.

C. botulinum toxin is transmitted most frequently through contaminated preserves and canned fish or meats. Strict controls in the food industry and the decreased practice of "home" preservation has reduced this already uncommon threat to an even more limited danger.

LABORATORY DIAGNOSIS

Specimens. Tissue, wound swabs or blood samples may reveal the organisms responsible in cases of gangrene. Toxin may be detected in tissue or wound swabs in tetanus, and in portions of the contaminated food in cases of botulism. Specimens should not be refrigerated or held more than two hours unless placed in a reducing medium.

Direct Examination. Gram-stained smears reveal *Clostridium*. The typical morphology of some species permits an early presumptive diagnosis in many cases.

Isolation. Specimens collected from cases of gangrene and tetanus often contain a number of aerobic bacteria, rendering primary isolation difficult because these aerobes may outgrow the *Clostridium* species. Heating a portion of the specimen at 80°C for 10 minutes will destroy most vegetating bacteria, thereby facilitating the isolation of spore-bearers. One should culture both a heated and a nonheated portion of the specimens on cooked meat broth and on two blood agar plates, one aerobic, one anaerobic. The media should be fresh and, once inoculated, incubated immediately under strict anaerobiosis (see Chapter 6).

11-4 DIFFERENTIATION

Sporolactobacillus, Desulfotomaculum and *Oscillospira* species are seldom encountered in the clinical laboratory and therefore need be of little concern to us. Gram-positive sporogenous cocci belong to the monotypic genus *Sporosarcina* and require no further identification.

Gram-positive, aerobic, spore-forming rods that are encountered in the clinical laboratory almost always belong to the genus *Bacillus*. Differentiation within this genus is difficult and serves no real purpose. When suspected, *B. anthracis* can be recognized as previously described. All other *Bacillus* isolates may be reported as "*Bacillus* species, no further identification."

Differentiation of *Clostridium* species is more involved. Of the

Table 11-1. Characteristics of the most common pathogenic *Clostridium* species.

	C. perfringens	*C. tetani*	*C. botulinum*	*C. novyi*	*C. septicum*
Microscopy	Sporulate only when grown with MgSO₄	Round, terminal spores, "drumsticks"	Round, subterminal spores, test at 25°C	Oval, central or subterminal spores	Oval, central or subterminal spores
Growth on cooked meat	Gas without digestion, but reddening of the meat	Little digestion, with darkening and a putrid odor	Gas with blackening of the meat	Gas without digestion, but reddening of the meat	Gas without digestion, but reddening of the meat
Dextrose	+	−	+	+	+
Lactose	+	−	−	−	+
Sucrose	+	−	−	−	−
Maltose	+	−	+	+	+
Litmus milk	Acid and gas, with rapid clotting, "stormy clot"	No change	No change	Acid and gas	Acid and gas, with slow clotting
Opalescence on L.E.Y. agar	Yes	No	Yes	Yes	No

61 species, at least five are commonly isolated in the clinical laboratory and are pathogenic to man. Generally speaking, all gram-positive, sporogenous, anaerobic rods isolated from clinical materials may be classified as *Clostridium* species. For further identification of the more common species, one may use a special fermentation medium (see p. 407), litmus milk, lactose-egg yolk-milk medium, and cooked meat broth. Typical reactions on these media are outlined in Table 11–1, which may be used as a guide in identifying the species listed. Clostridia that do not conform to any of these species may simply be labelled *Clostridium* species, or may be sent to a reference laboratory for differentiation, where more sophisticated techniques such as gas liquid chromatography may be available. A commercially available anaerobic multitest microsystem* appears to yield satisfactory results and may warrant adoption to allow the average clinical laboratory to expand its scope of identification of anaerobic isolates.

---

*Anaerobic Micromethod System, Analytab Products, Inc., New York, N.Y.

$MgSO_4$

FURTHER READING

1. Willis, A. T.: *Anaerobic Bacteriology in Clinical Medicine.* 3rd ed., London, Butterworth and Co., Publ. Ltd., 1977.
2. Dowell, V. R., Jr., and Hawkins, T. M.: *Laboratory Methods in Anaerobic Bacteriology,* Public Health Service, Publication No. 1803, Washington, D.C., U.S. Govt. Printing Office, 1968.
3. Smith, L. D.: *The Pathogenic Anaerobic Bacteria.* 2nd ed., Springfield, Ill., Charles C Thomas, 1975.
4. Holdeman, L. V., and Moore, W. E. C.: *Anaerobe Laboratory Manual.* 4th ed., Blacksburg, Virginia, Virginia Polytechnic Institute, 1977.

chapter 12
Gram-Positive Asporogenous Rods

12-1 CLASSIFICATION

Bergey's Manual, Part 16
Gram-positive, asporogenous, rod-shaped bacteria
    Family I. *Lactobacillaceae*
        Genus   I. *Lactobacillus*   Species: 25
    Genera of Uncertain Affiliation:
        Genus: *Listeria*   Species: *monocytogenes*
                                           3 others
                Erysipelothrix   *rhusiopathiae*
                Caryophanon   *latum*

Bergey's Manual, Part 17
Coryneform group of bacteria*

	Genus	I. *Corynebacterium*	Species:	*diphtheriae*
				38 others†
		II. *Arthrobacter*		7
		III. *Cellulomonas*		*flavigena*
		IV. *Kurthia*		*zopfii*
Family I. *Propionibacteriaceae*				
	Genus	I. *Propionibacterium*	Species:	8
		II. *Eubacterium*		28

DEFINITIONS

Lactobacillaceae. Straight or curved rods usually occurring singly or in chains. Generally nonmotile. Gram-positive aerobic or facultative anaerobes; catalase-negative.

Lactobacillus. Rods varying from long and slender to short coccobacillary. Chain formation is common. Carbohydrates are fermented; some strains are obligate anaerobes on isolation.

Listeria. Small coccoid rods with a tendency to produce short chains. Arrange in typical palisades as Y or V forms. Nonencapsulated, motile with peritrichous flagella at 20°C. Produce acid but no gas from glucose; hydrolyze esculin but not gelatin, casein or urea; are usually catalase-positive and oxidase-negative.

Erysipelothrix. Rod-shaped with a tendency to form long filaments. Nonencapsulated and nonmotile. Produce acid but no gas from glucose; do not hydrolyze esculin; are catalase-negative.

Corynebacterium. Straight to slightly curved rods with irregularly stained segments. May demonstrate granules, barring, or club-shaped swellings. Arrange in typical palisades. Generally nonmotile, facultative anaerobes. Ferment carbohydrates; are catalase-positive and oxidase-negative.

Arthrobacter. In complex media, these bacteria undergo a notable change in form. Do not ferment carbohydrates; are catalase-positive and oxidase-negative.

Cellulomonas. Similar to *Corynebacterium,* but occasional cells may show a rudimentary branching and metabolize primarily by oxidation.

---

*In *Bergey's Manual,* ed. 8, this group is included in Part 17, Actinomycetes and related forms. They present a number of unresolved problems in classification. For practical reasons, we have included them here and will refer to them and to *Listeria* and *Erysipelothrix* collectivelly as corynebacteria.
†*Corynebacterium* species other than *diphtheriae* are commonly referred to as diphtheroids.

Kurthia. Straight rods occurring in chains and parallel arrangements, ranging from 2 to 9 μm in length and 0.8 μm in diameter, fragmenting into coccoid cells in older cultures. Motile; catalase-positive and oxidase-negative; metabolize by oxidation.

Propionibacterium. Anaerobic to aerotolerant, pleomorphic rods. Ferment carbohydrates and produce propionic acid.

Eubacterium. Anaerobic rods, ferment carbohydrates and do not produce propionic acid.

12-2 LISTERIA MONOCYTOGENES

These microorganisms are short (2.0 by 0.5 μm), gram-positive rods, often appearing in pairs at an acute angle end-to-end to one another (see Fig. 12–1).

They are nonencapsulated, nonsporogenous, and lose their gram-positivity almost completely in cultures older than 48 hours. In broth cultures grown at 37°C, they are feebly motile, but when grown at 25°C they display a characteristic active tumbling motility.

Listeria grow fairly well on ordinary media at 37°C, but they grow even better on media containing liver extract, blood, serum, or glucose. Colonies first appear very small and dropletlike. In a few days, they may attain a 2-mm diameter, become smooth, transparent, and later opaque. A narrow zone of beta-hemolysis may be noted on blood agar.

Increasingly, cases of meningoencephalitis in man have been attributed to *L. monocytogenes.* Mononuclear or polymorphonuclear exudate in the cerebrospinal fluid and monocytosis are characteristically associated with this disease. The disease can be diagnosed by isolation of the organisms from the spinal fluid or the

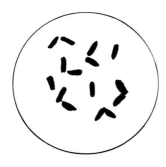

Fig. 12–1. *Listeria.*

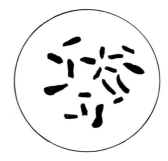

Fig. 12–2. *Corynebacterium.*

blood. The disease is often associated with corticosteroid or radiation therapy, which suggests that latent infections are activated by such treatments. In untreated cases, the mortality rate is about 70%. Treatment with ampicillin, penicillin, or tetracycline lowers the mortality rate considerably.

L. monocytogenes resembles the other corynebacteria in many respects. The fact that they may display tumbling motility offers the simplest means of identification.

Another type of disease apparently caused by these organisms is granulomatosis infantiseptica. This is an intrauterine infection in pregnancy that causes extensive focal necrosis of the spleen and liver of the fetus. Autopsy tissues, stored at 4°C for several days, more readily yield isolates than do fresh specimens. The reason for this peculiar phenomenon may be that the organisms replicate slowly at 4°C, or that they are released slowly from their intracellular location.

12-3 ERYSIPELOTHRIX RHUSIOPATHIAE

These are commonly found in a variety of animals, especially in hogs, poultry, fish, and crayfish. Handlers of these animals frequently develop abrasions on their hands or forearms. The abrasions may become infected with *E. rhusiopathiae,* causing the so-called erysipeloids. Typical lesions are associated with severe pain and swelling of the affected area and a dusky discoloration of the skin.

The organisms are slender (1 to 2 μm by 0.2 to 0.4 μm), gram-positive, nonmotile rods. They occur singly or in chains. *E. rhusiopathiae* grows well on routine media, even at 20°C, though much better at 37°C. Primary isolates are microaerophilic but they soon grow aerobically as well as anaerobically. Isolates from typical lesions offer little difficulty in identification when compared morphologically with other corynebacteria.

12-4 CORYNEBACTERIUM

Members of this genus were first described by Klebs in 1883, who investigated the pseudomembranes of patients suffering from diphtheria. Pure cultures of *C. diphtheriae* were isolated by Loeffler in 1884, but the association between the organisms and the disease were in doubt until Roux and Yersin discovered the action of diphtheria toxin in 1888.

MORPHOLOGY

Corynebacterium diphtheriae organisms appear as slender, straight, or slightly curved rods varying from 1.2 to 6.4 μm in length by 0.3 to 1.1 μm in width. They are rarely of uniform thickness and frequently show club-shaped thickenings at one or both ends. Occasionally they may be thickest at their center and taper off toward the ends. Internal structures and metachromatic granules are also noticed, particularly when the organisms are grown on Loeffler's medium (see p. 390). These structures become more apparent when the organisms are stained by Neisser's or Albert's technique (see p. 419). They are gram-positive (though more easily decolorized than most other gram-positive organisms), nonmotile, nonsporogenous, and noncapsulated.

C. pseudodiphtheriticum is shorter and thicker than *C. diphtheriae* and usually straight and slightly clubbed at one end, rarely at both. *C. xerosis* and other diphtheroids resemble *C. diphtheriae* more closely.

CULTURAL CHARACTERISTICS

Corynebacterium grow well on ordinary media within a temperature range from 15° to 40°C. Their optimal temperature lies between 34° and 37°C. On Loeffler's serum slants, minute, glistening, grayish white colonies appear in about 18 hours at 37°C. It has been suggested that Loeffler's medium is a starvation medium, and therefore enhances the development of bizarre forms, which are of some diagnostic help (see Morphology). *Corynebacterium* species grow well in the presence of small amounts of potassium tellurite incorporated in modified Tinsdale medium, a selective medium for *Corynebacterium* (see p. 395). This medium is also useful for differentiating between species and varieties, because the tellurite is reduced to variable degrees by different *Corynebacterium* species. Reduction of the tellurite results in darkening of the colonies. Differentiation on the basis of colonial variations does have limitations; the following should serve only as a general guide for identification and not be considered conclusive.

C. diphtheriae-gravis. Color ranges from battleship gray to black; flat, dull, dry, with radial striations; friable; may measure up to 4 mm in diameter.

C. diphtheriae-mitis. Black, smooth, convex, shiny, and butyrous; seldom measures more than 2 mm in diameter.

C. diphtheriae-intermedius. Dark-gray with an even darker center; umbonate, friable; relatively small (1 mm in diameter).

Diphtheroids. Generally grow more luxuriantly than *C. diphtheriae* and may display a variety of the foregoing characteristics.

RESISTANCE

Diphtheria bacilli have survived on dried pseudomembranes for up to 14 weeks. They are killed by boiling within two minutes and at 60°C in ten minutes. They are fairly resistant to drying and freezing, and are more resistant to sunlight than most other vegetative bacteria. Routine disinfectants destroy them with ease. They are sensitive to penicillin and tetracyclines.

PATHOGENICITY

C. diphtheriae is the only true pathogenic species of this genus and the cause of diphtheria in man. For diphtheria to occur, the bacteria must be able to produce a certain amount of exotoxin. The ability of different strains to produce this toxin seems to be related to several predisposing factors, one of which may be a certain balance of minerals. In vitro studies have demonstrated that toxin production is optimal in media that contain 0.14 μg of iron per ml, and is reduced to undetectable amounts when the iron content of the medium is 0.5 μg per ml. The disease is absent unless toxin is produced.

The toxin is readily absorbed by the mucous membranes and causes rapid destruction of the epithelium of the throat. The necrotic epithelium becomes embedded in exuding fibrin, erythrocytes and leukocytes, forming a grayish "pseudomembrane" that overlies the tonsils, pharynx, and larynx. Unless this pseudomembrane is removed or the air passage maintained by insertion of a tube, the patient may suffocate. Continued toxin production may result in damage to the heart muscles, nerve cells, kidneys, liver, and adrenal glands. Permanent paralysis and death frequently occur in untreated victims.

TREATMENT

Diphtheria antitoxin is the only effective treatment. Antitoxin must be administered early in the disease because it is inactive against cell-bound toxins. Epidemiologic studies have revealed that the fatality rate is virtually nil when antitoxin is given during the first day of the disease, but rapidly climbs to 5% when treatment is delayed until day two, and to 20% when delayed to day five.

Antibiotics such as penicillin, tetracycline and erythromycin have no effect on the disease process itself. Their use, however, will result in a more rapid destruction of the bacteria.

TRANSMISSION AND PREVENTION

Diphtheria is the ideal disease to use as an example in the study of principles of public health and preventive medicine. No other infectious disease offers all the following criteria necessary for such studies in such simple forms:

a. The isolation of the responsible organisms from patients and from healthy individuals is fairly simple.
b. The susceptibility or immunity of large populations can be ascertained by a simple test (Schick test).
c. Active immunization programs can be carried out safely and inexpensively with toxoids.
d. The effectiveness of the immunization program can be ascertained by the Schick test.
e. Passive immunization with antitoxin is possible for prophylaxis and treatment.
f. Man is the only host for the responsible organisms so that it is possible to reduce the number of carriers and ease the ultimate elimination of the disease.

Routine immunization in early life had almost completely eradicated diphtheria from North America, but recent evidence from some regions warns that a resurgence of this disease is possible. Improved efforts should be directed toward the continuing control of diphtheria.

The Schick Test. In 1913, Schick introduced a method by which small amounts of diphtheria toxin are inoculated into the skin in order to detect susceptibility or resistance to the toxin. A positive reaction appears as a red induration at the inoculation site in about 24 to 36 hours and will last for four days or more in susceptible individuals. A negative reaction will fail to show such redness and is evidence of the person's immune status. A control toxin heated to 60°C for 15 minutes should be inoculated in the opposite arm to determine nonspecific skin reactions.

LABORATORY DIAGNOSIS

Specimen. Throat secretions, throat swabs or the pseudomembrane are all suitable for isolation.

Direct Examination. Smears are diagnostically significant in only a small number of cases. Stained by Albert's or Neisser's methods, the smears may reveal large numbers of beaded rods in typical arrangements. The examiner should remember that *Pseudomonas* species may also demonstrate these characteristics when stained by the same methods. *Pseudomonas* are gram-negative, however, and differentiation by the Gram's stain must be made together with the Albert's or Neisser's stain.

Isolation. Swabs or the pseudomembrane should be rubbed over the surface of a Loeffler's serum slant, then dipped in the water of condensation at the foot of the slant. Next, the specimen may be planted on tellurite blood agar, blood agar, or both. Upon 12 to 18 hours' incubation at 37°C, characteristic colonies may be seen on both the Loeffler's and tellurite media. Smears made from growth on Loeffler's slants will further demonstrate a more characteristic microscopic morphology.

Identification. Apart from differentiating *Corynebacterium* species on the basis of biochemical, cultural and morphologic characteristics as outlined in Section 12–5, two other methods are particularly useful in distinguishing between pathogenic and non-pathogenic strains. These two methods are measures of the organisms' ability to produce diphtheria toxin.

a. The *animal virulence test*—in this test, one of two guinea pigs is inoculated with 1000 units of diphtheria antitoxin. Both animals are subsequently inoculated intracutaneously with pure cultures of the isolated strain under study. Virulent diphtheria bacilli will produce a well-defined area of inflammation about 15 mm in diameter surrounding the inoculation site within 24 to 48 hours. The inflammation will fade in about three to four days, resulting in a minor necrotic patch on the skin of the animal. If the isolate inoculated is indeed a toxigenic strain of *C. diphtheriae*, only the animal that did not previously receive the antitoxin will demonstrate the typical inflammation.

b. The *Elek diffusion test* is an in vitro test by which strips of filter paper are soaked in diphtheria antitoxin and placed on a special medium (see Elek's medium). The strain under study is inoculated on this plate in streaks perpendicular to the filter paper strips. The antitoxin diffuses into the medium away from the strip, and when the culture under study produces toxin corresponding to that antitoxin, the two will meet somewhere in optimal proportions and react to form a thin line of precipitation. A number of cultures may be tested simultaneously on one Elek plate.

Unless a *C. diphtheriae* isolate demonstrates toxin production, it should not be considered harmful.

12-5 DIFFERENTIATION

Most clinically significant bacteria covered within the scope of this chapter will be isolated on selective media or will be recognized by the skilled technologist on routine media once he is alerted by the clinical picture or by a specific request presented with the specimen. In such instances, differentiation is much simplified and requires only verification that a particular isolate indeed conforms with the suspected pathogen.

When it becomes necessary to identify other gram-positive rods, a more elaborate system must be followed. First, the primary characteristics listed in Chart 25–1 must be ascertained and compared with that chart (see p. 345). This will ensure that the isolate belongs to the Lactobacillaceae or to the corynebacteria group of bacteria. Subsequently, identification within these groups may be attempted as outlined below. *Eubacterium* and *Propionibacterium* species can be excluded if the isolate grows in air. Differentiation into species of either of these should not be required in a clinical laboratory. The characteristic difference between these genera, of course, is the production of propionic acid by the latter. *Caryophan, Arthrobacter* or *Kurthia* species are seldom encountered in a clinical laboratory. They can easily be distinguished by characteristic morphologic differences (see Chart 12–1). Of the remaining genera within this group, *Cellulomonas* is the only one that attacks carbohydrates oxidatively. *Listeria* demonstrates tumbling motility at 25°C; *Erysipelothrix* is catalase-negative and does not ferment maltose; and *Lactobacillus* species are catalase-negative and generally ferment maltose. (See also Chart 12–1 and Table 12–1.)

Table 12–1. Differentiation of corynebacteria

	Hydrolyse starch	Motility	Reduce nitrate	Ferment glucose	maltose	sucrose
C. diphtheriae-gravis	+	−	+	+	+	−
C. diphtheriae-mitis	−	−	+	+	+	∓
C. diphtheriae-intermedius	−	−	+	+	+	−
Diphtheroids	−	−	±	∓	−	±
L. monocytogenes	±	+	−	+	+	+
E. rhusiopathiae	−	−	−	+	−	−

Chart 12–1. Differentiation of gram-positive asporogenous rods.*

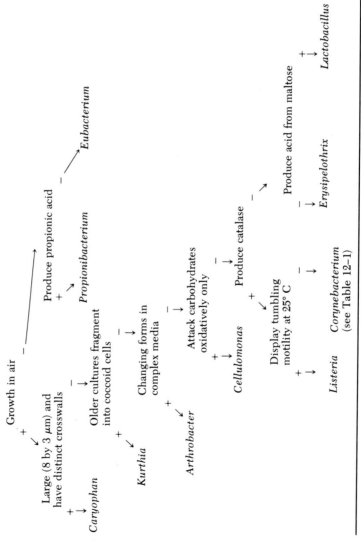

*See also Chapter 17.

FURTHER READING

1. Barksdale, W. L.: Corynebacterium and its relatives. Bacteriol. Rev., *34*:378–422, 1971.
2. Newton, S. V.: Listeriosis—a review. Canad. J. Med. Technol., *37*:88–93, 1975.
3. Bickham, S. T. and Jones, W. L.: Problems in the use of in vitro toxigenicity tests for *C. diphtheriae*. Amer. J. Clin. Path., *57*:244–246, 1972.

chapter 13
Gram-Negative Cocci

13-1 CLASSIFICATION

Bergey's Manual, Part 10
Gram-negative, aerobic, cocci and coccobacilli

Family	I. Neisseriaceae			
Genus	I. *Neisseria*	Species:	*meningitidis*	
			gonorrhoeae	
			14 others	
	II. *Branhamella*		*catarrhalis*	
	III. *Moraxella*		7	
	IV. *Acinetobacter*		*calcoaceticus*	
Uncertain genera:	*Paracoccus*		2	
	Lampropedia		*hyalina*	

Bergey's Manual, Part 11
Gram-negative, anaerobic cocci
Family   I. Veillonellaceae
    Genus   I. *Veillonella*   Species: *parvula*
                                           alcalescens
           II: *Acidaminococcus*   *fermentans*
          III. *Megasphaera*   *elsdenii*

DEFINITIONS

Neisseriaceae. Spherical or rod-shaped gram-negative aerobes that appear in pairs or short chains. In general, catalase- and oxidase-positive.

Neisseria. Gram-negative diplococci that characteristically occur in pairs with their adjacent sides flattened. They are non-motile.

Branhamella. Differs from *Neisseria* only in DNA base content and fatty acid composition.

Moraxella. Short, plump coccobacilli that appear in pairs or short chains. Strict aerobes; possess no flagella, but may demonstrate a twitching motility under special conditions. Produce oxidase and usually catalase.

Acinetobacter. Differs from *Moraxella* in its lack of oxidase production.

Veillonellaceae. Small to large gram-negative cocci; anaerobic. Oxidase- and catalase-negative; nonmotile.

Veillonella. Small cocci (0.3 to 0.5 μm) that appear in pairs, masses, and short chains. In pairs, adjacent sides appear flattened.

Acidaminococcus. Oval to kidney-shaped cocci that measure between 0.6 and 1.0 μm; appear largely as diplococci.

Megasphaera. Large cocci (2 μm or larger) that occur in pairs or chains.

13-2 NEISSERIA MENINGITIDIS

This microorganism was first isolated by Weichselbaum in 1887 from cases of epidemic meningitis.

MORPHOLOGY

These gram-negative diplococci measure approximately 0.8 μm in diameter. Individual organisms are somewhat bean-shaped; the adjacent sides flatten when they occur in pairs. In thick smears they retain crystal violet. They are nonmotile and may demonstrate a small capsule. In CSF smears, they appear characteristically as intracellular cocci, usually in pairs but also in larger aggregates. During the early stages of disease, most organisms are found extracellularly. In older cultures, the cells appear to be swollen.

CULTURAL CHARACTERISTICS

Neisseria are strict aerobes. Pathogenic species grow best on enriched media, chocolate agar or Thayer-Martin medium at a temperature of 35°C. Increased CO_2 (5 to 10%) enhances their growth, especially in primary isolation. They do not grow at temperatures below 22°C or above 42°C.

At 24 to 48 hours, colonies on chocolate agar appear smooth, moist, elevated, translucent bluish gray, approximately 1 to 2 mm in diameter. They autolyse quickly, even during development. This latter phenomenon may explain the swollen appearance described before.

BIOCHEMICAL CHARACTERISTICS

All *Neisseria* species produce the enzyme oxidase and can be further identified by their fermentative ability (see Table 13–2).

RESISTANCE

Neisseria species, especially the pathogenic ones, are rather delicate organisms. When dry, they are killed within 24 hours, even more quickly in sunlight. They are highly sensitive to heat (50°C for 10 minutes) and to the usual disinfectants.

They can be maintained on cystine trypticase agar for several weeks but should be lyophilized in serum broth in order to ensure preservation. Penicillins are usually effective against *N. meningitidis*.

VARIABILITY

Fresh isolates of Groups A and C (see Antigenicity) are usually encapsulated and produce typical colonies. Strains of Group B are often nonencapsulated and produce smaller, rather rough colonies. Virulent strains may develop into papillated colonies. Variants requiring streptomycin for growth have been developed by repeated subculture in media containing this antibiotic.

ANTIGENICITY

N. meningitidis may be separated on the basis of seven agglutinable antigens: A, B, C, D, X, Y, and Z.

PATHOGENICITY

Man, the only natural host for *N. meningitidis,* is usually infected through the nasopharyngeal area, where the organisms may be carried for months without causing any discomfort. In some predisposed individuals, the infection may progress and enter the lymph canal. Bacteremia may follow and can develop into metastatic lesions in the lungs, joints and middle ear, but particularly in the meninges. Symptoms of meningococcal meningitis usually occur suddenly, with intense headaches, associated with vomiting and a stiff neck, progressing to a coma within a few hours. Purpuric spots resulting from thrombosis of the capillaries of subterminal skin vessels are quite common. Without treatment, the disease is fatal in 85% of cases.

TREATMENT

Penicillin is the most effective drug. When signs of adrenal insufficiency are detected, hydrocortisone, pressor amines and parenteral fluids may also be required.

TRANSMISSION

Epidemics occur in waves. In some regions, they occur every 10 to 11 years. Epidemics often start in army camps, recruits appearing the more susceptible individuals, and from there may spread through civilian populations. Hospital personnel are frequently found to carry the organisms in their nasopharynx as apparent commensals. The exact mode of spread of virulent strains and hence the control of this disease is still much of a mystery.

LABORATORY DIAGNOSIS

Specimens. Blood and CSF cultures yield the best source of *N. meningitidis* in cases of meningitis due to this organism. Both these specimens should be taken before antibiotic treatment is initiated.

Direct smears have definite diagnostic value. Direct smears of the CSF often reveal large numbers of diplococci and pus cells. Smears may also aid differential diagnosis when streptococci, pneumococci or *Haemophilus*-like organisms are seen instead of diplococci. Isolation is best effected by inoculating the specimens as soon as possible onto a preheated (35°C) chocolate agar plate, which should be incubated under 5 to 10% CO_2 at 35°C. When specimens must be transported over any distance, the use of transport media may somewhat increase the chances of isolation.

An additional diagnostic test for meningococcal meningitis is the detection of bacterial products in the CSF or serum by serologic techniques.*

13-3 NEISSERIA GONORRHOEAE

Gonorrhea must have plagued man for quite some time. The name was introduced by Galen in 130 A.D. The disease, however, was known long before that time, as ancient Chinese and Hebrew scriptures bear testimony to.

Neisser, in 1879, described the diplococci in secretions from cases of acute vaginitis and urethritis. Leistikow and Bumm succeeded in cultivating them in 1885, and Bumm established the etiology of the disease by transmission of the organisms to human volunteers a year later. Following the appearance of antibiotics, a notable decrease in the incidence of gonorrhea occurred during the forties and fifties. However, more recent public health figures show a drastic increase in later years. Whether this increase can be attributed to the development of resistant strains or to a more relaxed attitude toward sexual activity remains to be proven. The fact remains that in North America about two million cases of gonorrhea are reported annually.

MORPHOLOGIC, CULTURAL AND BIOCHEMICAL CHARACTERISTICS

These are much the same as those described under *N. meningitidis*. Gonococci, however, do not produce a detectable capsule. They do exhibit four rather characteristic colonial forms: two types of heavily pigmented, somewhat friable colonies which are generally virulent, and two types of much larger, less pigmented colonies which are usually avirulent.†

RESISTANCE

This is the same as in *N. meningitidis*, but strains resistant to penicillin appear more frequently.

VARIABILITY

Resistant mutants develop both in vivo and in vitro. Cultural variations also occur, as mentioned previously.

---

*Lancet, 1:1277, 1976.
†J. Bacteriol., 96:596, 1968.

PATHOGENICITY

They are mainly pathogens of the uro-genital tract. Other areas, however, are fairly frequently invaded, so that gonococcal arthritis, osteomyelitis, endocarditis and even meningitis are not uncommon.

Typically, gonococci attack the mucous membranes of the genitourinary tract, producing acute suppuration and possibly tissue invasion. In the male, urethritis may develop, with yellow, creamy pus being discharged. Urination becomes painful, and the infection often spreads to the prostate and epididymis. In the female, the infection usually extends from the urethra and vagina to the cervix and may progress to the fallopian tubes and beyond. Gonococcal conjunctivitis of the newborn (ophthalmia neonatorum) was once a major cause of blindness, resulting from the baby's passage through an infected birth canal.

TREATMENT

Penicillin is the drug of choice; more intensive treatment is required in females than in males.

TRANSMISSION

Sexual intercourse is the main, if not the only, means of spread (other than neonatal conjunctivitis). Indirect transmission is technically possible, but the organisms survive so poorly outside the body that claims to this effect can usually be regarded as "likely stories."

PREVENTION

The fact that infected females frequently are free from clinical symptoms, and therefore go untreated, presents the greatest single difficulty in the control of gonorrhea. Prophylactic antibiotic treatment, 400,000 units of penicillin, does lower the incidence, but is not often practical.

Gonococcal ophthalmia can usually be prevented by applying two drops of a 1% silver nitrate solution into the conjunctival sacs of the newborn, or by applying ophthalmic penicillin ointment.

LABORATORY DIAGNOSIS

The most common specimens yielding gonococci are discharges from genital lesions. Culture, isolation and identification attempts should follow the same routine as described under *N. meningitidis*. The addition of Thayer-Martin medium as an isolating medium improves the rate of isolation.

13-4 OTHER NEISSERIACEAE

Other species of *Neisseria* and *Branhamella* are considered nonpathogenic to man. They are frequent commensals of the upper respiratory tract and are less frequently found in a variety of clinical specimens.

Moraxella species are often associated with urinary tract infections, but their pathogenicity has not been clearly established.

Acinetobacter is primarily found in water and soil and sometimes in specimens from debilitated individuals. Their role in the disease process is also uncertain.

13-5 VEILLONELLACEAE

Veillonella have been associated with tooth abscesses and even pulmonary infections. They are often completely ignored by laboratory workers, although they will probably gain more prominence in the future.

Acidaminococcus have been isolated from the intestinal tracts of man and pigs. They are considered nonpathogenic. *Megasphaera* are found only in the rumen of cattle and sheep.

13-6 DIFFERENTIATION

The true gram-negative cocci can simply be differentiated by their atmospheric requirements. Aerobic isolates belong to the family Neisseriaceae; anaerobic isolates are Veillonellaceae. The gram-negative coccobacillary forms require further differentiation from other gram-negative bacteria as outlined in Chart 25–1. Once grouped in their respective families, identification is fairly simple; Neisseriaceae can be subdivided into genera by checking the morphology, oxidase production and acid production in glucose (see Table 13–1). Differentiation of species of *Neisseria* and

Table 13-1. Differentiation of Neisseriaceae

	Cell morphology	Oxidase production	Produce acid in glucose
Neisseria	cocci	+	+
Branhamella	cocci	+	−
Moraxella	rods	+	−
Acinetobacter	rods	−	+

Table 13-2. Differentiation of *Neisseria* and *Branhamella*

	Growth at 22°C	Reduces nitrates	Produce acid from				Hemolysis
			Glucose	Lactose	Maltose	Sucrose	
N. gonorrhoeae	−	−	+	−	−	−	−
N. meningitidis	−	−	+	−	+	−	−
N. pharyngis*	+	−	+	−	+	±	−
N. elongata†	+	−	−	−	−	−	−
N. mucosa	+	+	+	−	−	+	−
N. animalis	+	+	+	−	−	−	−
N. caviae	+	+	−	−	−	+	α
N. ovis	+	+	−	−	−	−	β
N. lactamicus	−	−	+	+	+	−	−
B. catarrhalis	+	+	−	−	−	−	−

*Includes *N. flava, N. perflava, N. subflava, N. sicca* and some *N. flavescens.*
†Includes some *N. flavescens.*

Branhamella may then be accomplished by determining the characteristics listed in Table 13–2. (From a clinical point of view, there is no real value in attempting to differentiate between those species that are lumped together in Table 13–2.)

Neisseria, especially the pathogenic species, grow poorly in media usually employed to determine carbohydrate metabolism. The medium most commonly employed for this purpose is cystine tryptose agar (p. 402). We prefer guinea pig serum medium (p. 401). The pathogenic *Neisseria* species may also be characterized by fluorescence microscopy. Commercial antisera suitable to label gonococci or meningococci in specimen smears or from isolates are available.* It is recommended that fluorescence test results be corroborated with biochemical analyses.

The gram-positive *Gemella* are often confused with *Neisseria* because they usually appear as gram-negative (see also Chart 10–3). They may be differentiated from *Neisseria* by their ability to ferment rather than oxidize carbohydrates, and by their inability to produce oxidase or catalase.

Moraxella species are commonly found in specimens associated with the urinary tract and less frequently in some other specimens. Since their pathogenicity is not known, differentiation of these isolates serves no real purpose in the routine clinical laboratory.

Acinetobacter is a monotypic genus and therefore requires no further identification.

Paracoccus occurs in soils or meat-curing brines, and *Lampropedia*, in swamp waters and food industry effluent. Neither is of concern to the clinical microbiologist.

The Veillonellaceae may be placed in their respective genera on the basis of cell size (see Table 13–3). Little work has been done on these organisms. In fact, most manuals of clinical bacteriology group all anaerobic gram-negative cocci under *Veillonella*.

Table 13–3. Differentiation of Veillonellaceae

	Carbohydrate fermentation	*Lactate fermentation*	*Succinate decarboxylase*	*Average cell diameter*
Veillonella	−	+	+	0.4 μm
Acidaminococcus	∓	−	−	0.6–1.0 μm
Megasphaera	+	+	−	2.0 μm or more

Key: + = positive, − = negative, ∓ = some are positive.

*Difco Laboratories, Detroit, Mich.; Baltimore Biological Laboratories, Cockeysville, Md.

FURTHER READING

1. Balows, A., and Printz, D. W.: CDC program for diagnosis of gonorrhoeae. Letter, JAMA, 222:1557, 1972.
2. Reyn, A.: Recent developments in the laboratory diagnosis of gonococcal infections. Bull. WHO, 49:245–255, 1969.

chapter 14

Gram-Negative Aerobic Rods

14-1 CLASSIFICATION

Bergey's Manual Part 7 is described as gram-negative aerobic rods and cocci. To better differentiate between the organisms described here and those described in Chapter 13, and because the cocci classified in *Bergey's Manual* under Part 7 have no clinical significance, we will ignore the cocci altogether and consider only gram-negative aerobic rods.

Bergey's Manual, Part 7*
Gram-negative aerobic rods

Family	I: Pseudomonadaceae		
Genus	I. *Pseudomonas*	Species:	*aeruginosa*
			230 others
	II. *Xanthomonas*		5
	2 other genera		

---

*See Table 7–2 for full listing of families and genera.

Three other Families
Genera of Uncertain Affiliation

Alcaligenes	Species:	*faecalis*
		3 others
Acetobacter		3
Brucella		*melitensis*
		abortus
		suis
		3 others
Bordetella		*pertussis*
		parapertussis
		bronchiseptica
Francisella		*tularensis*
		novicida
Thermus		*aquaticus*

DEFINITIONS

Pseudomonadaceae. Gram-negative, aerobic rods usually motile with polar flagella. Do not ferment carbohydrates.

Pseudomonas. Oxidase- and catalase-positive; may denitrify nitrates.

Xanthomonas. Catalase-positive, oxidase-negative or weakly positive. Carry only one polar flagellum; are nitrate-negative.

Alcaligenes. Rods, coccal rods or cocci, 0.5 to 1.2 μm. Motile with one to four peritrichous flagella. Oxidase- and catalase-positive.

Acetobacter. Ellipsoidal to rod-shaped bacilli; grow at pH 4.5; oxidize ethanol to acetic acid; may be motile or nonmotile.

Brucella. Coccobacillary to short rods; nonmotile. They require thiamine, niacin and biotin, but not X or V factor (see p. 213). They are catalase-, urease- and usually oxidase-positive and reduce nitrate.

Bordetella. Minute coccobacilli; do not ferment carbohydrates. Require nicotinic acid, cystine and methionine, but not X or V factor (p. 213). Catalase- and oxidase-positive.

Francisella: Very small nonmotile coccoid bacilli. Catalase-negative and H_2S-positive. Require cystine, and will produce acid without gas from carbohydrates.

Thermus. Grow at a range of 40° to 70°C; are nonmotile rods or filaments.

14-2 PSEUDOMONADACEAE

PSEUDOMONAS

Members of this genus are mainly free-living bacteria and are widely distributed in soil and water. A relatively small number of species is frequently associated with disease in man. These can be classified as opportunistic pathogens.

In cultural and morphologic characteristics, the *Pseudomonas* resemble the *Enterobacteriaceae* closely (see p. 218). Biochemically, however, they differ considerably in that they fail to ferment carbohydrates and are oxidase-positive. The most common pathogen is *P. aeruginosa (P. pyocyanea)*, which because of its resistance to many antibiotics, often establishes itself as the predominant organism at various body sites. This organism is easily characterized by its peculiar bluish-green metallic sheen and its musty odor. *Pseudomonas* are frequently isolated from various lesions in man; the most common sites are the middle ear of patients suffering from chronic otitis media; wounds, particularly those associated with burns; the urinary tract; and the upper respiratory tract. Less commonly, *Pseudomonas* is associated with pneumonia or meningitis.

For treatment, polymyxin B, colistin, gentamicin, and more recently carbenicillin have been used successfully. Because some of these are toxic, particularly carbenicillin, treatment should be approached with caution. In cases of severe burns, immunotherapy has also been used effectively to reduce fatalities.

Of the other *Pseudomonas* species, *P. malei* and *P. pseudomalei* are the causative agents of glanders and melioidosis respectively. Glanders is a severe infectious disease of horses which on rare occasions can be transmitted to man. The disease is characterized by nodular, eventually necrotic, involvement of nasal mucous membranes, the lymphatics, or the skin. Melioidosis is a glanders-like syndrome that has appeared in America in soldiers returning from Southeast Asia. Isolation of *Pseudomonas* presents little problem in the diagnostic laboratory because the organisms grow well on most routine media.

XANTHOMONAS

Primarily pathogens of plants, these organisms may occasionally find their way into the diagnostic laboratory as contaminants.

ALCALIGENES

These organisms are generally harmless saprophytes that may sometimes contaminate intravenous and irrigation solutions and have thus been responsible for some cases of postoperative septicemia and urinary tract infection. Tetracycline and chloramphenicol appear to be the antibiotics of choice in such instances. In the laboratory, isolation is no problem.

ACETOBACTER

Members of this genus are of interest because they readily produce acetic acid from ethanol. Pasteur's classic "vinegar bacilli" belong to this genus. They have no medical importance and are mentioned here only because "they started it all."

14-3 BRUCELLA

The first *Brucella* organisms were isolated in 1887 by Bruce from patients suffering from undulant fever. The organisms were traced to goats, and found to be transmitted by goat's milk to peasants and visitors of Malta who drank raw milk. The disease became known as Malta fever, and the organism responsible, as *Brucella melitensis*. Other species were discovered later.

Brucella abortus frequently infects cattle; *Brucella suis* more frequently infects hogs. The organisms are stimulated by erythritol, which is found in high concentrations in the placental tissues of cattle, goats and pigs.

MORPHOLOGY

Microorganisms of the genus *Brucella* are very small, non-motile, nonsporogenous, gram-negative coccobacilli. *B. melitensis* measures approximately 0.6 μm in width and 2.2 μm in length; *B. abortus*, 0.4 μm and 2.5 μm; and *B. suis*, 0.6 μm and 3.0 μm.

In tissues and exudates, rather small, mainly coccobacillary forms are seen. Depending on the medium, they may appear entirely coccoid or bacillary in culture. Upon frequent subculture, both *B. suis* and *B. abortus* change to predominantly bacillary forms, whereas *B. melitensis* takes an almost completely coccoid form.

CULTURAL CHARACTERISTICS

All *Brucella* species are aerobes and grow best at a pH of 6.8 to 7.2 at 37°C. They grow well on relatively simple media, but *B. abortus* requires 10% CO_2 for primary isolation, and may require CO_2 supplementation for several subcultures. Peculiarly, *B. suis* appears to be slightly suppressed by CO_2. *Brucella* colonies grown on blood agar are round or semispherical, smooth, and opaque, white or dull creamy-colored. These colonies range from 2 to 4 mm in diameter at 24 hours. Blood cultures yield the best results when grown on enriched media. Serum, liver extracts, or whole rabbit blood in meat infusions give the best chances for isolation.

BIOCHEMICAL CHARACTERISTICS

Urease and H_2S production are somewhat useful in the differentiation of *Brucella*. The methods required for these estimations, however, differ from the conventional methods employed for the *Enterobacteriaceae*.

RESISTANCE

Brucella are readily killed by the usual disinfectants and by pasteurization. The organisms remain viable in whole milk at 4°C for up to ten days, in cheese for several months, and in meats for several weeks. They are generally resistant to penicillin but are sensitive to tetracycline and streptomycin.

PATHOGENICITY

Man is highly susceptible to brucellosis. Most infections, however, must be subclinical, since many more individuals demonstrate brucellar agglutinins in their serum than reported cases of brucellosis would suggest. Brucellosis may be differentiated into three phases; acute, subacute, or chronic.

Acute brucellosis may have an incubation period that ranges between four and thirty days. The classic undulating fever is seldom observed in North America. The symptoms of brucellosis are usually mild in all phases but, because of their persistence, are very disabling. Local and focal lesions may appear in skin, mouth and lung tissues. Some rare cases of abortion have been attributed to *Brucella*. Of late, pulmonary brucellosis has become more frequent.

The acute phase is often self-limiting within one to three months. During the second and third weeks of the disease, cultures from blood specimens are most likely to be positive.

A *subacute phase* may follow the acute phase, may be more or less severe, and may last for several months. When the disease lasts for over a year, we speak of *chronic brucellosis*. In some cases, brucellosis has lasted for 20 years or more.

TREATMENT

The disease usually responds to antibiotics. Because an endotoxin released by rapidly lysing bacteria may cause severe reactions, initial doses of antibiotics should be small. The eradication of organisms is further complicated by their intracellular location, which protects them from the action of antibiotics. Prolonged treatment may be required.

TRANSMISSION

Brucella may be contracted directly from infected animals, or indirectly from milk, water, manure, and soil. Laboratory workers are probably the group at highest risk. Extreme care should be taken in dealing with *Brucella* cultures, or with specimens suspected of containing *Brucella*.

PREVENTION

Pasteurization of all dairy products and strict control of farm animals can help prevent brucellosis. Animals infected with *Brucella* usually carry high titers of antibodies in their serum, which are easily demonstrated by the "ring test" for milk or the agglutination test for serum. Rigid control has rendered North American herds generally free from *Brucella*.

LABORATORY DIAGNOSIS

Specimens. Repeated cultures from blood specimens should be made since, at best, they give positive results in only 30 to 50% of attempts.

Isolation. At least two glucose-serum-broth bottles should be set up each time, one under 10% CO_2, the other without the CO_2. Because the organisms are believed to be more concentrated in leukocytes, some workers claim that sediments of lysed cells yield more isolates. For this purpose, blood may be prepared as follows:

a. Five milliliters of citrated blood is centrifuged at 2500 rpm for 10 minutes.
b. The supernatant is discarded in a disinfectant and the sediment resuspended in 5 ml of sterile distilled water.
c. The preparation is recentrifuged; the resulting sediment is used as an inoculum.

In combination with the above treatment, Castaneda's method is advocated:

a. Prepare four-ounce square bottles to contain a slant of trypticase soy agar.
b. These slants, with the bottle upright, should be half covered with trypticase soy broth.
c. Inoculate 5 ml of whole blood or the sediment described above, into the broth of two bottles.
d. Thoroughly mix the inoculum and the broth and supply CO_2 to one bottle.
e. Examine daily for the appearance of tiny colonies on the

surface of the agar. If undetectable, the slant may be reinoculated every two days by simply tilting the bottles.

This method eliminates the necessity of subculturing blood cultures daily and could be used more widely.

Serology. Sera of patients suffering from brucellosis usually contain antibodies, which may be detected by simple agglutination tests (see Febrile antibodies, page 371).

14-3 BORDETELLA

Bordetella pertussis, the causative agent of whooping cough, was first isolated by Gengou in 1906. The genus contains two other species: *B. parapertussis*, occasionally associated with acute respiratory infections, and *B. bronchiseptica*, frequently found in the respiratory tract of dogs and occasionally in man. The following discussion applies primarily to *B. pertussis*, unless otherwise noted.

MORPHOLOGY

Bordetella are small, ovoid rods, measuring 0.3 to 0.5 μm in width, and 1.0 to 1.5 μm in length. They are nonmotile but encapsulated in exudates and in primary isolation.

CULTURAL CHARACTERISTICS

Bordetella pertussis is a strict aerobe, grows best at 37°C and very slowly at slightly lower temperatures. The medium of choice is that of Bordet and Gengou, which is a glycerine-potato-blood agar. Even on this medium, colonies are barely visible at 24 hours. In 48 to 72 hours, they reach maximal size, which is still less than 1 mm in diameter.

Confluent growth has been compared to thin streaks of aluminum paint; the discrete colonies, to tiny drops of mercury. The growth is highly refractile to light, and colonies are so cohesive that they can often be "picked off" in their entirety. Subcultures do adapt to blood-free media. Colonies produced by *B. parapertussis* are much larger, 2 to 3 mm in diameter within 48 hours, and furthermore they display a brown pigment. *B. bronchiseptica* may be isolated on simple blood-free media.

RESISTANCE

Bordetella are readily killed by drying, by the usual disinfectants, and by heat, 56°C at 30 minutes. They are generally resistant to penicillin but are sensitive to tetracyclines.

PATHOGENICITY

Bordetella pertussis grows well in and on the mucous membranes of the upper respiratory tract. Following a one- to two-week incubation period, the catarrhal stage sets in, with coryza, sneezing and mild coughs. Organisms are most abundant and the patient is most infective at this stage.

The catarrhal stage develops into the spasmodic stage when large amounts of toxin irritate the bronchi, resulting in the characteristic "whoopy cough."

TREATMENT AND PREVENTION

Convalescence is usually slow but the disease responds well to tetracycline. With the advent of widespread vaccination during the first six months of life, whooping cough had become a rare occurrence. However, lax attitudes toward vaccination have resulted in outbreaks of whooping cough in some communities.

LABORATORY DIAGNOSIS

Specimens gathered from the pharyngeal mucosa by auger suction give the highest yield of isolates per specimen. Auger suction is a simple device composed of a soft catheter attached to a 20-ml syringe. The catheter is inserted into the nasopharynx, and gentle suction applied to the plunger of the syringe usually aspirates sufficient specimen for culture. The next best specimen is the so-called coughplate. A Bordet-Gengou-blood-agar plate is held about six inches away from the patient while he is going through his spasmodic cough. Since *B. pertussis* is resistant to penicillin, this antibiotic is sometimes incorporated into the medium to render it selective. The characteristic growth and moreover, the classic clinical syndrome should help in simplifying the diagnosis. For a rapid provisional diagnosis, a smear made from the pharyngeal mucosa may be examined by fluorescence microscopy using antipertussis conjugate.*

14-5 FRANCISELLA TULARENSIS

This organism is the causative agent of tularemia, a disease primarily affecting lagomorphs (hares and rabbits), rodents, less frequently birds and occasionally man.

---

*Available from Difco Laboratories, Detroit, MI.

MORPHOLOGY

Francisella tularensis is a pleomorphic ovoid bacillus. Organisms range from 0.2 to 1.0 μm in width, and from 1.0 to 3.0 μm in length. Bean-shapes, L-shapes, dumbbell shapes, spermlike shapes and other forms have been described. The bizarre forms sometimes give one the impression that these organisms reproduce by budding rather than by binary fission.

CULTURAL CHARACTERISTICS

Members of this species are obligate aerobes with a temperature growth range between 24° and 39°C (optimal 37°C). *Francisella tularensis* can be cultivated only on special media. Pure egg yolk medium, blood agar or serum agar supplemented with rabbit spleen (simply rubbing the agar surface with a sterile spleen seems to provide the essential growth requirement), or horse-serum agar containing 0.1% cystine and 1% dextrose, have all been used successfully. Increased CO_2 (5%) aids the primary isolation. Laboratory workers are at considerable risk when dealing with this organism. Relatively small doses of bacteria, having entered by way of the eyes, the mucous membranes, or abraded skin, have resulted in some fatal infections.

RESISTANCE

F. tularensis survives poorly in old cultures but has been isolated from frozen tissues following several years of storage. The organisms are killed by pasteurization. They are resistant to sulfonamides and penicillin but are sensitive to streptomycin.

PATHOGENICITY

Five different clinical types of tularemia have been recognized: oculoglandular, ulceroglandular (skin), glandular (bubonic), typhoidal, and pulmonary. In the first two types, the organisms usually pass through the lymph nodes and develop into septicemia, sometimes even into meningitis. Oculoglandular tularemia more commonly follows laboratory-acquired infections.

TREATMENT

Streptomycin and tetracyclines are the drugs of choice. Tularemia is often fatal unless treatment is initiated early.

TRANSMISSION

Tularemia may be transmitted indirectly by the bites of fleas, flies, lice, and ticks, transferring the organisms from infected rodents to man. Direct contact, bites and scratches more often result in infections of furriers, trappers, and other animal handlers.

PREVENTION

Care in the handling of animals—especially "lazy rodents"—and infective material minimizes the chances for infection. Lasting immunity seems to be conferred by a previous infection. Vaccines have not had much value.

LABORATORY DIAGNOSIS

Depending on the clinical type of tularemia, specimens may vary from eyeswabs to feces. Isolation is the most difficult phase of laboratory diagnosis (see Cultural Characteristics). Once isolated, identification becomes relatively simple.

SEROLOGY

A simple agglutination test can be utilized as a measure of the immune status of individuals (see Febrile antibodies, p. 371).

14-6 DIFFERENTIATION

The primary identification can be based on the gram stain, motility, growth in air or without, and the oxidase and catalase reactions (see Chart 25–1.) However, since many of the specimens from which these organisms are frequently isolated are not routinely cultured anaerobically, one may base the initial differentiation on secondary characteristics as listed in Table 15–1. For further differentiation, the Pseudomonadaceae are separated from the *Brucella-Bordetella-Francisella* group by their motility and their less fastidious nature (they grow on simple media). The various genera within the Pseudomonadaceae can be differentiated on the basis of: growth at pH 4.5 (if *Acetobacter* is expected);

Table 14–1. Differentiation of Pseudomonadaceae

	Growth at pH 4.5	F/O	Number of polar flagella
Pseudomonas	−	−/+	several
Xanthomonas	−	−/+	one
Alcaligenes	−	−/−	
Acetobacter	+		

F/O = Fermentation/Oxidation reaction Hugh-Leiffson.

Chart 14–1. Differentiation of *Pseudomonas*.

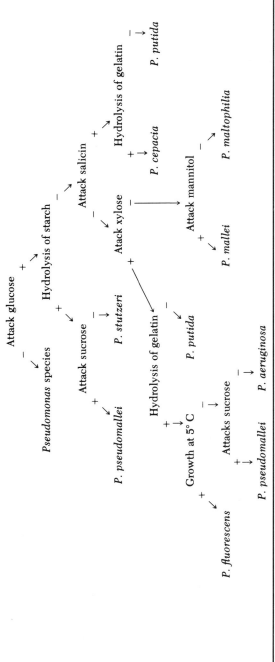

Guide to Chart 14–1: These organisms attack carbohydrates oxidatively rather than fermentatively. Inoculate glucose, starch, sucrose, salicin, xylose, gelatin, mannitol, and nutrient broths. Incubate nutrient broth at 5° C and all others at 35° C for 96 hours. Record your results and follow the chart.

failure to attack carbohydrates oxidatively (*Alcaligenes*); and location and number of flagella (*Xanthomonas* has only one polar flagellum, *Pseudomonas* has more than one) (see also Table 14–1). There is little clinical advantage in separating *Xanthomonas* from *Pseudomonas*. The cumbersome determination of flagellar location and count is not a common practice in the routine of clinical laboratories, but it should be recognized that without such determinations, some isolates reported as "*Pseudomonas* species" could in fact be *Xanthomonas*.

The differentiation of *Pseudomonas* species presents many problems. It is impossible to differentiate all known species, and even if this were possible, it would serve little purpose. Only eight species are commonly known as human pathogens. Chart 14–1 shows how to differentiate only these species; all others are designated as "*Pseudomonas* species" only.

All members of the *Brucella-Bordetella* group are strictly aerobic, fastidious, and nonmotile. Isolates that fit this group according to Chart 25–1 but grow well on simple media may be considered Pseudomonadaceae, or may be *Thermus* species. *Thermus* species, of course, are rarely encountered in the clinical laboratory; they grow at 65°C, as does none other discussed in this chapter.

The identification of *Brucella*, *Bordetella* or *Francisella* should be guided by the clinical findings and the following characteristics.

Table 14–2. Some differential characteristics of *Bordetella*

	Motility	*Growth characteristics*
B. pertussis	Nonmotile	Grows only on enriched media
B. parapertussis	Nonmotile	Produces a brown pigment
B. bronchiseptica	Motile	Grows on simple media

Table 14–3. Identification of *Brucella* species*

	melitensis	*suis*	*abortus*
Thionine 1:50,000	Resistant	Resistant	Sensitive
Basic fuschsin 1:25,000	Resistant	Sensitive	Resistant
Require CO_2 for primary isolation	No	No	Yes
Found mainly in	Sheep Goats	Pigs	Cattle

*Use dyes from the National Aniline Chemical Co., N.Y., or dyes standardized against theirs.

Francisella tularensis requires cystine (grows well on cystine-dextrose-blood agar), produces H_2S, is catalase-negative, and produces acid but no gas from fermentation of glucose, maltose, fructose, and mannose.

Bordetella require methionine and nicotinic acid in addition to cystine (all of which are provided by Bordet-Gengou medium); these organisms are nonfermenters.

Brucella require thiamine, niacin and biotin (all are provided by liver infusion agar), and they break down carbohydrates by oxidation. *Bordetella* species may be differentiated following the characteristics listed in Table 14–2. *Brucella* have variable resistances to thionine and basic fuchsin and may be differentiated on that basis (see Table 14–3).

FURTHER READING

1. Pickett, M. J. et al.: Nonfermentative bacilli associated with man, I, II, and III. Amer. J. Clin. Path., *54*:155–192, 1970.
2. Lautrop, H.: Laboratory diagnosis of whooping cough or *Bordetella* infections. Bull. WHO, *23*:15–31, 1960.
3. Quaife, R. A.: Brucellosis in man. J. Med. Lab. Techn., *26*:349, 1969.
4. Ruiz Castaneda, M.: Laboratory diagnosis of brucellosis in man. Bull. WHO, *24*:73–84, 1961.

chapter 15

Gram-Negative Facultatively Anaerobic Rods

15-1 CLASSIFICATION

Bergey's Manual, Part 8
Gram-negative facultatively anaerobic rods
    Family I.   Enterobacteriaceae
        Genus: *Escherichia*   Species: *coli*
                   Shigella   *dysenteriae*
                                            flexneri
                                          boydii
                                          sonnei
                   Edwardsiella   *tarda*
                   Citrobacter   *freundii*
                                            intermedius
                   Salmonella   *cholerae-suis*
                                            typhi
                                          enteritidis
                                          arizonae
                                          9 others
                   Klebsiella   *pneumoniae*
                                          2 others
                   Enterobacter   *cloacae*
                                          aerogenes
                   Hafnia   *alvei*
                   Serratia   *marcescens*
                   Proteus   *mirabilis*
                                          morganii
                                          vulgaris
                                          rettgeri
                                          inconstans
                   Yersinia   *pestis*
                                          pseudotuberculosis
                                          enterocolitica
                   Erwinia   13
    Family II.   Vibrionaceae*
        Genus: *Vibrio*   Species: *cholerae*
                                          4 others
                   Aeromonas   3
                   3 others

---

*Some genera have been deleted. For a complete listing of genera, see Table 7–2.

Genera of Uncertain Affiliation

Haemophilus	*influenzae*
	aegyptius
	aphrophilus
	ducreyi
	14 others
Pasteurella	*multocida*
	3 others
8 others	

DEFINITIONS†

Enterobacteriaceae. Gram-negative, nonsporing rods; grow on simple media; aerobic, but facultatively anaerobic. Ferment dextrose; reduce nitrates to nitrites; oxidase-negative; catalase-positive. Intestinal parasites of animals including man.

Escherichia. Produces indole; does not utilize citrate; sensitive to potassium cyanide (KCN); does not produce H_2S; ferments lactose and mannitol, but not adonitol or inositol.

Shigella. Nonmotile; do not utilize citrate; do not produce H_2S; sensitive to KCN; do not ferment lactose (few strains of *S. sonnei* do ferment lactose slowly); ferments neither adonitol nor inositol.

Edwardsiella. Does not ferment any carbohydrates other than dextrose; does not utilize citrate; motile; produces H_2S as well as indole.

Salmonella. Produce H_2S but not indole; sensitive to KCN; motile; lactose-negative and sucrose-negative; do not produce urease; decarboxylate lysine.

Citrobacter. Very similar to *Salmonella*, but less consistent; ferment lactose slowly and do not decarboxylate lysine.

Klebsiella. Do not produce indole or H_2S; lactose-positive; methyl red-negative; positive Voges-Proskauer's test; nonmotile; do not decarboxylate ornithine.

Enterobacter. Similar to *Klebsiella*; motile; decarboxylate ornithine.

Hafnia. Much like *Enterobacter*, but does not ferment adonitol or raffinose; generally lactose-negative.

---

†The characteristics described in this section are typical for species of the respective genera. Exceptions to these typical reactions are not uncommon. In most instances, however, the descriptions may be considered applicable without being exhaustive.

Serratia. Much like *Enterobacter* but may produce a nondiffusable red pigment; do not ferment arabinose.

Proteus. Lactose-negative and motile; resistant to KCN; deaminate phenylalanine.

Yersinia. Colonies generally much smaller than other Enterobacteriaceae; nonmotile at 37°C; produce acid but no gas from carbohydrate fermentation; do not utilize citrate.

Erwinia. Plant pathogens, seldom encountered in specimens of human origin.

Vibrionaceae. Rigid gram-negative rods, straight or curved. Generally motile by polar flagella; oxidase-positive; usually found in fresh or sea water, occasionally in fish or man.

Vibrio. Curved or straight rods; motile by a single polar flagellum; grow at alkaline pH, range 6.0 to 9.0.

Aeromonas. Motile by polar flagella; may form filaments up to 8 μm long; produce acid or acid and gas by fermentation.

Haemophilus. Minute rods or coccobacilli; may form threads as filaments. Nonmotile; require special growth factors.

Pasteurella. Ovoid to rod-shaped; nonmotile; catalase-, oxidase-, and nitrate-positive; ferment carbohydrates.

15-2 ESCHERICHIA COLI

E. coli is a normal inhabitant of the intestine. It probably serves a useful purpose by suppressing the growth of certain proteolytic organisms and by synthesizing large amounts of vitamins. Until recently, the importance of *E. coli* as an etiologic agent of disease was greatly underestimated. Coliformlike organisms served mainly as an index of fecal contamination of water; thus, they have long played a role in public health. The term "coliform" is a collective one and should be used with care. Most references define it as describing *E. coli*-like organisms. This "likeness" is based on colonial morphology only, so that, when estimated on blood agar culture, so-called coliforms could include any or all members of the *Enterobacteriaceae* and other families as well. On MacConkey agar, "coliform" would mean any lactose fermenter.

MORPHOLOGY AND STAINING

E. coli are short, plump rods, measuring 0.4 μm to 0.7 μm wide, and 1.0 to 4.0 μm long. They uniformly stain gram-negative. Coccoid forms and short chains may be found in fresh broth cultures. Some strains produce capsules. Their motility varies from active to sluggish to nonmotile.

CULTURAL CHARACTERISTICS

E. coli is aerobic but facultatively anaerobic. Members of this species grow well on routine media, producing large, moist, convex-to-domed, entire, opaque, butyrous colonies on blood agar within 24 hours. For optimal growth, the temperature should lie between 20° and 40°C; the pH, between 6 and 8. Growth may be inhibited by brilliant green, and by a mixture of sodium desoxycholate and sodium citrate (see Salmonella-Shigella (SS) agar, p. 398, and desoxycholate citrate agar, p. 399).

BIOCHEMICAL CHARACTERISTICS

The following are main characteristics that would allow rapid identification of most strains. Glucose, lactose, maltose and various other carbohydrates are fermented with the production of both acid and gas. *E. coli* is indole-positive, citrate-negative, methyl-red-positive and Voges-Proskauer-negative. It does not liquefy gelatin.

RESISTANCE

These bacilli will survive in culture at room temperature for several weeks, as can most Enterobacteriaceae. They may be maintained on egg-saline for up to one year. They are fairly sensitive to most disinfectants, and can be killed in broth cultures at 60°C in 20 minutes. To purify drinking water, 0.5 to 1.0 part per million of chlorine is an effective bactericide in most instances (see Chapter 4).

VARIABILITY

Smooth and rough types of colonies occur. Most fresh isolates appear in the S phase and are motile. Some strains (some say subspecies) grow well in the presence of lactose, but take up to seven days to demonstrate fermentation.

ANTIGENICITY

The antigenic composition of the Enterobacteriaceae is rather complex; this topic is discussed further in Section 15–16. Most members of this family possess at least three distinct types of antigens.

a. The *somatic* or *"O" antigens* are closely bound to the organism itself and are heat stable at 100°C for 30 minutes.
b. The *envelope, capsule,* or *"K" antigens,* of course, occur mainly in capsular organisms. These antigens can be destroyed by boiling the organisms for 30 to 60 minutes. Some

workers believe that these antigens mask or cover many of the O antigens, and that removing the K antigens by boiling renders the O antigens more accessible to antibody.

c. The *flagellar* or *"H" antigens* also are thermolabile at 100°C for 30 minutes.

In addition, some species possess a "Vi" antigen that is believed to be associated with the virulence of the organism; it too is a surfacelike antigen. *E. coli* are typed on the basis of their O and K antigens. Three varieties of K antigens have been described for *E. coli*: L, A and B. Most pathogenic strains of *E. coli* possess at least one K antigen of the B variety (see Section 15–16).

PATHOGENICITY

E. coli is the most frequent cause of urinary tract infections, which may take the form of cystitis, pyelitis, pyelonephritis, or nephritis. It is also a frequent cause of appendicitis, peritonitis, and postoperative wound infection. Infantile diarrhea is the more classic *E. coli* infection. Sporadic "summer" diarrhea in older children may also be caused by these common bacilli.

TREATMENT

E. coli is generally sensitive to sulfonamides, ampicillin, cephalosporin, carbenicillin and tetracyclines. For long-term suppression of urinary tract infections, nitrofurantoin or nalidixic acid are commonly used.

TRANSMISSION AND PREVENTION

One study has revealed that 45% of the *E. coli* infections were acquired in hospital. Poor feeding techniques of the newborn are a frequent cause of infantile diarrhea.

Good surgical techniques and proper training programs for *all* hospital personnel will reduce hospital-acquired infections to a minimum. Breast feeding not only eliminates contamination from improperly sterilized bottles but also induces immunity by passing maternal antibodies to the infant.

LABORATORY DIAGNOSIS

Of course, stool and urine specimens yield *E. coli* most frequently. Because this organism is present in the stools of even normal individuals, there is little point in isolating it from stools except under special circumstances. Depending on protocol, laboratory workers would seek to isolate *E. coli* from stool specimens of infants under six months of age and only upon special request for adults. Isolation of *E. coli* from materials other than stool is governed by the general methodology outlined in Section 15–15. Final identification of *E. coli* depends on serology (Section 15-16).

15-3 SHIGELLA

Four species of *Shigella* are known: *dysenteriae, flexneri, boydii* and *sonnei*. They are the most common cause of dysentery in man and are listed in order of decreasing virulence.

MORPHOLOGY AND STAINING

Members of the genus *Shigella* are short, nonmotile, nonencapsulated rods, measuring 0.5 to 0.7 μm in width and 2.0 to 3.0 μm in length. They stain uniformly gram-negative.

CULTURAL CHARACTERISTICS

Shigellae are aerobes but facultatively anaerobic; they grow readily on routine media. On blood agar their colonies resemble those of *E. coli*. The temperature growth range is from 10° to 40°C, except for *S. sonnei*, which grows up to 45°C. The optimal temperature is 37°C. The pH range is 6 to 8. They are partially inhibited by bismuth sulfite and by brilliant green, and partially favored by other substances (see p. 398).

BIOCHEMICAL CHARACTERISTICS

Except for some strains of aerogenic *S. flexneri*, all shigellae produce acid without gas when fermenting carbohydrates. Salicin, inositol and adonitol are not fermented. They do not grow on citrate agar, are urea-negative, methyl-red-positive, and Voges-Proskauer-negative.

RESISTANCE

Shigellae have been found to remain viable for up to six months in tap water. Milk supports their growth. They have been isolated from soiled clothing several weeks following contamination. They are killed in broth cultures at 55°C in one hour. Pasteurization and chlorination are effective in controlling these organisms. They are sensitive to sulfonamides, streptomycin, oxytetracycline and chlortetracycline, but resistant strains frequently develop.

ANTIGENICITY

Most *Shigella* strains contain two major somatic antigens and a number of minor antigens. The major antigens are specific, the minor antigens may be shared by several *Shigella* as well as by some *Escherichia*. Hence, cross reactions may occur with all of these organisms unless carefully prepared antisera are used.

PATHOGENICITY

All *Shigella* species can cause dysentery in man, varying in severity from *S. dysenteriae* to the relatively mild *S. sonnei*. Infection is usually acquired by ingestion. It is believed that small numbers of shigellae can initiate an infection, in contrast to salmonellosis, which requires relatively large numbers of organisms.

Symptoms associated with dysentery are extremely variable, even when the same species is responsible for infections among different individuals. Incubation periods vary from one to four days. The onset is usually sudden, and manifests itself by fever, cramps, and severe diarrhea. Some patients suffer only mild discomfort with a few loose stools. Others suffer from nausea, vomiting and severe prostration. The diarrhea, which at first appears as a thin watery discharge, soon loses its fecal character and is later composed mainly of pus, mucus, and blood. Severe colicky pains usually occur at this stage.

The mortality rate with dysentery due to *S. dysenteriae* is approximately 20%. A soluble neurotoxin that acts mainly on small blood vessels is probably responsible for this high rate.

The organisms appear sparsely in the stool itself or in the liquid portion, but are present in large numbers in pus and mucus. They rarely invade the blood stream.

TREATMENT

Dehydration needs to be treated physiologically by introducing intravenous fluids, glucose, and electrolytes. The infection may be controlled by appropriate antibiotic therapy.

TRANSMISSION

In well-organized civil life, *Shigella* causes only a minor nuisance. In war times and other disasters, it constitutes a major hazard owing to frequent fecal contamination of water supplies. Many a battle has been lost because of dysentery. Since man is the sole source of *Shigella*, it could conceivably be eradicated.

PREVENTION

Antitoxins have been prepared but are not readily available. Antibacterial sera do not seem to be effective against disease. Prevention, therefore, depends entirely on hygienic measures, of which chlorination of water supplies is the key factor. Patients should be isolated as much as possible until their stools appear negative on culture.

LABORATORY DIAGNOSIS

For successful isolation of *Shigella* from fecal matter, it is more important to select proper material for inoculation than to select a proper medium. Bits of pus or tinged mucus should be used for inoculation. Serum-coated rectal swabs have also been recommended, but successful isolations from these specimens are less frequent. Some workers find microscopic examination of wet films valuable. Abundant cellular exudates, mainly those containing polymorphonuclear cells and erythrocytes, are said to be characteristic of *Shigella* dysentery by some. For identification schemes, consult Section 15–15. Final identification of the species rests on serology, using A, B, C and D group antisera respectively; it is described under Section 15–16.

15-4 EDWARDSIELLA

This is the most recently-established genus of the Enterobacteriaceae. Its sole member, *E. tarda,* was first reported in 1959. It has been associated with diarrhea and has been isolated from normal stools, from blood and urine, and from warm- and cold-blooded animals. *E. tarda* can be differentiated from other Enterobacteriaceae fairly easily in that it does not attack any carbohydrates other than dextrose and maltose.

15-5 SALMONELLA

Only 13 species of *Salmonella* should be recognized; all other types should be listed as serotypes (ser) or biological serotypes (bioser) of the species *S. enteritidis.* There are approximately 1400 known serotypes of *Salmonella.*

SALMONELLA TYPHI*

This is the cause of typhoid fever.

Morphology and Staining. Members of this species are short, plump rods, measuring 0.5 to 0.8 μm in width, and 1.0 to 3.5 μm in length. They are actively motile and stain uniformly gram-negative.

---

*Much what is described under *S. typhi* also applies to most other *Salmonella.* Specific differences are listed under *Salmonella enteritidis.*

Cultural Characteristics. *Salmonella typhi* organisms are aerobic but facultatively anaerobic, grow well on routine media at a pH range between 6 and 8 and at temperatures between 15°C and 41°C. Their optimal temperature is 37°C. In 24 hours, the colonies are somewhat smaller and more delicate than those of typical *E. coli*. Sodium tetrathionate and selenite favor the growth of *Salmonella* (and *Shigella**) at the expense of most other Enterobacteriaceae. These substances are not inhibitory to the other Enterobacteriaceae, but when reduced by *Salmonella* or *Shigella*, they can be utilized as additional sources of energy. Sodium deoxycholate may be incorporated in media to render them selective for *Salmonella* and *Shigella*.

Biochemical Characteristics. *S. typhi* produces acid but no gas from dextrose, maltose, mannitol, dextrin, and trehalose by fermentation. It does not ferment lactose or sucrose, does not grow in KCN or on malonate, but will decarboxylate lysine.

Resistance. *S. typhi* survives for months in moist cultures and ice, and for weeks in sewage and water. It is killed in broth cultures heated at 56°C for one hour, and it is usually destroyed by pasteurization and chlorination. It is resistant to sulfonamides and penicillins but sensitive to chlortetracyclines. Because *Salmonella* are somewhat more dye-resistant than most Enterobacteriaceae, certain dyes may be incorporated in some media to render them selective for *Salmonella* (malachite green, brilliant green).

Variability. Variations are mainly confined to antigenic differences. However, the following cultural variations may occur: smooth motile, smooth nonmotile, rough motile, and rough nonmotile. Rough cultures are generally less virulent than smooth cultures. Both virulence and smoothness can be regained by repeated subculture in mice.

Antigenicity. *Salmonella* possess both O (somatic) and H (flagellar) antigens. Moreover, many types possess two forms of flagella which may occur at different phases. Originally, the antigens occurring in these phases were called group and specific antigens; the phases, group and specific phases. Of late, the phases are simply listed as phase one and two. In addition to the O and H antigens, some salmonellae, particularly *S. typhi*, have the so-called Vi antigen. The Vi antigen is directly related to the virulence of the organism. It is a surface antigen that can mask the O antigen

---

*Most workers will agree that *Salmonella* species are more benefitted by sodium tetrathionate and selenite than are *Shigella*.

in a manner similar to K antigens in *Escherichia coli.* Its presence can be detected by means similar to those employed to detect K antigens (see p. 230). Because patients suffering from S. *typhi* often develop anti-Vi antibodies, detection of high levels of such anti-bodies in a patient's serum is diagnostic of exposure to S. *typhi.* The test used for detecting such antibodies is the Widal test (p. 371).

Pathogenicity. As mentioned earlier, the disease caused by S. *typhi* is typhoid fever. Infection is by ingestion; the incubation period is usually 14 days, but varies from 3 to 21 days. From the small intestine, the organisms may pass by way of the lymphatics to the mesenteric glands, where they may invade the circulation by way of the thoracic duct. The liver, gallbladder, spleen, kidney and bone marrow usually become infected during this bacteremic phase, which occurs over the first seven to ten days of the disease.

From the gallbladder, a further invasion of the intestine results, involving primarily lymphoid tissue (Peyer's patches—the whitish, flat, lymphatic follicles in the mucosal and submucosal layers of the small intestine). Necrosis results with characteristic typhoid ulcers. Hemorrhage and perforation of the Peyer's patches may further complicate this condition. Typhoid fever can last for several weeks.

Transmission. As these are primarily intestinal parasites, they are found most frequently in sewage. From there, they may contaminate the water supply and hence food. Human carriers may shed typhoid bacilli for 2 to 12 months following their initial infection. Chronic carriers shed the organisms much longer, often until they have undergone surgery to remove their gallbladder.

Prevention. Because of the wide distribution and the ease of spread of the *Salmonella,* typhoid and other salmonelloses are difficult to control. Vaccines are available and seem to be effective. They are recommended for those who travel to areas where typhoid is endemic. Detection, control and treatment of carriers, in particular the screening of personnel involved with foods, is mandatory to limit typhoid. Pasteurization and chlorination undoubtedly reduce the numbers infected.

Laboratory Diagnosis. Salmonellae are isolated most frequently from stools. When the disease is complicated by nephritis, the organism can be isolated from the urine, chiefly between the third and sixth weeks of infection. When complicated by enteric fever, the blood offers another source.

If one always suspects *Salmonella,* isolation and identification offer little difficulty (see Section 15–15). When one's guard is down, isolates may often be missed or lost by misdirection. A more detailed laboratory approach is outlined in Section 15–15. Demonstration of a rise in antibodies as detected by the Widal test (p. 371) is a further aid in diagnosing salmonellosis.

SALMONELLA ENTERITIDIS

This is by far the most frequently occurring species of *Salmonella*. Some 1400 different types are recognized, mainly on the basis of antigenic analyses. Of these types, *bioser Paratyphi A* and *ser Paratyphi B* cause a milder form of typhoid fever, which is called paratyphoid. All other types have been associated with enteritis or food poisoning.

Morphology. See *S. typhi*, although some are nonmotile. Motility and pathogenicity are not related.

Cultural Characteristics. See *S. typhi*.

Biochemical Characteristics. These are generally the same as those of *S. typhi*. Some variations occur, but these are not consistent enough for a species to be identified purely on the basis of biochemical analysis.

Resistance. See *S. typhi*.

Variability. See *S. typhi*.

Antigenicity. See *S. typhi*. Vi antigens are seldom encountered.

Pathogenicity. Diseases caused by *S. enteritidis* are generally referred to as salmonelloses. Apart from paratyphoid, already mentioned, salmonellosis may take several different forms:

  a. *Enteritis* is an inflammation, usually of the small intestine. Stools may vary in consistency from solid to liquid.
  b. In *enteric fever* the patient develops a fever followed by enteritis. The fever may be caused by the presence of bacteria or their toxins in the blood.
  c. The enteric fever may terminate in meningitis, encephalitis, osteomyelitis, endocarditis, nephritis, or a combination of these.

Most *Salmonella* infections occur as a nasty enteritis of a relatively short duration.

Treatment. Bed rest with convenient access to bathroom, commode or bedpan is recommended. Light liquid diets and antibiotic therapy cure most cases in one to two weeks.

Transmission. The same as *S. typhi*, although *S. enteritidis* is even more widely distributed among animals, particularly in fowl, swine, fish, and clams.

Prevention. Good hygiene; particular care should be taken in the food industry to prevent contamination of packaged or processed foods.

Laboratory Diagnosis. See *S. typhi*.

SALMONELLA ARIZONAE

This organism may frequently be isolated from sick and healthy reptiles; it is less frequently associated with infections in man, dogs and a variety of fowl. In man, it has been incriminated as the cause of enteric fever and enteritis of varying severity.

15-6 CITROBACTER

These organisms were formerly placed in two groups under the names *Bethesda-Ballerup* and *Escherichia freundii*. They are presently grouped together under one genus. Their association with disease is uncertain. *Citrobacter* will grow in the presence of KCN.

15-7 KLEBSIELLA PNEUMONIAE

K. pneumoniae can cause severe enteritis in children, as well as pneumonia and upper respiratory tract infections in man generally. Less frequently, it may cause septicemia, peritonitis, and even meningitis.

Some workers differentiate *Klebsiella* organisms into three species: *K. pneumoniae; K. rhinoscleromatis*, which is associated with nodules in the nose; and *K. ozenae*, which causes a disorder of the smelling faculties. Other workers only differentiate between types of *K. pneumoniae* on the basis of capsular antigens. Seventy-two types have been identified.

MORPHOLOGY AND STAINING

These are short to fairly long bacilli, ranging in size from 0.5 to 1.0 μm in width and 1 to 4 μm in length. They all produce capsules, are nonmotile, and stain uniformly gram-negative.

CULTURAL CHARACTERISTICS

Cultures of *K. pneumoniae* are much like *E. coli*, but on MacConkey agar the colonies appear to be a light pink rather than red. Furthermore, most strains are viscid to mucoid rather than butyrous. Many strains produce a "yeasty" odor.

BIOCHEMICAL CHARACTERISTICS

K. pneumoniae can be differentiated from other Enterobacteriaceae fairly easily because they ferment lactose, are methyl-red-negative, Voges-Proskauer-positive, and grow on citrate.

15-8 ENTEROBACTER

These may be encountered in the soil, in water and in dairy products. They are frequently isolated from patients suffering from urinary tract infections or septicemia. Their isolation and identification should offer little more difficulty than that of *Klebsiella* or *E. coli* (see Section 15–15).

15-9 HAFNIA-SERRATIA

These organisms occur naturally in water bodies and in soil. They have been associated with pneumonia, empyema, meningitis, septicemia, pulmonary abscess, urinary tract infection, and wound infection. These infections are believed to be acquired mainly in the hospital.

Some strains of *Serratia marcescens* produce a characteristic brick red or amber pigment, particularly on nutrient agar at room temperature: this aids in their diagnosis. Further identification is reasonably simple, following Section 15–15 as a guide.

15-10 PROTEUS

Five species of this genus are recognized: *P. vulgaris, P. mirabilis, P. morganii, P. rettgeri,* and *P. inconstans.*

MORPHOLOGY AND STAINING

Proteus are generally rod-shaped, measuring 1.5 μm in width and 3.0 to 5.0 μm in length. Pleomorphic forms are quite common, particularly in young, swarming cultures, when curved or filamentous forms may reach up to 30 μm in length. They are nonencapsulated and stain uniformly gram-negative.

CULTURAL CHARACTERISTICS

Proteus are aerobic but facultatively anaerobic, and grow well on routine media. Several *Proteus* strains, particularly *P. vulgaris* and *P. mirabilis,* spread or swarm over the entire surface of moist agar plates. When swarming, the culture appears as a thin film, which is easily missed by careless screeners and therefore often the cause of difficulty in obtaining pure cultures. Swarming may be prevented by one of the following: increasing the agar concentration to 5% or by incorporating 0.01 to 0.04% of tellurite, or 1:500 chloral hydrate, or 1:5000 sodium azide into the medium. *Proteus* produce a strong seminal odor, which may aid screening.

BIOCHEMICAL CHARACTERISTICS

Proteus can be more easily identified than any of the other Enterobacteriaceae by the fact that only they deaminate phenylalanine. *P. inconstans* fails to produce urease; the other four do so within four to six hours. Two species only, *P. vulgaris* and *P. mirabilis*, produce H₂S rapidly. Of these, only *P. vulgaris* converts tryptophan to indole. Only *P. rettgeri* grows on citrate agar.

PATHOGENICITY

Proteus species are second only to *E. coli* in frequency of causing infections of the urinary tract. Because of their urease activity, they are usually more destructive, particularly to the kidneys.

Proteus are also frequently found in the stools of individuals receiving antibiotic therapy; they have been isolated from acute cases of dysentery, and even from the blood.

TREATMENT

Streptomycin and tetracyclines are usually effective, but resistant strains are not uncommon and appear to be increasing.

15-11 YERSINIA (PASTEURELLA)

This genus has been created only recently, partly to accommodate a relative newcomer, *Y. enterocolitica,* and partly to reshape the somewhat chaotic *Pasteurella* genus. The former *Pasteurella pestis* and *P. pseudotuberculosis* have been placed in this new genus; *Pasteurella tularensis* was placed in a genus by itself *(Francisella);* and the other *Pasteurella* species have remained under that name (see Section 15–14).

YERSINIA PESTIS

This organism is responsible for the historic black death. It is estimated that during the 14th century, approximately 25 million people died from this disease in Europe and Asia Minor. At one time, 50% of all people in the Roman Empire died of the plague. More recent figures record 523 cases in the United States between 1900 and 1951; sporadic cases are still reported.

Morphology. The organisms are generally short, plump rods that measure 0.5 to 0.7 μm in width and 1.5 to 7.5 μm in length. Particularly in older cultures, the organisms can be pleomorphic. They are gram-negative with bipolar staining, nonmotile, and nonsporogenous. In fresh cultures and in clinical material, they are often encapsulated.

Cultural Characteristics. *Yersinia pestis* is aerobic but facultatively anaerobic. It grows well on ordinary media, even media containing bile salts, gentian violet, or both. For primary isolation, blood agar is probably most suitable. Growth temperature ranges from 0°C to 43°C, with an optimal temperature of 28°C. The pH range is 6.6 to 8.0, with the optimum between 7.2 and 7.4. Colonies on blood agar are nonhemolytic, round, transparent, and shiny; they measure about 2 mm in diameter at 24 hours.

Biochemical Characteristics. Carbohydrate fermentation reactions are variable. Nitrates are reduced to nitrites. Neither indole nor urease is produced, but catalase is.

Resistance. *Y. pestis* is readily killed by common disinfectants and by pasteurization. Often, however, the organisms are embedded in protein or pus, which enhances their chance for survival.

Pathogenicity. Three clinical types of plague can be produced in man: bubonic, septicemic and pneumonic. Bubonic plague is characterized by an infection of the lymph nodes, which swell and develop into the typical buboes. In septicemic plague, small hemorrhages in the skin and mucous membranes result from a generalized invasion. Pneumonic plague spreads mainly through the lymphatics of the lungs, until both lungs become hemorrhagic.

Treatment. Sulfadiazine appears to be as effective if not superior to the often recommended antiplague serum. However, streptomycin, chloramphenicol, and tetracycline are much more effective, particularly when administered at the onset of fever.

Transmission. Transmission occurs directly by droplets from infected persons and indirectly from rat fleas. Laboratory infections are easily contracted by careless workers who create aerosols, particularly while handling tissues at necropsy of experimentally infected animals.

Prevention. Prevention includes proper care of patients and specimens. During epidemics, rat and flea control should be the first defense.

Laboratory Diagnosis. In bubonic plague, the buboes should be punctured with a hypodermic needle and the exudate withdrawn with a small syringe. A methylene blue or gram-stained smear should reveal numerous bipolar rods. For septicemic plague, the blood should be cultured, and for pneumonic plague, the sputum.

Colonies appear by 24 hours on blood agar culture at 25° to 30°C (although the organisms also grow well at 37°C). In broth cultures, a chainlike growth appears. When the broth is overlaid with a film of oil, an even more characteristic stalactite growth forms. Direct fluorescence microscopy offers a rapid diagnostic tool. For further identification, see Section 15–15.

OTHER YERSINIA SPECIES

Yersinia pseudotuberculosis and *Y. enterocolitica* are relatively large coccobacilli (0.5 to 1.0 μm by 1.0 to 2.0 μm). They are motile at 22°C but not at 37°C. They are widely established in animals such as rabbits, mice, and guinea pigs, and can cause major outbreaks of fatal septicemia in laboratory animal populations. They have been associated with disease in man, in particular, *Y. enterocolitica.* More than 1000 cases of enterocolitis caused by this organism were reported in the U.S. between 1966 and 1970.

These species may be isolated on ordinary media. On MacConkey agar they grow reasonably well, demonstrating pinpoint lactose-negative colonies that are often disregarded. Cultures from stool specimens should be incubated for 48 hours before one discards them as "no lactose-negative organisms isolated." Differentiation from other Enterobacteriaceae is fairly simple (see Section 15–15). *Y. enterocolitica* is generally susceptible to chloramphenicol, colistin, gentamicin, kanamycin, and streptomycin. *Y. pseudotuberculosis* is susceptible to kanamycin, streptomycin, and tetracycline.

15-12 VIBRIONACEAE

Ten genera of simple, curved, twisted rods belong to this family. The genus *Vibrio* is the only one of interest because it contains *V. cholerae,* the cause of cholera in man.

VIBRIO CHOLERAE

Cholera, a major concern in some areas (Burma, China, India, Nepal, Bangladesh and Pakistan), has spread much wider in recent years than it had 50 years ago.

Morphology and Staining. The organism is comma-shaped, measuring about 1.5 to 3.0 μm in length and 0.5 μm in width over its widest point. It is gram-negative and motile.

Cultural Characteristics. *Vibrio cholerae* is aerobic, grows best at a pH of 8.0 and at 37°C; temperature may range from 16° to 40°C. Colonies are usually moist and mucoid, particularly on media containing bile salts.

Biochemical Characteristics. *V. cholerae* ferments dextrose, sucrose, mannitol, maltose and mannose, producing acid but no gas. It does not ferment lactose, dulcitol, arabinose, sorbitol, adonitol or salicin. It produces indole and nitrites, detectable by the cholera-red reaction. In this test, a few drops of sulfuric acid added to overnight cultures in peptone water will produce a red to pink color owing to the formation of "indole-nitrose."

Pathogenicity. An incubation period lasting from two to five days is usually followed by a sudden onset of nausea, vomiting, and profuse diarrhea with abdominal cramps. The stool contains mucus, epithelial cells and large numbers of *V. cholerae*. Rapid loss of fluids and salts leads to profound dehydration, circulatory collapse, and anuria.

Cholera is not invasive; organisms are confined to the intestinal tract where they multiply rapidly, producing endotoxins that are liberated by dead cells and other harmful products. These substances irritate and damage the mucosa of the intestinal walls, resulting in the characteristic diarrhea. Cholera is fatal in 25 to 50% of cases, depending largely on the type of treatment received by its victims.

Laboratory Diagnosis. Large numbers of *Vibrio* in stools of suspect cases can easily be recognized by their characteristic movements. They "dart" across the microscopic field because of their single flagellum. This motility can be inhibited by specific antiserum.

V. cholerae is readily cultured on alkaline media (pH 8.0 to 9.0). Peptone broth at a pH of 8.4 is frequently used as an enrichment medium to allow for the isolation of small numbers of *Vibrio* mixed with Enterobacteriaceae. The alkalinity slows the Enterobacteriaceae down, allowing the *Vibrio* to grow in a membrane-like pellicle at the top of the broth. Following incubation at 37°C for six to eight hours, subcultures of the pellicle or surface film usually result in isolation of the *Vibrio*. Identification may be made on the basis of biochemical or serologic characteristics.

Treatment. The response to prompt and adequate intravenous replacement of lost fluid and electrolytes is dramatic. Together with tetracycline administration, which causes a significant reduction of fluid loss, this treatment will rapidly reverse the patient's severe condition. Continued oral administration of large amounts of glucose and electrolyte solutions may be necessary when the supply of intravenous solutions is limited.

Prevention and Transmission. Since cholera spreads primarily by way of contaminated water and foods, it can be contained by maintaining good sanitary conditions.

15-13 HAEMOPHILUS

H. influenzae was isolated as early as 1892 by Pfeiffer from people suffering from influenza. Until 1933, when the influenza virus was isolated, it was believed to be the sole cause of influenza. It is presently regarded as a secondary invader of the upper respiratory tract.

H. ducreyi is the cause of soft chancre, chancroid, a fairly common venereal disease. *H. aegyptius*, the historic "Koch-Weeks bacillus," may frequently be isolated from cases of conjunctivitis. *H. aphrophilus* has been associated with rare cases of endocarditis, pneumonia, and lately meningitis. Other *Haemophilus* species are less frequently associated with disease in man. *H. parainfluenzae* appears to be a commensal of the upper respiratory tract of some individuals.

The following discussions pertain to *H. influenzae* only unless specific reference to the contrary is made.

MORPHOLOGY

Members of the genus *Haemophilus* are generally very small rods measuring 0.2 to 0.3 μm in width and 1.0 to 1.5 μm in length. In the Gram stain, carbol fuchsin should be used as a counterstain. In smooth cultures and in exudates, the small regular forms are predominant. In rough cultures and in exudates from healing lesions, pleomorphic forms are more frequently encountered, ranging from coccoid forms to long filamentous forms. In broth cultures and in cerebrospinal fluid, long filamentous forms are the rule rather than the exception. Some filaments may reach to 30 μm or more in length. *Haemophilus* are nonmotile and nonsporogenous but usually produce capsules.

CULTURAL CHARACTERISTICS

Haemophilus are aerobic but facultatively anaerobic. These organisms grow best at 37°C, with a growth range from 20° to 42°C, and a pH of 7.2 to 7.6. The most peculiar growth characteristic of medically important species is that they require one or both of two substances found in whole blood, hemin and nicotinamide-adenine-dinucleotide (NAD), which have been labelled X and V factors respectively. Hemin is related to hemoglobin, and it is more readily available to organisms growing on chocolated agar than on blood agar. It is heat stable at 120°C for 30 minutes.

NAD is a heat-labile (120°C for 30 minutes) coenzyme. In addition to being present in the blood, it is also produced by many bacteria, yeasts, and plant cells. *Staphylococcus* and *Streptococcus faecalis* in particular produce extra amounts of V factor. Thus, when colonies of these organisms are allowed to grow in the proximity of *Haemophilus*, excess factor V diffuses into the planted medium, providing the *Haemophilus* with the extra growth factor. *Haemophilus* therefore often grow as "satellite colonies" in the proximity of *Staphylococcus* or other colonies supplying the V factor. The dependence on either X, V or both factors of different *Haemophilus* species is indicated in Table 15–2.

On chocolated agar, *Haemophilus* colonies reach a diameter of 1 to 2 mm in 24 hours. these colonies are transparent, colorless and shiny; they resemble dewdrops. Special enriched media for the growth of *Haemophilus* have been developed (see Levinthal's medium, p. 392).

RESISTANCE

Haemophilus are killed by heat at 56°C in 30 minutes, fairly rapidly by drying, and by the usual disinfectants. They are susceptible to ampicillin and tetracyclines.

ANTIGENICITY

Several antigens are shared by *H. influenzae* and *H. aegyptius*, but some specific antigens are found in members of each species. *Haemophilus* has been classified into serotypes on the basis of capsular polysaccharides, employing the Quellung reaction (p. 138). Six types of *H. influenzae*, *a* to *f*, have been recognized thus far.

PATHOGENICITY

H. influenzae may cause primary and secondary respiratory infections of varying severity. In children, and occasionally in adults, it may also cause meningitis. Influenzal meningitis in adults is usually associated with chronic sinusitis, mastoiditis, or middle ear infections. Subacute bacterial endocarditis is a less frequent complication of *H. influenzae* infections. Diseases caused by other *Haemophilus* species have already been mentioned.

TREATMENT AND PREVENTION

Ampicillin, chloramphenicol, and tetracyclines are the drugs of choice. These are frequently administered prophylactically to high risk groups, such as inhabitants of homes for the elderly who are most susceptible to respiratory infections during influenza outbreaks.

LABORATORY DIAGNOSIS

The clinical type of infection dictates the selection of the specimen—sputum, cerebrospinal fluid, or blood. Urethral swabs would be taken for chancroid; eye swabs, for conjunctivitis.

Chocolated blood agar plates, prewarmed to 37°C with a so-called *Staph.* streak to supply extra V factor, offer the most practical means for isolation. The *Staph.* streak should be applied to a plate inoculated with the specimen in the usual manner by running a single streak from the main inoculum to the other side of the plate. *Haemophilus* will grow most abundantly near this streak.

Once isolated and recognized, identification can be completed by an estimation of V and X factor dependency. By using X and V factor strips* on hemin- and NAD-free media and consulting Table 15–2, this is a fairly simple procedure.

15-14 PASTEURELLA

This historically important genus has recently been reduced to one of relatively little importance (see *Yersinia*, p. 209). The remaining *Pasteurella* are small cocoid bacilli, nonmotile, catalase-, oxidase-, and nitrate-positive, that ferment carbohydrates.

Pasteurella multocida is the cause of hemorrhagic septicemia in animals, and occasionally it causes a variety of infections in man: local soft tissue infections, bacteremia, meningitis, and respiratory tract infections.

15-15 DIFFERENTIATION

In most instances, of course, the clinical picture, or at least the type of specimen submitted for analysis, guides the microbiologist toward the differentiation of specific bacteria. Since this is such a primary factor in clinical bacteriology, we offer here a system that allows differentiation of most gram-negative bacteria that might be encountered in clinical specimens. Understand that such a system may not always correctly identify every isolate, but it will provide clinically relevant data in most instances, and furthermore, will do it economically and rapidly.

---

*Available from Baltimore Biological Laboratories, Cockeysville, Md.

Facultatively anaerobic gram-negative bacilli can be differentiated from other bacteria fairly easily if all primary characteristics as listed in Chart 25-2 are known. Determining atmospheric requirements, however, is not practical for isolates from many specimens. When doubts arise about whether an isolate belongs to the organisms assigned to Part 8 in *Bergey's Manual* or to some other group, the first step toward differentiation should be based on the characteristics listed in Table 15–1. *Brucella, Bordetella, Francisella,* and *Haemophilus* species are readily differentiated because they require special growth requirements that will be provided only when these organisms are suspected. Differentiation of the first three species has already been considered in Chapter 14; *Haemophilus* species can be differentiated on the basis

Table 15–1. Secondary differentiation of gram-negative bacilli.

	Oxidase reaction	Nitrate reduction	Growth on MacConkey agar	O/F* reaction	Refer to section
Enterobacteriaceae	−	+	+	+/+	15–15
Vibrio or Aeromonas	+	+	+	+/+	15–15
Pasteurella	+	+	−‡	+/+	15–15
Pseudomonas or					
Xanthomonas	+†	±	+	+/−	14–6
Alcaligenes	+	+	+	−/−	14–6
Brucella	+	+	−	−/−	14–6
Bordetella	−	−	∓	−/−	14–6
Acinetobacter	−	−	+	+/−	13–6
Moraxella	+	±	±	−/−	13–6

Key: + = positive; − = negative; ± = most strains are positive;
     ∓ = most strains are negative; +/+ = fermentative; +/− = oxidative;
     −/− = do not attack carbohydrates

*O/F = oxidative/fermentation Hugh-Leiffson reaction.
†*Pseudomonas maltophilia* is oxidase-negative.
‡*Pasteurella haemolytica* grows on MacConkey agar.

Table 15–2. Some differential characteristics of *Haemophilus.*

	Requires X factor	Requires V factor	Affects mainly the:
H. influenzae	Yes	Yes	Respiratory tract, also conjunctiva and meninges
H. aegyptius	Yes	Yes	Conjunctiva
H. ducreyi	Yes	No	Genitalia
H. aphrophilus	Yes	No	Blood and heart valves
H. parainfluenzae	No	Yes	Respiratory tract

Chart 15–1. Differentiation of *Pasteurella* species.

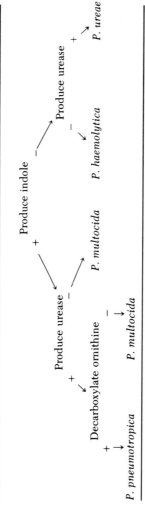

Guide to Chart 15–1: Inoculate peptone water, urea agar, and ornithine decarboxylase broth. Incubate at 35° C for 48 hours. Complete tests, record you results, and follow the chart.

Chart 15–2. Identification of *Vibrio* and *Aeromonas*.

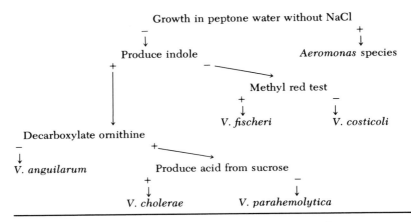

Guide to Chart 15–2: Inoculate peptone water without NaCl, peptone agar, and methyl red, sucrose and ornithine decarboxylase broths. Incubate at 35°C for 48 hrs. Complete tests, record your results, and follow the chart.

of their factor X and V requirements. This is a fairly simple procedure if one uses factor X and V strips* and a medium that is free of NAD and hemin, and consults Table 15–2.

Pasteurella, once the genus has been recognized (see Table 15–1), can be further identified on the basis of production of indole, urease, and ornithine decarboxylase (see Chart 15–1). *Pasteurella haemolytica* is differentiated from *Vibrio* and *Aeromonas* by its lack of motility.

There is little reason to try to differentiate species of *Vibrio* or *Aeromonas* except when the presence of *V. cholerae* is suspected. In that case, the isolate should be subjected to the cholera-red test and to specific antisera that would inhibit motility (see Section 15–12). Should more complete differentiation be warranted, further aids in identification are listed in Chart 15–2.

ENTEROBACTERIACEAE

Since this is such a large and important group of bacteria, we shall discuss their laboratory diagnosis in more detail.

Realizing that most Enterobacteriaceae are isolated from the feces, we shall confine our discussion to isolation from this source

---

*Available from Baltimore Biological Laboratories, Cockeysville, Md.

only. The student must remember that these organisms may be found in many other specimens as well. In fact, it is doubtful whether one could name any type of human specimen from which Enterobacteriaceae of one form or another have never been isolated. Stool specimens should be cultured immediately upon arrival in the laboratory, lest the "normal flora" outgrow or "overshadow" possible pathogens. If specimens have to be transported or stored for any length of time, they should be refrigerated.

Most workers agree that little value lies in the microscopic examination of stool specimens, other than that already discussed under *Shigella* and screening for ova or cysts of parasites (p. 321).

For primary culture or isolation, a variety of media can be chosen. Usually, one differential medium [MacConkey agar or eosin-methylene blue (EMB) agar], one selective medium [Salmonella-Shigella agar (SS) or deoxycholate-citrate agar (DCA)], and one enrichment medium (selenite or tetra-thionate broth) are used in conjunction with one another. My choice has always been MacConkey-SS-selenite media, but other combinations may give equal results or even better, according to some workers.

(To allow isolation of possible gram-positive organisms, blood agar may be included. This has the added advantage that when *E. coli* is expected and isolated in apparently pure culture, serologic studies may be performed directly from the blood agar culture, although the results must be corroborated by follow-up studies. When *Staphylococcus aureus* is suspected, a salt mannitol agar should also be included to facilitate isolation.)

The advantages of using three different types of media should be explained: when fairly large numbers of *Salmonella* and *Shigella* organisms are mixed with normal flora in a specimen, both pathogens can be isolated readily on MacConkey and SS agar. However, when only a few of these pathogens are mixed with large numbers of normal flora, the inoculum size may be insufficient to allow their isolation on these media. That is why an enrichment broth is used. For example, suppose that a relatively large inoculum, about 1 gram, is added to selenite broth. The selenite will suppress the large numbers of lactose-fermenters and possible *Proteus* species, while simultaneously enhancing the growth of *Salmonella* and *Shigella*. This usually permits one to isolate *Salmonella* or *Shigella* by subculturing the selenite broth onto MacConkey or SS agar. MacConkey agar is useful for isolating all the Enterobacteriaceae that are neither *Salmonella* nor *Shigella*.

Having isolated Enterobacteriaceae on either SS or MacConkey agars, one can usually differentiate between lactose-fermenters

Chart 15–3. Further identification of lactose-fermenters taken from MacConkey agar culture.

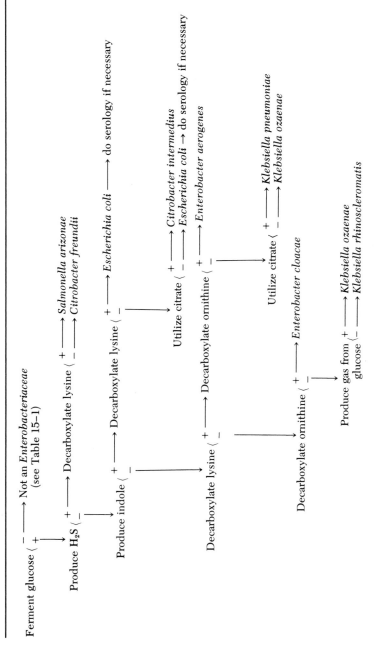

Guide to Chart 15–3: Inoculate glucose, lysine and ornithine broths, and SIM and citrate agar; incubate at 35° C for 48 hrs. Complete and record reactions; follow the chart with the results.

Chart 15–4. Further identification of nonlactose fermenters from MacConkey agar.

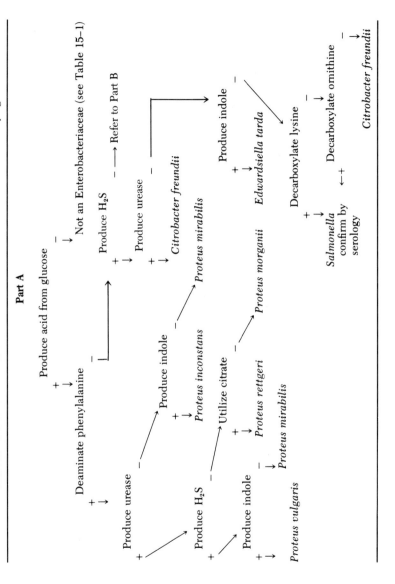

Chart 15–4 continued (Part B)

Part B

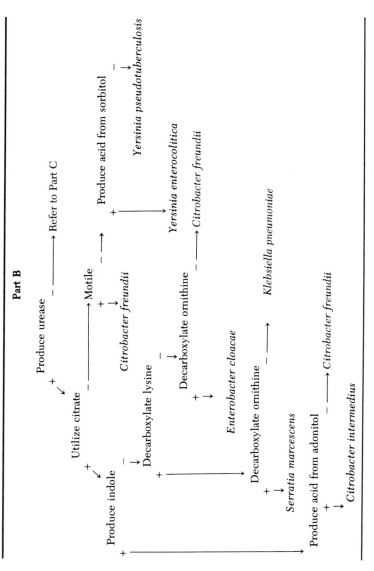

Chart 15–4. continued (Part C)

Part C

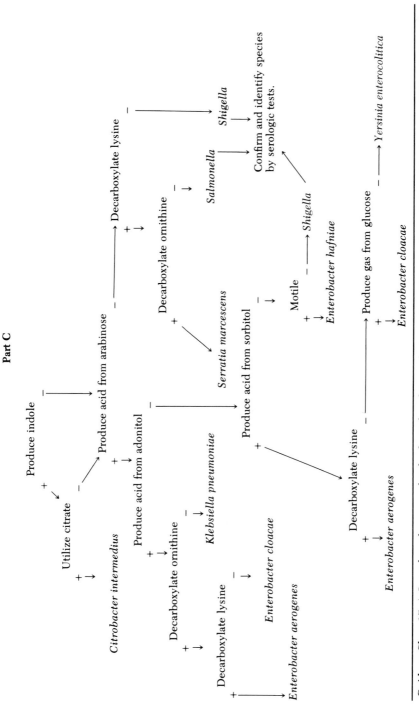

Guide to Chart 15–4: Inoculate glucose, sorbitol, adonitol, arabinose, lysine and ornithine broths, and phenylalanine, urea, SIM and citrate agar; incubate at 35°C for 48 hrs. Complete, read and record reactions; follow the chart with the results.

Table 15–3. Identification of lactose fermenters by IMViC reaction pattern.

	Indole	Methyl red	Voges-Proskauer	Citrate
E. coli	+	+	−	−
Citrobacter	−	+	−	+
Enterobacter*	−	−	+	+
Klebsiella*	−	−	+	+

Enterobacter is motile, *Klebsiella* is not.

and nonlactose-fermenters, after which the isolate may be identified further according to the routes outlined in Charts 15–3 and
15–4.*

Several other approaches, of course, give equally satisfactory or
more scientifically accurate results. The relative cost of each
approach and the technical competence of the laboratorian responsible for the results must be weighed against the clinical benefits
derived from the system used. One popular approach proceeds as
follows:

    1. Inoculate a sulfide indole motility (SIM) agar, a methyl-
red-Voges-Proskauer broth (MR-VP), and a citrate agar with
each apparent lactose-fermenter.

    2. Inoculate a triple sugar iron (TSI) agar, a urea, and a
phenylalanine agar slant with each apparent nonlactose-
fermenter.

The more common lactose-fermenters can be identified with reasonable accuracy by their so-called IMViC reaction pattern: Indole,
Methyl-red, Voges-Proskauer, and Citrate respectively (see Table
15–3). (The "i" in IMViC is included for euphonics only.) To
follow-up the apparent nonlactose-fermenters, consult Table 15–4
for the various TSI reactions and their interpretation. Further
identification of these species can be obtained by consulting Charts
15–5 to 15–11 as indicated in Table 15–4. Note that some apparently nonlactose-fermenters prove to be typical lactose-fermenting
species upon further analysis.

Several commercial systems have been developed for so-called
rapid identification of Enterobacteriaceae. The merits of some of
these systems in the hands of relatively inexperienced laboratorians are questionable, as may be the claims for "rapid identification." No doubt, a commercial system will be developed that will

---

*The media referred to in these charts are fully explained in Chapter 29.

Table 15–4. Possible results of cultures grown on triple-sugar iron (TSI) agar.

Column Recording	A −/−	B −/+	C −/⊕	D −/+ H₂S
Interpretation	No sugars fermented.	Glucose only fermented.	As B; gas also produced.	As B; H₂S also produced.
Possible organisms	Alcaligenes Pseudomonas Acinetobacter	Proteus morganii Proteus rettgeri Proteus inconstans Salmonella typhi Serratia Shigella Yersinia pestis Yersinia pseudotuberculosis	Proteus rettgeri Proteus morganii Proteus inconstans Shigella	Citrobacter Edwardsiella Proteus mirabilis Proteus vulgaris Salmonella typhi Salmonella arizonae
For further identification see	Chapter 14	Chart 15–5	Chart 15–6	Chart 15–7

Column Recording	E −/⊕ H₂S	F +/+	G +/⊕	H +/⊕ H₂S
Interpretation	As B; gas and H₂S also produced.	Acid slope and butt; glucose and lactose or sucrose fermented.	As F; gas also produced.	As G; H₂S also produced.
Possible organisms	Citrobacter Edwardsiella Proteus mirabilis Proteus vulgaris Salmonella	Erwinia Hafnia Klebsiella Serratia Staphylococcus Streptococcus Yersinia enterocolitica	Enterobacter Escherichia coli Klebsiella Proteus inconstans Proteus rettgeri	Citrobacter Proteus mirabilis Proteus vulgaris Salmonella arizonae
For further identification see	Chart 15–8	Chart 15–9	Chart 15–10	Chart 15–11

−/ = negative slant
/− = negative butt
O = gas produced
H₂S = Hydrogen sulfide produced

Chart 15–5. Differentiation of organisms listed under B, Table 15–4.

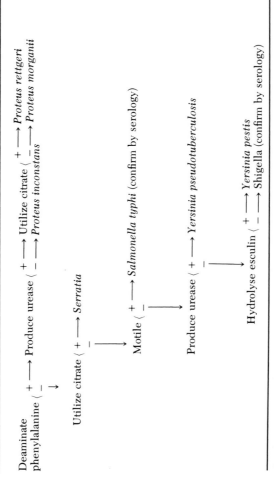

Guide to Chart 15–5: Inoculate phenylalanine, urea, citrate, esculin, and motility agar media; incubate at 35°C for 48 hrs. Complete tests and read reactions; follow the chart with your results.

Chart 15–6. Differentiation of organisms listed under C, Table 15–4.

Deaminate
phenylalanine $\langle$ + ⟶ Produce urease $\langle$ − ⟶ *Proteus inconstans*
  + ⟶ Utilize citrate $\langle$ + ⟶ *Proteus rettgeri*
  − ⟶ *Proteus morganii*
  −
  ↓
  Shigella (confirm by serology)

Guide to Chart 15–6. Inoculate phenylalanine, urea and citrate agar media; incubate at 35° C for 48 hrs. Complete tests and read reactions; follow the chart with your results.

Chart 15–7. Differentiation of organisms listed under D, Table 15–4.

Deaminate
phenylalanine $\langle$ +
  −
  ↓
  Grow in KCN $\langle$ + ⟶ *Citrobacter freundii*
    + ⟶ Produce indole $\langle$ + ⟶ *Proteus vulgaris*
      − ⟶ *Proteus mirabilis*
    −
    ↓
    Produce H$_2$S $\langle$ + ⟶ *Salmonella arizonae*
      − ⟶ *Citrobacter intermedius*
    Produce indole $\langle$ + ⟶ *Edwardsiella*
    Produce malonate $\langle$ + − ⟶ *Salmonella typhi* (confirm by serology)
      −
      ↓

Guide to Chart 15–7. Inoculate phenylalanine and SIM agar, and KCN and malonate broth media; incubate at 35° C for 48 hrs. Complete tests and read reactions; follow the chart with your results.

Chart 15–8. Differentiation of organisms listed under E, Table 15–4.

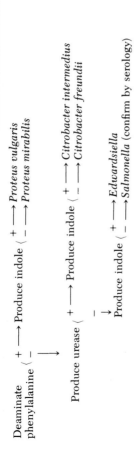

Deaminate phenylalanine $\langle$ + → Produce indole $\langle$ + → *Proteus vulgaris*
$\qquad$ − → *Proteus mirabilis*

− →

Produce urease $\langle$ + → Produce indole $\langle$ + → *Citrobacter intermedius*
$\qquad$ − → *Citrobacter freundii*

− →

Produce indole $\langle$ + → *Edwardsiella*
$\qquad$ − → *Salmonella* (confirm by serology)

Guide to Chart 15–8: Inoculate phenylalanine and urea agar, and peptone water; incubate at 35° C for 48 hrs. Complete tests and read reactions; follow the chart with your results.

Chart 15–9. Differentiation of organisms listed under F, Table 15–4.

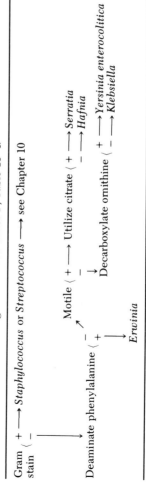

Gram $\langle$ + → *Staphylococcus* or *Streptococcus* → see Chapter 10
stain − →

Motile $\langle$ + → Utilize citrate $\langle$ + → *Serratia*
$\qquad$ − → *Hafnia*

−
↓

Deaminate phenylalanine $\langle$ − → Decarboxylate ornithine $\langle$ + → *Yersinia enterocolitica*
$\qquad$ − → *Klebsiella*

+ →

Erwinia

Guide to Chart 15–9. Do Gram's stain; if negative, inoculate phenylalanine, citrate, motility and ornithine media; incubate at 35° C for 48 hrs. Complete tests and read reactions; follow the chart with your results.

Chart 15–10. Differentiation of organisms listed under G, Table 15–4.

Deaminate
phenylalanine ⟨ + ⟶ Produce urease ⟨ + ⟶ *Proteus rettgeri*
⟨ − ⟶ *Proteus inconstans*
⟨ −

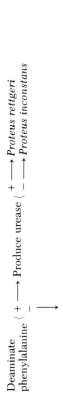

Decarboxylate ornithine ⟨ + ⟶ Utilize citrate ⟨ + ⟶ *Enterobacter*
⟨ − ⟨ −
Klebsiella
Produce indole ⟨ + ⟶ *Escherichia coli*
⟨ − ⟶ *Enterobacter*

Guide to Chart 15–10: Inoculate phenylalanine, urea, citrate and ornithine media, and peptone water; incubate at 35° C for 48 hrs. Complete tests and read reactions; follow the chart with your results.

Chart 15–11. Differentiation of organisms listed under H, Table 15–4.

Deaminate
phenylalanine ⟨ + ⟶ Produce indole ⟨ + ⟶ *Proteus vulgaris*
⟨ − ⟨ − ⟶ *Proteus mirabilis*
⟨ −
Decarboxylate lysine ⟨ + ⟶ *Salmonella arizonae*
⟨ −
⟶ Produce indole ⟨ + ⟶ *Citrobacter intermedius*
⟨ − ⟶ *Citrobacter freundii*

Guide to Chart 15–11: Inoculate phenylalanine and lysine media, and peptone water; incubate at 35° C for 48 hrs. Complete tests and read reactions; follow the chart with your results.

229

be accurate, dependable, and economical, but at the time of this writing, no such system is available.

15-16 THE SEROLOGY OF ENTEROBACTERIACEAE

By serology, we usually mean the study of antibodies in patient's serum. Here we are concerned with the identification of bacteria and should rightly refer to this area of study as "reverse serology," since we employ known antisera to distinguish between unknown antigens carried by organisms whose biochemistry is partially known.

ANTIGENIC COMPLEXITY OF ENTEROBACTERIACEAE

Members of this family possess a variety of different antigens or, as the word goes, a mosaic of antigens. The main varieties can be placed in the following four categories:

The "O" Antigens. From the German "ohne hauch" or nonspreading. These are heat stable at 100°C for 30 minutes, are located within the cell or near its surface, and are polysaccharides.

The "H" Antigens. From the German "hauch" or spreading (meaning that organisms possessing these antigens are usually motile). These are located in the flagella and are proteins. They are called flagellar antigens, and are heat labile at 100°C for 30 minutes.

The "K" Antigens. From the German "kapsel," or envelope. These surround the cell, and are usually heat labile. They are called capsular antigens and can be destroyed by boiling in 30 to 60 minutes.

The "Vi" Antigen. This is a poorly understood antigen which often masks the true somatic antigens, thus rendering them inagglutinable. This phenomenon may be made inactive because these antigens are also heat labile to boiling for 30 minutes. They are said to be related to the virulence of the organisms, hence their designation as "Vi."

TEST PROCEDURE

The usual procedure employed in the serologic identification of Enterobacteriaceae is the slide agglutination test:

    a. To saline in a test tube, add a smooth culture from a TSI or nutrient agar slant; this will form a milky suspension.

    b. Mark off an area on a glass slide with a grease pencil; add a
small drop of antiserum* to this area.

    c. To the drop of antiserum, add a similar drop of the culture
suspension and mix it with the antiserum by gently rocking
the slide.

When the antigens on the cells match the antibodies in the
antiserum, agglutination should occur promptly and be macroscopically recognizable by the appearance of fine granules or larger
aggregates.

If isolates fail to agglutinate in any of the O antisera, heat the
culture suspension at 100°C for 30 minutes, cool, and repeat steps *B*
and *C* before reporting the test as negative. As explained earlier,
masking capsular or Vi antigens may render O antigens inagglutinable until they are removed by heat.

SEROLOGIC IDENTIFICATION OF ESCHERICHIA COLI

Members of *E. coli* are all alike biochemically, but may be
divided into 150 groups according to their "O" antigens, and may
be further typed by their "K" and "H" antigens.†

The system is basically similar to that used in the identification
of the *Salmonella*, except that the serologic types of *Escherichia* are
designated by the formula of their antigenic structures, and not by
different names as are *Salmonella*. Furthermore, only 16 serotypes
of *E. coli* are associated with disease and therefore, the clinical
microbiologist needs to be concerned only with these.‡

Table 15–5. Antigenic structures of *E. coli* serotypes.

Poly A	Poly B	Poly C
O26 :B6	O86 :B7	O18 :B21
O55 :B5	O119:B14	O20 :B7
O111:B4	O124:B17	O20 :B84
O127:B8	O125:B15	O28 :B18
	O126:B16	O44 :K74
	O128:B12	O112:B11

---

*Antisera to type *E. coli* and *Salmonella*, and to group *Shigella*, are commercially
available from Difco Laboratories, Detroit, Mich.; Baltimore Biological Laboratories, Cockeysville, Md.; Lederle Laboratories, Pearl River, N.Y.
†According to *Bergey's Manual*, 8th ed., 150 O, 90 K, and 50 H antigens have been
recognized.
‡The value of serotyping *E. coli* strains is questionable, since a lack of correlation
between virulence properties and serotypes has been demonstrated. J. Infect. Dis.,
133:153–156, 1976.

The antigenic structures of these 16 serotypes are listed in Table 15-5. The first number in each column represents somatic (O) antigens; the second, the capsular (K) antigens (which have been further grouped as B-type capsular antigens).

The three columns of serotypes (Poly A, Poly B, and Poly C) represent groups of serotypes for which polyvalent antisera have been pooled and made commercially available.* By first testing a suspected *E. coli* isolate with one of these three polyvalent antisera, one can place the isolate in group A, B, or C. The next step would entail using specific sera prepared against individuals of each type within the particular group. This two-step method spares the time and expense incurred if one had to test each isolate with 16 antisera.

SEROLOGIC IDENTIFICATION OF SHIGELLA

Shigella is divided antigenically into four subgroups: A, B, C, and D. Each group is designated by a species name as well as by a letter: A—*Shigella dysenteriae,* B—*Shigella flexneri,* C—*Shigella boydii,* and D—*Shigella sonnei.*

Members of each group share certain O antigens that are not found in members of the other groups. By preparing antisera to these antigens, four so-called polyvalent group antisera (A, B, C and D) can be employed to differentiate between the four species of *Shigella.* If a suspected *Shigella* isolate fails to agglutinate with any of these antisera, it is possible that some of the K antigens are "blocking" or "masking" the O antigens, rendering them inagglutinable. Such isolates should be suspended in 0.5% formalin in saline, boiled for one hour, and cooled, at which time agglutination tests may be repeated. If still negative, the isolate is unlikely to be a *Shigella.* If the isolate reacts with one of the antisera listed, for example, D, it can be identified as *Shigella sonnei.* If more than one of the antisera cause agglutination, it is wise to check another batch of antisera. If inconsistencies still prevail, consult your reference laboratory.

Shigella species can be further typed by using type-specific sera corresponding to antigens that may be carried by different members of a group. Ten types of group A, eight of group B, fifteen of group C, and two of group D have been recognized. Typing of *Shigella* is not a routine procedure.

---

*Difco Laboratories, Detroit, Mich.

SEROLOGIC IDENTIFICATION OF SALMONELLA

The distribution of antigenic components is used in a "natural" scheme to classify different types of *Salmonella*. This scheme is known as the Kauffman and White scheme. However, different serologic types should no longer be classified as different species. Since *Salmonella* has previously been given different species names on this basis, there will be contradictions between current and less recent literatures. If you remember that under the current system all but 13 *Salmonella* species are serotypes of *S. enteritidis*, the confusion will be short-lived.

As may seem reasonable, the antigenic structures of the cell itself, the somatic antigens, have been regarded more fundamental than those of the flagella or the capsules. Therefore, the somatic antigens are used to classify the *Salmonella* into groups, each member of a group sharing a particular O antigen in common with other members of the same group.

In addition to these group antigens, salmonellae may possess up to three other O antigens, which they may share indiscriminately with members of other groups. For example, in Table 15–6, O antigen 2 is the group antigen for group A; O antigen 4, for group B; O antigen 7, for group C; O antigen 9, for group D; and O antigen 3, for group E. As can be seen, O antigens 1 and 12 may be found in members of other groups.

Some groups of salmonellae are further subdivided into subgroups, each member of a subgroup sharing a subgroup-specific somatic antigen. For example in Table 15–7, O antigen 6 is the

Table 15–6. Relationship of group antigens of salmonellae.

Group	Serotype	O antigens	H antigens	
			Ph. 1	*Ph. 2*
A	Paratyphi-A	1-2-12	a	—
B	Paratyphi-B	1-4-5-12	b	1-2
B	Typhimurium	1-4-5-12	i	1-2
B	Abortus-bovis	1-4-12-27	b	e-n-x
C_1	Paratyphi-C	6-7-Vi	c	1-5
D	Zega	9-12	d	z-6
E_1	London etc.	3-10	1-v	1-6

Table 15-7. Relationship of subgroup antigens.

Group	Serotype	O antigens	H antigens Ph. 1	Ph. 2
C_1	Parathyphi-C	6-7-Vi	c	1-5
C_1	Thompson	6-7	k	1-5
C_1	Amersfoort	6-7	d	e-n-x
C_2	Manhattan	6-8	d	1-5
C_2	Newport	6-8	e-h	1-2

group antigen for group C, and O antigens 7 and 8 are subgroup antigens for subgroups C_1 and C_2 respectively. More than 30 groups and subgroups have thus far been recognized. The first five groups contain more than half the total number of types of *Salmonella*, and nearly all those associated with disease in man. Most isolates of *Salmonella* can be grouped by using commercially available polyvalent O antiserum that contains antibodies to all the commonly occurring types of *Salmonella*, and group antisera to groups A, B, C_1, C_2, D, E, and E_2.

Once *Salmonella* has been placed within its appropriate group or subgroup, further typing, based on flagellar (H) antigen composition, is relatively simple. H antigens may belong to one of two phases. The exact nature of these two phases is purely academic to the average technologist. To type *Salmonella*, one simply looks up the H antigens that members of a designated group may possess (Tables 15-6 and 15-7). By selecting H antisera containing antibodies to these antigens, typing should present little difficulty. Tables 15-6 and 15-7, of course, represent only a few examples of *Salmonella* types. The complete Kauffman and White scheme must be consulted when typings are attempted. The typing of *Salmonella* is usually performed only by the regional or state reference laboratory.

FURTHER READING

1. Edward, P. R., and Ewing, W. H.: *Identification of Enterobacteriaceae.* 3rd ed. Minneapolis, Burgess Publishing Co., 1972.
2. Smith, P. B., et al.: A.P.I. system; a multitube micromethod for identification of *Enterobacteriaceae.* Applied Microbiol., 24:449–452, 1972.
3. Hirschhorn, N., and Greenough, W. B.: Cholera. Sci. Amer., 225:2, 15–21, 1971.
4. Balows, A., Hermann, G. J., and Dewitt, W. E.: The isolation and identification of *Vibrio cholerae*—a review. Health Lab. Sci., 8: 167–175, 1971.
5. Baltazard, M. et al.: Recommended laboratory methods for the diagnosis of plague. Bull. WHO, 14: 457–509, 1956.
6. Kilian, M.: A taxonomic study of the genus Haemophilus, with the proposal of a new species. J. Gen. Microbiol, 93:9–62, 1976.

chapter 16
Gram-Negative Anaerobic Bacteria

16-1 Classification
16-2 *Bacteroides*
16-3 *Fusobacterium*
16-4 Differentiation

16-1 CLASSIFICATION

Bergey's Manual, Part 9
Gram-negative anaerobic bacteria

Family	I: Bacteroidaceae	
Genus	I. *Bacteroides*	Species: *fragilis*
		21 others
	II. *Fusobacterium*	*nucleatum*
		(fusiforme)
		15 others
	III. *Leptotrichia*	*buccalis*

Six genera of uncertain affiliation are also listed in *Bergey's Manual,* 8th edition. Since none of these appear to be associated with disease in man, they have been excluded here. Refer to Table 7–2 for a complete listing.

DEFINITIONS

Bacteroidaceae. Gram-negative, anaerobic, pleomorphic or uniformly shaped rods. Nonmotile or motile with peritrichous flagella.

Bacteroides. Produce mixtures of acids from glucose fermentation without any product being predominant.

Fusobacterium. Butyric acid is a major product from glucose fermentation. Does not produce isobutyric or isovaleric acids.

Leptotrichia. Produce primarily lactic acid from glucose fermentation.

16-2 BACTEROIDES

In the majority of human specimens, species of this genus are present more abundantly and more often than any other types of organisms. Since they require rather enriched media (they grow best on 25% ascitic fluid in blood agar) and anaerobic conditions, they are not isolated as frequently as their ubiquity would indicate.

Members of the genus *Bacteroides* are normal inhabitants of the intestinal, genital and respiratory tracts of man. They constitute 95% or more of the normal flora of the intestine. *Bacteroides* has been associated with gangrenous infections, abscesses of the brain, liver or lungs, ulcerative lesions of mucous membranes, peritonitis, bacteremia, and endocarditis. About 10% of gram-negative bacteremias in the United States have been attributed to *Bacteroides* species. Infections by *Bacteroides* usually respond to massive doses of tetracycline or penicillin, but may require surgical drainage in addition to chemotherapy.

The most commonly encountered species are *B. fragilis* and *B. melaninogenicus.* They may be differentiated on the basis of colonial and biochemical characteristics, as well as on antibiotic sensitivity patterns. Most routine laboratories do not attempt their diagnosis to the species level.

16-3 FUSOBACTERIUM

Of the six species in this genus, only *F. nucleatum* is associated with disease in man. *F. nucleatum* are large (5 to 14 μm by 1 μm), spindle-shaped, nonmotile, gram-negative, anaerobic rods. They may be found in the saliva and in throats of normal individuals. More commonly, they are found in ulcerative infections of the mouth and of the mucous membranes of the lungs and intestines. Most commonly, however, they occur in association with *Tre-*

ponema vincentii in the mouths of patients with Vincent's infection (see p. 260). *F. nucleatum* is cultured more easily than *Bacteroides.*

16-4 DIFFERENTIATION

Infections caused by anaerobic bacteria, once thought to be rather infrequent occurrences, are presently encountered with increasing frequency. This increase is primarily due to the improved technology of anaerobic culture and identification, and it has sparked an acute awareness of anaerobes among recent medical graduates. The improvement in technology, however, has not kept pace with its practical implementation. It is fair to say that as far as their ability to identify anaerobes is concerned, most clinical laboratories remain in the "Dark Ages." Since this text is fairly elementary, and since the technology that allows full differentiation of anaerobes is highly sophisticated, the following should be considered an elementary guide only. The titles listed under "Further Reading" must be consulted before one attempts any serious efforts in anaerobic techniques.

Gram-negative anaerobic bacilli of medical importance belong to either the *Bacteroides* or the *Fusobacterium* genera. Without such sophisticated equipment as gas liquid chromatographs, differentiation of isolates into species would be difficult if not impossible. Novice bacteriologists must therefore limit themselves to a crude differentiation based on such characteristics as morphology and culture. Older texts generally describe the *Bacteroides* as anaerobic gram-negative bacilli with rounded ends, and the *Fusobacterium* as anaerobic gram-negative bacilli with tapered or pointed ends.

One can also identify the most common isolate, *B. fragilis*, on the basis of kanamycin susceptibility and its ability to grow on 20% bile. Gram-negative anaerobic bacilli that are resistant to 1000 μg of kanamycin and grow on 20% bile usually are *B. fragilis*. The average technologist can do little more, and must consult a reference laboratory in order to determine the species of any gram-negative anaerobic rod he may isolate. Without such further consultation, one must realize the limitations of such general classifications as *"Bacteroides* species" and *"Fusobacterium* species," and exercise caution in attributing infections to these organisms on the basis of such limited information.

FURTHER READING

1. Willis, A. T.: *Anaerobic Bacteriology in Clinical Medicine.* 3rd ed. London, Butterworth and Co., Publ. Ltd., 1977.

2. Dowell, V. T., Jr. and Hawkins, T. M.: *Laboratory Methods in Anaerobic Bacteriology*, Public Health Service, Publication No. 1803, Washington, D. C., U.S. Gov't. Printing Office, 1968.
3. Smith, L. D.: *The Pathogenic Anaerobic Bacteria.* 2nd ed. Springfield, Ill., Charles C Thomas, 1975.
4. Holdeman, L. V., and Moore, W. E. C.: *Anaerobic Laboratory Manual.* 4th ed. Blacksburg, Va., Virginia Polytechnic Institute, 1977.

17-1 CLASSIFICATION

Bergey's Manual, Part 17
The Actinomycetes and related forms*
  I. The Coryneform group of bacteria
 II. Family I: Propionibacteriaceae
III. Order I: Actinomycetales
   Family   I: Actinomycetaceae
     Genus   I. *Actinomyces*   Species: *bovis*
                                          4 others

    Four other genera†

---

*I and II have been considered in Chapter 12 for reasons explained there. A more complete listing of III may be found in Table 7–2. Here we list only those members of known medical significance.
†*Thermopolyspora polyspora* and *Micromonospora vulgaris* are two thermophilic actinomycetes that have been incriminated in "farmer's lung," an allergy caused by inhaling moldy dust.

Family	II: Mycobacteriaceae	
Genus	I. *Mycobacterium*	*tuberculosis*
		leprae
		28 others
Family	IV: Nocardiaceae	
Genus	I. *Nocardia*	31 species
Family	VII: Streptomycetaceae	
Genus	I. *Streptomyces*	463 species

DEFINITIONS

Actinomycetales. Bacteria that have a tendency to form branching filaments, which may develop into a mycelium.

Actinomyces. Nonacid-fast; mainly anaerobic to microaerophilic. Produce true filaments, but rapidly fragment into irregularly sized elements.

Mycobacterium. Acid-fast or acid- and alcohol-fast; aerobic, gram-positive rods. Have a rather long gestation period compared to other bacteria.

Nocardia. Produce filaments that develop into a true mycelium which easily fragments. Aerobic and only partially acid-fast.

Streptomyces. Produce a true mycelium that remains intact. (*Streptomyces* are important to medical microbiology because several species produce antibacterial agents that are used in therapy.)

17-2 MYCOBACTERIUM TUBERCULOSIS

The earliest evidence of tuberculosis appears in Egyptian mummies. The organism was first isolated by Koch in 1882.

Tuberculosis is no longer the most common cause of death as it was in the early nineteenth century, when the urban death rate from this disease in the United States was 440 per 100,000 population. In 1975, the death rate due to tuberculosis was 2 per 100,000 in the United States. However, it is still a significant disease factor, especially when considered on a global basis. The WHO reports figures of 20,000,000 cases, with up to 2,000,000 deaths annually, and these figures are considered conservative by some experts. Indians are affected 10 times more often than whites; Eskimos, 30 times more.

Improved methods of treatment have reduced the length of stay in sanatoria tremendously, which has created the false public belief that tuberculosis is no longer a disease to be reckoned with.

MORPHOLOGY

Owing to the high lipid coat in their cell wall, mycobacteria stain rather poorly with ordinary stains. To stain successfully, a mordant such as phenol should be used; furthermore, the application of heat is required for the stain to penetrate. A number of stains and staining methods have been developed, but the method by Ziehl-Neelsen, which uses basic fuchsin in combination with phenol (carbol fuchsin), is the most popular. Once stained over heat, the organisms retain this stain, even when flooded with mineral acids and alcohols. This ability to retain stains after acid washings has led to the term "acid-fast bacilli," which is used to designate these organisms collectively.

Mycobacteria are usually straight or slightly curved, with rounded ends. They appear singly or in small groups of three to four. They vary from the usual length of 1 to 4 μm to as long as 8 μm. Typical forms are between 0.3 and 0.6 μm wide. (Long filamentous forms sometimes described in the literature most probably belong to the genus *Actinomyces.*) Older cultures usually display much shorter forms. Human strains more often appear as long, thin, curved forms with granular staining. They are gram-positive when heated; gentian violet in alcohol with aniline oil is used instead of the conventional crystal violet.

Fluorescent Staining Technique. In this technique, fluorochrome dyes (auramine) are used, which accept the high energy of ultraviolet light and then emit light of a longer wave length, in the visible spectrum. The acid-fast organisms, having a high affinity for these dyes, appear as luminescent objects against a dark background when viewed through a microscope fitted with the correct optical system (see Chapter 3).

Cording. Virulent strains of human tuberculosis and eugonic strains of bovine tuberculosis often form characteristic microscopic cords in liquid media. These cords are formed by parallel arrangements of bacilli in a long strand, side by side and end to end.

CULTURAL CHARACTERISTICS

With the exception of *M. leprae*, all mycobacteria grow to some extent on ordinary media. To initiate growth on these media, however, a heavy inoculum should be used, because long-chain fatty acids contained in these media somewhat inhibit *Mycobacteria*. The inhibitory effect may be nullified by incorporating egg yolk, albumin, charcoal, or serum. The most satisfactory media are solid, inspissated serum, egg, or potato media. The more common media in use today are Loewenstein-Jensen medium, Petragnani's medium, Middlebrook's 7H9 liquid medium, Middlebrook's 7H10 solid medium, and Tarshis medium.

The generation time of mycobacteria is far in excess of that of most other bacteria, and ranges from one hour for the so-called "rapid growers," to 20 to 30 days for *M. leprae*. Most pathogenic species require a minimum of three to four weeks before colonies become visible to the naked eye. Substances such as glycerol and Tween 80 have a tendency to shorten the generation time of some strains. Organisms that show enhanced growth in the presence of these substances are said to be eugonic; those that are retarded in their presence are called dysgonic. The pH range is 6.0 to 7.8. The virulence of pathogenic mycobacteria is best maintained at a pH of 6.8. At a pH of 6.0, attenuation occurs in a small number of subcultures.

Optimal temperatures for growth of *Mycobacteria* vary among species, depending on their natural habitat or hosts that they parasitize. For example, for avian strains, those that parasitize birds primarily, the optimal temperature is 40°C; for human and animal strains, around 37°C; for strains affecting cold-blooded creatures such as fish and reptiles, 25°C.

Mycobacteria are strict aerobes. The pathogenic species require added CO_2 concentrations for optimal growth, although some authorities maintain that this does not hold true for all strains. A higher rate of isolation on primary culture is obtained when two cultures are set up, one with and one without added CO_2. This seems to indicate that some strains require added CO_2, but that others grow better without it.

COLONIAL CHARACTERISTICS

Colonies of mycobacteria cultures are usually dry and wrinkled, with highly irregular edges. *M. tuberculosis*, particularly, looks like dry cake crumbs scattered over the surface of the medium. Most colonies are extremely difficult to emulsify. Many cultures produce a rather pleasant "fruity" odor, though it is obviously inadvisable to encourage "sniffing" of cultures.

Saprophytic species produce colonies that vary from those described above to shiny, butyrous colonies with an even periphery.

All mycobacteria produce opaque colonies with varying degrees of pigmentation, from cream to various shades of lemon or orange, to many shades of red. The pigments, as other colonial characteristics, are useful in differentiating species. Pigments may

develop in the presence of light, a feature that further aids identification.

VARIABILITY

Most variants appear to be little more than cultural adaptations.
Smooth and rough cultures may be encountered on the same
medium. Little is known about the relationship between the S and
R types and their respective degrees of virulence. However, most S
types are avirulent and most R types are virulent. For easy reference, it is best to follow Steenken's designations, which are
regarded by many as standard:

H = human variety

Number designates the strain

R or S = rough or smooth

A or V = avirulent or virulent

Hence, strains may be recorded, and usually are, such as H37RV or
H37SA.

RESISTANCE

Mycobacteria are generally more resistant to chemicals than
are other vegetative bacteria, probably because of the high lipid
content of their cell walls. Their increased resistance, together with
their high pathogenicity rates, warrant extreme care in handling
specimens that might contain these organisms. In routine laboratory practice, the following precautions should be taken, over and
above those already practiced in any bacteriology laboratory:

   a. An inoculating hood equipped with U.V. light or a proper
      exhaust system should always be used.
   b. Masks, gowns and gloves should be worn, and once worn
      should be disposed of as contaminated material.
   c. Pipetting by mouth should never be attempted.
   d. Shielded bunsen burners should be used to prevent en-
      vironmental contamination by "spattering" materials.
   e. Work areas should be irradiated by U.V. light for at least 12
      hours after each use, or should be washed down with 5%
      phenol.
   f. Cultures should always be disposed of by autoclaving at
      126°C for 20 minutes.

ANTIGENICITY

Agglutination, precipitation and complement fixation tests
have all been used to distinguish between the mycobacteria. To

date, however, these tests are still experimental rather than diagnostic.

BIOCHEMICAL CHARACTERISTICS

None of the usual carbohydrates are fermented. Mycobacteria produce varying amounts of catalase; the hominis variety of *M. tuberculosis* and some bovine strains produce excessive amounts of niacin. Both semiquantitative catalase tests and niacin detection are useful diagnostic measures.

PATHOGENICITY

The organisms usually enter the body by inhalation or ingestion, and less frequently through the skin. Most organisms are phagocytosed rapidly and therefore do not enter into the infective stage. Typically, tuberculosis develops first in the lymph nodes of the trachea and bronchi and in the lungs as an acute inflammation. Within a few weeks, one or more events may happen:

    a. Caseous necrosis: infected tissue cells die off en masse, producing the characteristic microscopic tubercles.

    b. The organisms simply lyse, thereby limiting the infection to a minor scar.

    c. The organisms spread to neighboring tissues and other body sites, where they develop into a variety of infections such as osteomyelitis, nephritis, and even meningitis.

Organisms may enter the bloodstream, but they have never been isolated from the blood. When large numbers of bacilli enter the bloodstream, the disease is called miliary tuberculosis and is often fatal. At the early stage of the infection, the patient develops a hypersensitivity to tuberculo-protein. This condition may be detected by the tuberculin test.

Some diseases that may be caused by mycobacteria other than tuberculosis or leprosy are:

    a. Pulmonary infections: *M. fortuitum*, photochromogens and some nonchromogens

    b. Skin lesions: *M. fortuitum, M. ulcerans*

    c. Cervical adenitis: scotochromogens

Rapidly growing species are generally considered nonpathogenic.

TREATMENT

Streptomycin, isonicotinic acid hydrazide (INH), para-aminosalicylic acid (PAS), ethambutol, rifampin, viomycin, and other drugs have been used. The emergence of resistant strains warrants careful administration of a combination of these drugs over a prolonged period of time.

PAS appears to reduce the rate of elimination of INH from the body and reduces the number of resistant strains produced. Of course, treatment such as plenty of fresh air, good food, and pleasant surroundings contribute much toward rapid convalescence of patients.

TRANSMISSION

Man appears to be far more resistant to the disease tuberculosis than to milder infections by *M. tuberculosis*, as may be borne out from the fact that in some areas where evidence of infection, as measured by the tuberculin test, is demonstrated in up to 90% of the population, few or no active cases of tuberculosis are reported from these same areas. As most bacilli enter the body by inhalation, droplets spread directly from patients who have tuberculosis are the most frequent modes of transmission. Ingestion of foods contaminated by droplets or milk from tuberculous cows are the second most frequent means of transmission.

PREVENTION

Certain factors definitely predispose persons to tuberculosis, because the incidence of disease increases when living conditions deteriorate (e.g., as in urban ghettos). The incidence of tuberculosis among miners and other occupational groups exposed to inorganic dust that causes silicosis is rather high. Control of infective cases, slaughter of tuberculin-positive cattle, and pasteurization of milk products, have proven successful in limiting the spread of tuberculosis.

Vaccination. The bacillus of Calmette and Guérin (BCG bacillus), a bovine strain of *M. tuberculosis*, has been used extensively as a vaccine against tuberculosis. This vaccine should be administered only to individuals who are tuberculin-negative; the acquired immunity is relative rather than absolute.

Tuberculin Test. With this test, a delayed type of hypersensitivity to *M. tuberculosis* can be detected. A preparation of tuberculo-protein (old tuberculin, OT, or purified protein derivative, PPD) is used. The protein is inoculated intracutaneously (Mantoux test) and various degrees of induration to this protein can be ascertained. In most instances, a positive reaction is indicative of the presence of tubercle bacilli at some recently past period. In that event, of course, there is a possibility that the organisms are still around. False negative results may occur in patients suffering from an involved tuberculosis; in these cases, however, tuberculosis can be diagnosed easily by other means. The value of the tuberculin test lies in the fact that it may generally be assumed that healthy individuals who demonstrate a negative tuberculin reaction are not infected with mycobacteria. The prognosis of active tuberculosis among those who demonstrate a strongly positive tuberculin test is enhanced during the first year following the positive result. These persons are said to be hypersensitive to the disease.

LABORATORY DIAGNOSIS

In the laboratory, the safety measures outlined on page 243 should be practiced at all times.

Specimens. The wide variety of pathologic syndromes caused by these organisms allows the isolation of mycobacteria from several different specimens. The most common are sputa, laryngeal swabs, tissues, urine, and gastric lavage.

The safest way to collect sputum specimens, which also permits easy treatment, is to use a special sputum collection system distributed by B.B.L.* Extreme care should be taken in the collection, transport, storage, and treatment of all specimens. Early morning urine specimens are preferred over the more commonly requested 24-hour collections. (Amer. J. Clin. Path. 37: 347, 1967).

Direct Examination. Sputum smears should be made from small flecks of sputum or from caseous material. These materials should be teased out gently with a pair of applicator sticks, and a tiny piece applied to a clean, new slide. Placing another similar slide over this one and applying gentle pressure will produce two smears of the required thickness.

These smears should then be stained by Ziehl-Neelsen's (ZN) method or, as is becoming more popular, with auramine stain. Smears stained by ZN should be examined for at least 10 minutes before reporting a negative result. Smears stained with auramine and examined under the fluorescence microscope require only a few minutes of scanning by the experienced technologist.

Specimen Treatment. More often than not, mycobacteria are encased by mucoid or caseous materials, so that specimens have to be treated to dislodge the mycobacteria from mucus and to concentrate them before inoculation. Several methods have been employed for this purpose. One that is both fairly simple and effective follows:

Reagents
A. A 1 M solution of trisodium citrate, 29.4 g in 100 ml of H_2O, autoclaved at 121°C for 15 minutes.

---

*Baltimore Biological Laboratories, Cockeysville, Md.

B. A 20% w/v solution of N-acetyl-L-cystine in H_2O. This is self-sterilizing.

C. A 10% brain-heart infusion broth in 100-ml volumes, autoclaved at 121°C for 15 minutes.

D. Digestion mixture: aseptically, add 5.0 ml of reagent A and 2.5 ml of reagent B to reagent C. Mix well, date, and store at 4°C. This mixture is stable for 48 hours.

E. A 0.2% solution of bovine albumin in saline at pH 7.0, Seitz-filtered.

Procedure

1. Carry out all manipulations in a safety cabinet.
2. Add an equal volume of digestion mixture (reagent D) to the sputum sample to be tested.
3. Mix on a Vortex mixer until liquified (15 to 30 seconds).
4. Allow to stand for 10 to 15 minutes to facilitate digestion and decontamination.*
5. Fill the tube with sterile distilled water, to decrease the specific gravity and to facilitate centrifugation.
6. Decant the supernatant into a 5% phenol solution.
7. Add 1.0 ml of bovine albumin solution (reagent E).
8. Resuspend the pellicle.
9. Proceed with culture.

Isolation. Inoculate the foregoing preparation onto a minimum of two Loewenstein-Jensen slants and one Middlebrook's 7H10 agar plate. Extending the variety of media by including additional slants of Petragnani's and Tarshis' media will increase the chances of isolating mycobacteria. Incubate at least two Loewenstein-Jensen slants (cover one with three layers of tinfoil) and the agar plate at 37°C for up to six weeks. At first, cultures should be incubated horizontally to allow inoculation of the entire slant. After one day, the slants may be placed upright.

Identification. Incubated media should be examined after 48 hours, after five days, and then once a week. When significant growth first appears on the unwrapped slant, examine the Middlebrook agar plate for the presence of single colonies. If more than one type of colony appears on this medium, the slant cultures probably contain mixed growths and should be discarded. Prepare a new set of slants and inoculate from each type of colony; identify each type of colony separately. If only one type of colony is evident

---

*If contamination is particularly worrisome, 2 to 4% NaOH may be incorporated in reagent D.

on the agar plates, proceed with identification on the incubated slants as follows:

1. Make a smear, stain for acid fastness (Ziehl-Neelsen or Auramine O stains), and examine. If no acid-fast bacilli (AFB) are detected, simply report "AFB not isolated." If AFB are seen, proceed with step 2.
2. Perform niacin and nitrate tests from culture on one un-wrapped slant. If both tests are positive, report immediately as "M. tuberculosis isolated" and proceed with step 8. If one or both are negative, proceed with step 3.
3. Unwrap the covered slant, examine for pigmentation, amount of growth, and length of time of incubation. Scoto-chromogens demonstrate pigmentation initially. If no pig-ment was formed, expose the slant to incandescent light for one hour and reincubate for 24 hours; photochromogens will produce pigment following this process. Nonchromo-gens remain colorless. Record all findings and follow Chart 17–1.

Chart 17–1. Primary identification of Mycobacteria.

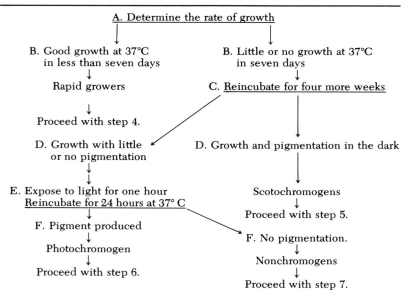

4. If the isolate is a rapid-grower, determine pigmentation.
   a. If pigment was produced in the light, report as *M. vaccae.*
   b. If pigment was produced in the dark only, report as *M. phlei.*
   c. If no pigment was produced, transfer to a MacConkey agar plate, incubate at 37°C for five days, and check for growth.
   d. If no growth has occurred, report as *M. smegmatis.*
   e. If growth is evident, check the nitrate result (step 2).
   f. If nitrate is positive, report as *M. fortuitum.*
   g. If nitrate is negative, report as *M. chelonei.*
5. If the isolate is a scotochromogen, check the nitrate result (step 2).
   a. If nitrate is positive, report as *M. flavescens.*
   b. If nitrate is negative, determine the catalase activity.
   c. If catalase activity is < 45 mm, report as *M. xenopi.*
   d. If catalase activity is > 45 mm, determine urease activity, using 3 ml of urea broth, a heavy inoculum, and three days' incubation at 37°C.
   e. If urease is positive, report as *M. scrofulaceum.*
   f. If urease is negative, report as *M. gordonae.*
6. If the isolate is a photochromogen, check the nitrate result (step 2).
   a. If nitrate was positive, report as *M. kansasii.*
   b. If nitrate was negative, report as *M. marinum.*
7. If the isolate is a nonchromogen, repeat the niacin test.
   a. If niacin is positive, report as *M. tuberculosis* and proceed with step 8.
   b. If niacin is negative, determine NaCl tolerance.
   c. If tolerant to NaCl, report as *M. triviale.*
   d. If intolerant to NaCl, check the nitrate result (step 2).
   e. If nitrate is positive, report as *M. terrae-complex.*
   f. If nitrate is negative, determine tellurite reduction within three days and catalase activity at 68°C.
   g. If both tests are negative, report as *M. bovis.*
   h. If either one or both are positive, report as *M. avium-intercellulare-complex.*
8. When a culture has been identified primarily as *M. tuberculosis,* submit the culture to a reference laboratory for sensitivity testing and corroboration of result.

The foregoing steps are summarized in Table 17–1; they provide a simplified approach to a complicated problem. They will provide accurate identification of all acid-fast isolates in 90% of all

Table 17-1. Identification of Mycobacteria.

− = usually negative + = usually positive ∓ = sometimes positive ± = sometimes negative v = variable	Growth in less than 7 days	Pigment in the light	Pigment in the dark	Growth on MacConkey agar in 5 days	Nitrate	Niacin	Catalase in mm²	Catalase at 68°C	Growth on 5% NaCl	Tellurite reduction in 3 days
M. vaccae	+	+	+	−	v	−	>45	+	+	v
M. phlei	+	−	+	−	v	−	>45	+	+	+
M. smegmatis	+	−	−	−	v	−	>45	+	+	+
M. fortuitum	+	−	−	+	+	−	>45	+	+	v
M. chelonei	+	−	−	+	−	∓	>45	+	v	v
M. flavescens	∓	+	+	−	+	−	>45	+	±	−
M. xenopi	−	+	+	−	−	−	<45	+	−	−
M. scrofulaceum	−	+	+	−	−	−	>45	+	−	−
M. gordonae	−	+	+	−	−	−	>45	+	−	−
M. kansasii	−	+	−	−	+	−	>45	+	−	−
M. marinum	−	+	−	−	−	∓	<45	∓	−	−
M. tuberculosis	−	−	−	−	±	+	<45	−	−	−
M. bovis	−	−	−	−	−	−	<45	−	−	−
M. triviale	−	−	−	−	∓	−	>45	+	+	−
M. terrae-complex	−	−	−	−	+	−	>45	+	−	±
M. avium-intracellulare- complex	−	−	−	∓	−	−	<45	+	−	±

cases, and will always detect and identify *M. tuberculosis* accurately. Table 17-1 also lists additional characteristics that might be helpful to more experienced workers in identifying atypical isolates, which comprise less than 10% of all cases.

17-3 MYCOBACTERIUM LEPRAE

The WHO advocates the use of the term "Hansen's disease" for this infection instead of "leprosy," to help deter much of the unnecessary social pressure that burdens victims of this disease. The physical discomforts resulting from this disease could be better treated when its victims are considered sick people in need of medical attention rather than social outcasts.

Because this organism is a true parasite and it has not been possible to cultivate it on artificial media, we limit our study to a brief look at the disease and the laboratory diagnosis.

PATHOGENICITY

Hansen's disease is most common in central Africa. It is also found in North America, as the leprosaria in Tracadie, New

Brunswick and Carville, Louisiana attest.* Intimate contact appears to be a prerequisite for infection, and the incubation period is two to four years. The disease is chronic, and the mortality rate is high.

Two types of infection have been recorded:

    a. The lepromatous type, characterized by gross deformation, with many organisms detectable within the lesions.

    b. the tuberculoid type, also known as "macula anesthesia," in which less dramatic lesions occur which contain fewer organisms and are insensitive to such stimuli as heat and touch.

An effective cure has not been developed as yet. Prolonged therapy with diaminodiphenyl sulfone may suppress the disease to a point of convalescence, but complete cures are indeed uncommon.

LABORATORY DIAGNOSIS

Many bacilli may be demonstrated in aspirates from lesions or from biopsy materials. These materials may be boiled to ensure the safety of laboratory workers without losing their diagnostic usefulness.

M. leprae is more acid-fast than the other *Mycobacterium* species. Therefore, one should use 1 to 40% H_2SO_4 as a decolorizer in the Ziehl-Neelsen staining method. The organisms tend to arrange intracellularly in large groups or pockets. This arrangement is retained even if the cells should rupture.

17-4 ACTINOMYCES AND NOCARDIA

The genus *Actinomyces* contains two pathogenic species, *A. bovis* and *A. israelii*, both obligate parasites that live in carious teeth and in tonsillar crypts of man. *A. bovis* is also frequently found in the mouths of cattle and is the cause of "lumpy jaw" in these animals. They are anaerobic and are not acid-fast. Infection occurs only when the organisms gain entry to the deeper tissues through injured mucus membranes, causing infection of the face and neck; when they are aspirated into the lungs, resulting in pulmonary actinomycosis; or when they are ingested, causing intestinal infection.

The genus *Nocardia* contains several species pathogenic for man (*N. asteroides, N. madurae, N. pelletieri,* etc.). All species are aerobic and some are acid-fast. A few species produce a limited

---

*A leprosarium is a hospital for lepers.

mycelium in culture. They produce disease similar to the *Actinomyces*.

LABORATORY DIAGNOSIS

Collection of Specimen. Pus is usually obtained from draining sinuses or fistulae in the cervicofacial region, the thorax, or the abdomen. Tissue removed at surgery is also satisfactory. Pus should be collected in a sterile tube or syringe from the sinuses; if these are not draining sufficiently to provide a good specimen, a gauze dressing from the wound should be submitted for examination. In suspected pulmonary actinomycosis, sputum should be examined.

Direct Examination. Examine the test tube or syringe in a good light for the presence of small yellow granules. Sputum should be spread in a Petri dish and examined carefully against a black background for granules. Place a granule on a slide, apply cover slip and examine for branching and intertwined filaments with club-shaped ends. Further slides should be prepared and stained with the Gram and acid-fast stains.

Isolation. Specimen should be inoculated into thioglycolate broth and on blood agar; the agar plates should be incubated anaerobically at 37°C. In addition, the specimen should be inoculated on Sabouraud's agar, because *Nocardia*, which gives an identical appearance on direct examination to *Actinomyces*, grows best on Sabouraud's medium.

FURTHER READING

1. Runyon, E. H. et al.: *Classification of Mycobacterial Pathogens*, Trans. 21st Research Conference in Pulmonary Diseases, Veterans Administration-Armed Forces, Washington, D.C., 1962.
2. *Handbook of Tuberculosis Laboratory Methods*, Veterans Administration-Armed Forces, Washington, D.C., 1962.
3. Rees, R. J. W.: New prospects for the study of leprosy in the laboratory. Bull. WHO, *40*:785-800, 1969.
4. Kubica, G. P. et al.: Laboratory services for mycobacterial diseases. Am. Rev. Resp. Dis., *112*:773–787, 1975. Reprinted in: Publ. H. Lab., *34*:129–156, 1976.
5. Vestal, A. L.: *Procedures for the Isolation and Identification of Mycobacteria*. DHEW Publication No. (HSM) 75-820, Center for Disease Control, Atlanta, 1975.

chapter 18

Spirochetes

18-1 CLASSIFICATION

Bergey's Manual, Part 5
Spirochetes

Family	I. Spirochaetaceae		
Genus	I. *Spirochaeta*	Species:	5
	II. *Cristispira*		*pectinis*
	III. *Treponema*		*pallidum*
			pertenue
			carateum
			vincentii
			7 others
	IV. *Borrelia*		*recurrentis*
			18 others
	V. *Leptospira*		*interrogans*

DEFINITIONS

Spirochaetaceae. Slender, flexuous, helically coiled unicellular organisms. They may measure from 3 to 500 μm in length.

Treponema. Anaerobic; stain with difficulty except with Giemsa stain or silver nitrate impregnation.

Borrelia. Anaerobic; stain readily with aniline dyes.

Leptospira. Aerobic; stain with difficulty except with Giemsa stain or silver nitrate impregnation.

Spirochaeta and *Cristispira* (Of no medical importance)

18-2 TREPONEMA

This genus includes the organisms responsible for: syphilis, *T. pallidum;* yaws or framboesia, *T. pertenue;* pinta, *T. carateum;* Vincent's infection, *T. vincentii;* and several other species.

TREPONEMA PALLIDUM

These delicate organisms are only 0.15 μm in diameter and range in length from 5 to 20 μm. They may be seen under darkfield microscopy or following silver nitrate impregnation.

T. pallidum has not been cultured on artificial media. Members of the species may be maintained by inoculation of the testis of live rabbits. In rabbit culture, it is extremely difficult to dissociate *T. pallidum* from *T. cuniculi*, an organism that frequently causes chronic infections of the genitals of rabbits.

Antigenicity. The importance of the antigenicity of *T. pallidum* can be understood only when seen in the full light of diagnostic measures for syphilis. An historical outline of developments in the field of syphilis control by serologic methods seems to offer the best approach. The student might wish to scan briefly the first sections of Chapter 28 before reading further. The first point to remember is that no *exclusively specific* treponemal antigens have been isolated or identified thus far.

Studies on the antigenicity of *T. pallidum* were initiated by Wasserman in 1906. He used an aqueous extract from syphilitic livers as an antigen in a complement fixation test and thus developed a fairly useful test to detect antibodies in the serum of syphilitics. Unfortunately, many of the later tests for syphilis antibody studies were also labelled "Wasserman tests." Let us remember that the Wasserman test is the test that employs syphilitic liver extracts as the antigen in the complement fixation test.

Michaels, in 1907, discovered that extracts from normal livers gave similar if not identical reactions to those from syphilitic livers.

This fact immediately raised questions whether liver extracts contain an antigen similar to one carried by *T. pallidum*, and whether syphilitics produce antibodies to substances other than the antigens of *T. pallidum*. These questions remain to be resolved. After Michaels' discovery, it was found that alcoholic extracts yielded more potent antigens than aqueous extracts. These findings led to the development of a precipitation test by Kahn in 1922. He used alcoholic solutions of ether-insoluble beef-heart lipids, which would precipitate in the presence of syphilitic sera. (Another unrelated antigen?)

Between 1920 and 1950, several minor variations in laboratory methods were developed by a score of workers, resulting in mass confusion on the part of laboratory workers and diagnosticians alike. In 1948, the Venereal Disease Research Laboratory set out to compare all the tests, one with another, in an effort to recommend the best method available. The VDRL studies revealed that even some of the more commonly used methods of those days were sadly lacking in sensitivity and specificity. They proposed a new test, known as the VDRL test and presently universally accepted as a screening test for syphilis. In the VDRL test, a purified cardiolipin is mixed in specific proportions with lecithin and cholesterol and used as an antigen to detect syphilitic antibodies (see Chapter 28). Tests that are more simple and just as useful as the VDRL test have since been developed. The most popular of these newer tests is the Rapid Plasma Reagin test (RPR test).* This test uses the same basic reagents as the VDRL test, but links these to tiny carbon particles. When they react with "reagin," the particles clump together in aggregates that are easily detected by the naked eye.

None of the foregoing pertains to the antigenicity of *T. pallidum* per se. All the antibodies detected by any of the methods discussed thus far are of the "reagin" type, and may or may not be associated with *T. pallidum*. Presently, we are aware of the existence of three distinct types of antibodies, any one or all three of which may be present in the sera of syphilitics:

   a. The *"reagin"* type, already discussed.
   b. The *T. pallidum immobilizing (TPI) antibody*; these are specific treponemal antibodies. They may be detected by the *Treponema pallidum* immobilization test developed by Nelson and Mayer in 1949. The TPI test is a rather tricky test by which living organisms of a motile strain of *T. pallidum* are mixed with syphilitic serum. When antibodies to *T. pallidum* react with the motile organisms, the organ-

*Available from Hynson, Westcott & Dunning, Inc., Baltimore, Md.

Chart 18–1. The triple test plan for syphilis serology

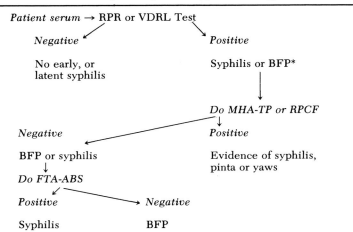

Patient serum → RPR or VDRL Test

Negative   *Positive*

No early, or   Syphilis or BFP*
latent syphilis

                                                             Do MHA-TP or RPCF

Negative   *Positive*

BFP or syphilis   Evidence of syphilis,
↓   pinta or yaws
Do FTA-ABS

Positive ——————→ *Negative*

Syphilis   BFP

*BFP = biologic false positive

isms become immobile. The TPI antibody appears to be
identical to that which reacts in the Fluorescent Treponema
Antibody test (FTA). Some products are available that yield
more specific results by FTA than by TPI. These products
use a "Reiter-like protein" to absorb nonsyphilitic antibodies before fluorescence conjugate is applied. Thus, the
test is known as the FTA absorption test or FTA-ABS. The
FTA-ABS test has largely replaced the TPI test as the final
confirmatory test in the triple test plan (see Chart 18–1).

   c. The *Reiter protein complement fixation (RPCF) antibodies*;
      these are antibodies to a protein extracted from a non-
      pathogenic strain of *T. pallidum*. The antigen is not specific
      for *T. pallidum*, since patients recovering from pinta or
      yaws, and even unrelated disease, may also produce an-
      tibodies that react in the RPCF test. The RPCF-type an-
      tibodies may also be detected by the less complex Micro-
      Hem-Agglutination test (MHA-TP).†

   Until specific treponemal antigens have been isolated and
identified, the serologic determination of treponemal antibodies
will remain a confusing issue. However, this discussion should

†Available from Miles Laboratories, Elkhart, Ind.

help to bring into perspective the current status of antibody-antigen reactions in the control of syphilis.

For further elaboration on this subject, the reader is again referred to Chapter 28 and the section on laboratory diagnosis in this chapter, and particularly to reference 1 in the bibliography.

Pathogenicity. *T. pallidum* is almost exclusively transmitted through sexual contact. Following exposure, a primary lesion may develop within a period of two to nine weeks. Early lesions release a serous exudate that abounds in spirochetes, which can be easily detected by darkfield microscopy. Because the lesions cause only mild discomfort and, furthermore, occur mainly on the vulva or cervix or on the penis, they often go unnoticed. Even without treatment, the primary lesions will heal. The spirochetes leave the lesions and invade neighboring mucous membranes and epithelial tissue. They multiply for a period ranging from two to six months, at which time more generalized, secondary lesions manifest themselves. These secondary lesions may cover the entire body as a red maculopapular rash. Like the primary lesions, the secondary lesions abound in spirochetes and are highly infectious.

The secondary lesions may recur within the first five years of infection, the disease may subside spontaneously or remain latent, or the patient may develop tertiary syphilis.

About 25% of untreated syphilitic patients develop tertiary syphilis. During this stage, the patient is no longer infectious, but the disease progresses to a chronic infestation of vital organs (liver, bones, heart, meninges, etc.). Massive distortions of the body often result, with advanced mental retardation in cases of neurosyphilis.

Transmission and Prevention. Except for congenital syphilis and rare occupational infection of medical personnel, syphilis is acquired by sexual contact.

In congenital syphilis, the spirochetes are transmitted from the infected mother to the fetus through the placenta.

The downward trend in syphilis during the early 1950s was attributed to the effectiveness of penicillin. Later figures have demonstrated that syphilis is still a threat and, as many other venereal diseases, is increasing rapidly in incidence. Infected individuals may remain contagious for years unless treated promptly. Early detection of all cases with follow-up treatment, investigation of contacts, prophylactic treatment, and proper education about sex hygiene could again reduce the incidence of or even eliminate syphilis.

Laboratory Diagnosis. *Specimens.* Exudate from lesions during the primary and secondary stage reveals many spirochetes when

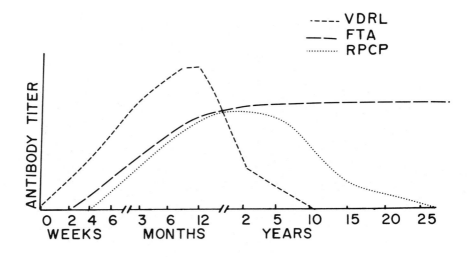

Fig. 18–1. Appearance and decline of various syphilis antibodies following the onset of infection.

examined by darkfield microscopy. These specimens are highly contagious.

Serology. The various antibodies will appear and persist independently of one another (see Fig. 18–1). Hence, VDRL "antibodies" (reagin) appear earliest, drop during the latent stage, and cannot be detected during the tertiary stage. Furthermore, a positive VDRL test does not *necessarily* indicate that the patient has syphilis. In fact, since so-called biologic false positive results (BFP) may indicate that the patient may be suffering from malaria, systemic lupus erythematosus, leprosy, rubella, or a number of other diseases, the patient may well wish he had the more readily curable syphilis. The VDRL test, however, is a useful screen test because it is highly sensitive. A positive VDRL result should be corroborated with a follow-up test. The triple test plan (see Chart 18–1) probably offers the most logical approach.

The triple test plan utilizes the simplest and most sensitive method first to reduce the number of specimens that must be tested by more cumbersome methods to a minimum. It then subjects the remaining number of positives to the next least cumbersome method, reducing the numbers to be tested by the more expensive FTA methods to an absolute minimum. A more objective analysis of the triple test plan reveals that it makes good diagnostic sense as well. Details of some individual tests in this plan are discussed in Chapter 28.

Treatment. All forms of syphilis respond to penicillin.

TREPONEMA PERTENUE

This organism is the cause of yaws, or framboesia, a rather mutilating chronic disease limited to the tropics. It is particularly endemic in parts of New Guinea and is more widespread among children than among adults.

The disease is almost exclusively contracted from person to person, although some insects have been incriminated as vectors.

The primary, ulcerating lesions usually appear first on the arms and legs. These develop into more generalized superficial lesions, which become increasingly destructive.

T. pertenue is virtually indistinguishable from *T. pallidum,* and yaws has been referred to as a variant of syphilis. Reagin type antibodies also develop in the sera of patients with yaws. Penicillin treatment fortunately gives a dramatic response.

TREPONEMA CARATEUM

The cause of pinta, a disease seemingly restricted to the darker-skinned races, *T. carateum* occurs frequently in Mexico and Central America, less frequently in the Caribbean and South America, and occasionally in the Philippines and Pacific regions. The disease characteristically infects the skin. From a primary, nonulcerating lesion, a lichen type of growth spreads, developing into depigmented and hyperpigmented patches. The disease pattern responds favorably to penicillin treatment. In the laboratory, large numbers of spirochetes may be demonstrated by examination of primary lesions under darkfield microscopy.

TREPONEMA VINCENTII

Treponema vincentii, in association with *Fusobacterium nucleatum,* is the cause of Vincent's infection (trenchmouth) and a number of similar lesions on the mucous membranes of the mouth and other body regions.

T. vincentii measures 7 to 18 μm long and 0.2 to 0.6 μm thick. Members of this species are actively motile with coarse lashing movements; they appear to be true symbionts that require the presence of other bacteria to grow. They can be cultured anaerobically on ascitic-fluid-enriched broth. Following primary, mixed growth culture, it is almost impossible to isolate *T. vincentii* from

Fusobacterium. Mixed cultures, however, can seemingly be sub-cultured ad infinitum.

Besides being symbionts, *T. vincentii* and *F. nucleatum* appear to be opportunists. Vincent's infection occurs most frequently when the gums are damaged, and the patient lacks vitamin B or C or has such infections as herpes simplex or mononucleosis. *T. vincentii* is sensitive to penicillins and tetracyclines. The laboratory diagnosis of Vincent's infection depends almost exclusively on microscopic examination of smears from swabs of mouth lesions. Large numbers of fusiform bacteria and spirochetes together with a number of pus cells and the clinical syndrome are conclusive evidence of this disease.

18-3 BORRELIA

Members of *Borrelia* are motile, refractile spirochetes, from 6 to 20 μm long and 0.3 to 0.7 μm wide, with few irregular coils. Several *Borrelia* species are pathogenic to man; others occur as commensals on various mucous membranes, particularly of the mouth and genitalia.

BORRELIA RECURRENTIS

B. recurrentis is the cause of relapsing fever. These spirochetes resemble delicate threads and have four to ten spirals per organism. They may vary from 10 to 20 μm in length and from 0.3 to 0.5 μm in width. They are actively motile by rotary or oscillating movements and have been cultured with considerable difficulty.

B. recurrentis is transmitted either from rodents to man by means of soft ticks (*Ornithodoros* species) or from man to man by means of head and body lice *(Pediculus humanus)*. An incubation period of three to ten days is followed by a sudden onset of fever, which may last for three to four days. During these four days, organisms may be detected in the blood in large numbers, which decrease with the fever. The cycle may be repeated again and again, hence the term relapsing fever. The disease responds well to penicillin.

The organisms are best detected in the blood under darkfield microscopy of direct smears or when stained by Giemsa's method. Animal pathogenicity tests are also helpful, because mice will demonstrate large numbers of spirochetes in their blood following intraperitoneal injection with 1 ml of blood from a person with relapsing fever.

18-4 LEPTOSPIRA

Leptospira are thin spirochetes about 0.1 μm in diameter and 6 to 20 μm long, with many fine coils. Examination of wet preparations by darkfield microscopy will demonstrate lashing movements of individual organisms.

The saprophytic strains can be grown on simple broths. Parasitic strains require a medium containing 5% to 10% enrichment. Bacto Leptospira Enrichment* is best suited, but rabbit, guinea pig, sheep and calf sera are all satisfactory. Most strains grow best at 25° to 32°C, but primary isolation of pathogenic strains is best attempted at 37°C. Cultures should be incubated in the dark for at least two weeks.

Some workers list several different pathogenic species, others list only *L. icterohaemorrhagiae* (now called *L. interrogans*) and ascribe various serologic types to this species.

Diseases caused by *Leptospira* are collectively called leptospiroses. The most common leptospirosis is Weil's disease or infectious jaundice. Marsh fever, pretibial fever and others occur far less commonly. Infectious jaundice is characterized by an incubation period of six to twelve days, followed by a high fever, nausea, vomiting, headache and muscular pains.

During the first week of illness, the leptospires are distributed throughout the body. Isolation of the organisms from the blood is possible during that first week, but none will be seen in bloodsmears. Urine samples may reveal leptospires for five weeks following the first symptoms.

Penicillin is the drug of choice for treatment. However, since recognizing the disease in its early stages is difficult, antibiotic therapy is often delayed. Vaccines or chemical prophylactic agents are not available. Leptospires gain entrance mainly through skin abrasions. Prevention of direct contact with contaminated water reservoirs is the only effective public health measure.

Stable, formalinized suspensions of different serotypes of *Leptospira* are commercially available.* These may be used to detect antibodies in a simple and rapid slide agglutination test. Antibodies may first appear in the patient's serum towards the end of the first week of illness.

---

*Available from Difco Laboratories, Detroit, Mich.

FURTHER READING

1. *Manual for Tests for Syphilis*, Public Health Service, Publication No. 411, Washington, D.C., U.S. Gov't. Printing Office, 1969.
2. Carpenter, C. M. et al.: A triple test plan for the serologic diagnosis of syphilis—a modern day approach. New Eng. J. Med., 263:1016–1018, 1960.
3. Felsenfeld, O.: Borreliae, human relapsing fever, and parasite-vector host relationships. Bacteriol. Rev., 29: 46, 1965.
4. Kohn, F. S.: Laboratory diagnosis of leptospirosis. J. Amer. Med. Technol., 35:223–225, 1973.

chapter 19

Mycoplasmas

19-1 Classification
19-2 *Mycoplasma*

19-1 CLASSIFICATION

Bergey's Manual, Part 19
The Mycoplasmas
Class Mollicutes

Order	I. Mycoplasmatales		
Family	I. Mycoplasmataceae		
Genus	I. *Mycoplasma*	Species:	*mycoides*
			pneumoniae
			hominis
			fermentans
			neurolyticum
			gallisepticum
			salivarium
			orale
			28 others
Family	II. Acholeplasmataceae		
Genus	I. *Acholeplasma*	3	
Uncertain genera:	*Thermoplasma*		
	Spiroplasma		

DEFINITION

Organisms in this class lack a true cell wall and are bounded by a single triple-layered membrane. Only some species of the genus *Mycoplasma* are of medical interest.

19-2 MYCOPLASMA

Only seven of the 36 species of this genus have been associated with disease in man.

MORPHOLOGIC AND CULTURAL CHARACTERISTICS

Members of the genus *Mycoplasma* are believed to include the smallest free-living organisms that can be cultured on artificial media. They do not possess a firm cell wall, hence their extreme pleomorphism; they require protein-enriched media for growth.

The smallest units observed range from 0.125 to 0.15 μm in width, which is smaller in diameter than the larger viruses. In culture, they form colonies that resemble the classic "fried egg" appearance. Despite what some textbooks state, their culture requires a great deal of patience and experience, and is far from a routine procedure. Because its complexity is beyond the scope of this text, the interested student should consult the bibliography or a more experienced colleague for further information on this topic.

PATHOGENICITY

As the name suggests, *M. pneumoniae* has been associated with pneumonia in man, more specifically, with primary atypical pneumonia (PAP). It should be realized that PAP is a syndrome which is probably caused by a number of infectious organisms. *M. hominis* and so-called T-strain organisms are frequently isolated from the genitourinary tract, and are more frequently associated with infections such as cervicitis, urethritis and prostatitis. T-strain organisms are able to hydrolyze urea, and it has been suggested that they be placed in a separate genus, *Ureaplasma*. *M. hominis* has also been isolated from cases with respiratory ailments. *M. orale* and *M. salivarium* are only known as commensals of the upper respiratory tract. *M. neurolyticum* and *M. gallisepticum* have been associated with disease of animals.

SEROLOGY

Patients suffering from infections with *M. pneumoniae* usually develop antibodies in their serum. These antibodies can be detected by the complement fixation test, for which satisfactory antigens are commercially available.* A demonstration of a rise in *M. pneumoniae* antibody titer is probably the most satisfactory diagnostic tool at our disposal to date to indicate exposure to these organisms. Cases of PAP usually develop cold agglutinins as well as agglutinins to a nonhemolytic strain of *Streptococcus*, M.G.

TREATMENT

Mycoplasmal infections are usually self-limiting. In general, mycoplasmas are resistant to penicillin, but mycoplasmal pneumonia responds to tetracycline, and genitourinary infections due to T-strains respond to tetracycline and erythromycin.

TRANSMISSION AND PREVENTION

Mycoplasmal infections appear to spread only from person to person; they are more prevalent among children and young adults. Several small epidemics have been recorded, which have indicated the existence of an incubation period of 9 to 12 days. No effective vaccine has been developed to date.

FURTHER READING

1. Stanbridge, E. J.: A reevaluation of the role of mycoplasmas in human disease. Ann. Rev. Microbiol., **30:** 169–187, 1976.
2. Hayflick, L. (ed.): *The Mycoplasmatales and the L-phase of bacteria.* Appleton-Century-Crofts, New York, 1969.

*Microbiological Associates, Bethesda, Md.

chapter 20

Rickettsias

20-1 CLASSIFICATION

Bergey's Manual, Part 18
The Rickettsias*

Order	I. Rickettsiales		
Family	I. Rickettsiaceae		
Genus	I. *Rickettsia*	Species:	*prowazekii*
			typhi
			canada
			rickettsii
			sibirica
			conorii
			australis
			akari
			parkeri
			tsutsugamushi
Genus	II. *Rochalimaea*		*quintana*
Genus	III. *Coxiella*		*burnetii*

---

*A complete listing of genera of this Part appears in Table 7–2. Here, we list only those genera containing members of medical importance.

Family	II. Bartonellaceae	
Genus	I. *Bartonella*	Species: *bacilliformis*
Order	II. Chlamydiales	
Family	I. Chlamydiaceae	
Genus	I. *Chlamydia*	*trachomatis*
		psittaci

DEFINITIONS

Rickettsiales. Parasitic or mutualistic microorganisms with a typical bacterial cell wall, which multiply only within certain host cells. They divide by binary fission and are gram-negative. Exceptions to the above are listed.

Rickettsiaceae. Intercellular, or intimately associated with tissue cells other than red blood cells.

Rickettsia. Unstable when separated from the host material; grow mainly in the cellular cytoplasm.

Rochalimaea. Resemble *Rickettsia*, but may be cultured in cell-free media.

Coxiella. Highly resistant to environmental changes; grow mainly in the vacuoles of the host cell.

Bartonellaceae. Characteristically found in or on red blood cells; have been cultured on artificial media.

Chlamydiales. Obligate intercellular parasites that are metabolically limited. They divide by fission of a noninfectious, thin-walled phase, which develops from a thick-walled infectious phase of the organism.

20-2 RICKETTSIALES

The organisms in this taxon are small, pleomorphic coccobacilli. They are obligate intracellular parasites, and survive only briefly when removed from their host. Two genera have been separated from the original *Rickettsia* because they are significantly different in some key characteristics: *Rochalimaea* may be cultured in cell-free media, and *Coxiella* are highly resistant to heat, drying, and sunlight. Rickettsiae are naturally found in a variety of mammalian and arthropodan hosts. Man is usually infected by an arthropod vector, except for *Coxiella*, which is transmitted by inhalation of infectious particles from contaminated sources.

The different species, their geographic distribution, main vectors, and disease patterns appear in Table 20–1. Because of their true parasitic nature, the rickettsiae were long considered inter-

Table 20–1. Distribution diseases, and vectors of Rickettsiales

Species	Diseased Produced	Geographic Distribution	Main Vector
R. prowazekii	Epidemic typhus, Brill's disease	Worldwide	Lice
R. typhi	Endemic murine typhus	Worldwide	Fleas
R. canada	Spotted fever	North America	Ticks
R. rickettsii	Rocky Mountain Spotted fever	Americas	Ticks
R. sibirica	North Asian tick fever	Siberia, Central Asia	Ticks
R. conorii	Mediterranean fever	Africa, Europe, India, Middle East	Ticks
R. australis	Queensland tick fever	Australia	Ticks
R. akari	Rickettsial pox	Europe, N. America	Mites
R. parkeri	Rocky Mountain spotted fever	North America	Ticks
R. tsutsugamushi	Scrub fever	Asia, Australia, Oceania	Mites
R. quintana	Trench fever	Africa, Europe, North America	Mites
C. burnetii	Q fever	Worldwide	Inhalation
B. bacilliformis	Oroya fever	South and Central America	Sandflies

mediary forms of organisms that should be placed between bacteria and viruses. Clear evidence is now on hand to include them with the bacteria:

1. They multiply by binary fission.
2. They contain both DNA and RNA.
3. They possess a number of metabolic enzymes.
4. They are susceptible to antibacterial agents.

PATHOGENICITY

Following the bite of the infected vector, rickettsiosis usually begins in the vascular system where the organisms multiply in the endothelial cells. They spread widely by way of the blood, and usually establish focal areas of obstruction in small blood vessels owing to hyperplasia of infected cells or tiny thrombi. An abrupt onset of disease usually follows an incubation period of one to four weeks. This onset is associated with headaches, chills, and fever, and is often followed by a hemorrhagic rash. In severe cases, delirium and shock may occur, as well as patchy gangrene of the skin and subcutaneous tissues. Different disease patterns may be fatal in 1% to 90% of cases, depending on treatment and severity of the infection. More specific details of some of the typical diseases caused by rickettsiae follows.

Epidemic Typhus. One to two weeks following the bite of an infected louse, illness begins with chills, headaches, fever, and exhaustion. The fever may run to 40°C or more by day three, and may remain for three weeks when recovery may ensue, or until death. A rash usually appears first on the trunk by day six, and spreads to the extremities but not on the face, palms or soles. Doxycycline is the most effective treatment. Vaccination or delousing are effective preventive measures.

Brill's Disease. This disease is generally milder than epidemic typhus. The rash is usually not evident, recovery is faster, and the fatality rate is low. It may follow a dormant phase that lasts several years after infection.

Endemic Murine Typhus. This is a mild form of typhus that seldom reaches epidemic proportions. The disease responds well to either chloramphenicol or tetracycline.

Spotted Fevers. These diseases are all transmitted by ticks and are caused by a group of antigenically related *Rickettsia* species. The onset resembles that of typhus, but the rash usually starts on the ankles, wrists, and forehead and then spreads to the trunk. Different strains and species result in variations in severity, the primary reservoir, and hence the geographic distribution. A number of disease syndromes have been described that relate to different areas or outbreaks (see Table 20–1).

Rickettsial Pox. Caused by *R. akari* and transmitted by mites, this disease varies from spotted fever in that the rash starts at the site of the bites and results in distinctive red papules and enlarged regional lymph nodes. The disease may be severe, but it is usually self-limited. It responds well to tetracycline.

Scrub Typhus. Like epidemic typhus, this disease is also associated with pneumonitis and pronounced stupor and prostration. Erythematous papules topped with multiple vesicles are typical. Tetracycline is highly effective in limiting the disease.

Trench Fever. Characteristic of this disease are its repeated cycles of chills and fever that last three to five days.

Q Fever. This disease is transmitted by inhalation of contaminated dust and aerosols associated with infected cattle and sheep. Pneumonitis is common but a rash is unusual. The disease responds well to tetracycline.

Oroya Fever. This disease manifests itself as a severe, febrile, hemolytic anemia. The organism is susceptible to penicillin, streptomycin, and chloramphenicol. The organism is characteristically found in red blood cells, and can be differentiated from *Protozoa* by the absence of a eukaryotic nucleus.

LABORATORY DIAGNOSIS

Only *Bartonella* and *Rochalimaea* can be cultured on blood agar; all other rickettsiae may be isolated using embryonated hen's eggs. Neither isolation nor identification of these organisms are routine procedures, and specimens usually must be submitted to a reference laboratory. A more simple laboratory diagnosis is the detection of a rise in antibodies by either complement fixation or the Weil-Felix test. The Weil-Felix test is the easiest to perform and can easily be adopted by laboratories of limited scope (see p. 372). The complement fixation test provides more specific results, but usually necessitates the use of a reference laboratory.

20-3 CHLAMYDIALES

Chlamydia are generally similar to rickettsiae except for the characteristics listed under Definitions. They are responsible for such diseases as trachoma, lymphogranuloma venereum, inclusion conjunctivitis, and ornithosis (psittacosis). They share an antigen, which is useful in their differentiation from other similar forms and in the detection of chlamydial antibodies by the complement fixation test.

TRACHOMA

This disease, caused by *Chlamydia trachomatis*, has plagued man since biblical times. It is limited to man, and seems to infect only the epithelial cells of the eye and perhaps the nasopharynx. Trachoma is the most frequent cause of blindness worldwide. An estimated 400 million people suffer from this disease, of which six million are totally blind. Characteristic follicles and scars in the conjunctiva, and vascularization and infiltration of the cornea develop. Sulfonamides and tetracycline are curative if used early.

LYMPHOGRANULOMA VENEREUM (LGV).

This disease manifests as herpetic lesions at the infective site, usually the genitals. Severe damage of the regional lymph nodes may follow primary lesions, which are often missed. The disease is uncommon except in highly promiscuous individuals, and it is limited largely to warmer climates. Inclusion conjunctivitis, which may occur in newborns 5 to 12 days after birth, is a consequence of

LGV. Both LGV and inclusion conjunctivitis respond well to tetracycline.

ORNITHOSIS (psittacosis).

C. psittaci is commonly found in wild psittacine birds (such as parrots). In man, the infection results from inhalation of infected dust or bird droppings. After one to three weeks, abrupt chills, fever, headaches, and an atypical pneumonia may develop. If diagnosed early, the disease responds well to tetracycline.

LABORATORY DIAGNOSIS

Chlamydia may be isolated from the yolk sac of embryonated hen's eggs. Such isolation is not simple and does take time. Antibody detection by the complement fixation test is also difficult, but is more reliable and therefore more conclusive.

FURTHER READING

1. Storz, J.: *Chlamydia and Chlamydia-Induced Diseases.* Springfield, Ill., Charles C Thomas, 1971.
2. Lennette, E. H., et al.: *Manual of Clinical Microbiology,* 2nd ed., Chapters 87–88, Washington, D.C., American Society for Microbiology, 1974.

chapter 21

Viruses

21-1 HISTORIC BACKGROUND

The first account of viral diseases may be found in ancient Chinese writings, in which smallpox is clearly described. Hippocrates was well acquainted with mumps, and Shakespeare gave reference to herpes of the lips in *Romeo and Juliet.* That viruses are not confined to animals but may also infect plants was first observed in the 16th century. Pictures by Rembrandt show rare varieties of colors of tulips. These tulips were actually infected by viruses and would only survive for one generation, hence their rarity and value. The first virus studied in a scientific manner was also a plant virus. Mayer, in 1886, showed that the sap of certain tobacco plants, suffering from tobacco mosaic disease, could be used to infect other healthy plants. Iwanowski confirmed this finding in 1892 and added that the sap lost its infectivity on boiling. He also showed that the sap remained infective after passage through a Chamberland filter. He concluded that the disease was caused by a "very small submicroscopic bacterium." The agent was later called "a filterable virus" by Beijerinck in 1899. Here we are interested mainly in the human viruses and therefore will not consider the plant and animal viruses.

Physicians had worked with viral agents long before the discovery of any specific virus. Vaccinations against smallpox, developed by Jenner, and against rabies, developed by Pasteur, are prime examples. The first virus disease to be definitely known as such was yellow fever, which was isolated in 1901 by Walter Reed in human volunteers during the Cuban war. In 1909, Landsteiner and Popper published their studies of poliomyelitis in monkeys.

In 1918, the world was plagued by the greatest outbreak of infectious disease in history. Five hundred million people contracted influenza, of whom 15 million died. However, the influenza virus was first isolated in 1930. These isolates were obtained by inoculating embryonated hen's eggs with specimens thought to contain virus. Effects on the infected chick embryo, ranging from death to minor lesions, could thus be studied. It was later noted, in 1942, that the fluid surrounding the infected embryo contained large amounts of virus and, even more important, that this fluid, or the virus in suspension in this fluid, was able to agglutinate red blood cells in vitro. The importance of this break-through may be appreciated when one realizes that this was the first method by which viruses could be demonstrated by other than infective means. Further studies soon revealed that the hemagglutination could be prevented by an antibody produced by patients suffering from influenza.

The greatest advances in virology, however, took place in 1953 or shortly thereafter. During 1953, Scherer developed a method by which cells could be grown in single layers in a test tube. Scherer's method was the culmination of the work of earlier workers who also deserve our attention. In 1928, Maitland and Maitland, a husband and wife team, grew tissue fragments in suspension and subsequently infected these "tissue cultures" with a number of viruses. Enders and coworkers, in 1949, advanced this method by growing the tissue fragments onto the surface of the tubes, by embedding them in a plasma clot. These tissue fragments could now be studied while they were still living, without interrupting their growth cycle as was necessary when studying infected suspended tissues. Scherer went one step further than this and used trypsin to digest the intercellular cement. Thus he obtained single cells in suspension, which grew out in sheets of cells only one cell thick. This method is commonly known as "monolayer cell culture," which allows continuous study of infectious processes of the single cells. In a relatively short period following Scherer's discovery, many new viruses were isolated using his method of cell culture. The rapid growth in the number of newly discovered viruses continued for several years but gradually slowed down until today few new viruses are being discovered. This slowdown is probably due to the fact that most viruses able to grow in cell strains presently at our disposal have been discovered.

21-2 BASIC VIROLOGY

Viruses are generally regarded the outlaws of nature. They may be defined in some lay dictionaries as "morbid poisons of contagious disease," or in differently worded descriptions that are equally elusive and inadequate. The scientist searching for a more precise and detailed definition does not fare much better. Various descriptions may be found in the literature, depending on whether one is guided by plant, animal, or medical virologists. The simplest definition suitable for our purpose is probably this: "A virus is a mass of infectious genetic material surrounded by a capsid or outer coat." The genetic material is composed of either DNA or RNA. The capsid protects the viral material from the environment, and serves as a vehicle of transport between different hosts.

THE VIRUS GROWTH CYCLE

Viruses replicate in a much more complex manner than do bacteria, primarily because they lack the necessary metabolic enzymes, for which they must depend on their host cells. A large number of viruses follow this cycle:

- a. *Adsorption:* Before a virus can enter the cell it must first come in contact with that cell and attach itself to it. This step is mainly effected by electrostatic forces, and depends on the presence of specific receptor sites on the cell surface.
- b. *Penetration:* Once the virus has become attached to the cell it will start to penetrate the cell. This may be achieved by several processes:
  1. Viropexis, a phagocytic-like process.
  2. Fusion and interaction of the virus envelope and the cell membrane.
  3. Interaction of the virus with receptor sites.
- c. *Eclipse phase or noninfective stage*: At this stage, the virus disintegrates by enzymatic removal of the envelope and subsequent unwinding of its coil of nucleic acid. If the cell

is disrupted at this stage, no infectious virus can be detected.

d. *Replication*: During this stage, the virus material directs the cell to manufacture new viral nucleoproteins and to synthesize the enzymes required for this manufacture. No complete infectious virus is detectable at this stage. It is believed that, in changing the genetic codes of the cells, some viruses may cause cells to become malignant without causing them to produce all the materials necessary for new virus synthesis. In other words, the virus causes damage in changing the cell's genes, but no virus will be detectable in the altered cell.

e. *Recombination*: Newly produced nucleic acid and proteins assemble into new, mature, infectious viruses.

f. *Release:* The completed virus leaves the cell. This may occur in one of two general ways:
   1. The cell wall may be destroyed, resulting in lysis of the cell and release of virus at a rapid rate.
   2. The virus may be slowly excreted from the cell, which remains intact.

THE DETECTION OF VIRUS GROWTH

Depending on whether animals, eggs, or cell cultures are used, the presence of a virus may be demonstrated by one or more of the following means:

a. *In animals*: Death, lesions, paralysis, or tissue damage.

b. *In embryonated eggs*: Death, pocks, lesions in the embryo's tissues or membranes surrounding those tissues, or hemagglutinating properties of various embryonic fluids.

c. *In tissue or cell-culture*
   1. *Cytopathogenic effects (CPE)*: When viruses damage and finally destroy cells, visible changes may become apparent in those cells. In many instances, more or less specific changes may indicate the type or group of virus with which one is dealing.
   2. *Hemagglutination or hemadsorption*: Some viruses may be released from cells without inflicting any apparent change on those cells. When the virus in question has hemagglutinating properties, it may be demonstrated by one of two methods. First, the cell-culture medium into which the virus has been released may be tested for hemagglutinating activity. A second similar but far more sensitive technique can be used, by which the culture

medium is aspirated from the cell sheet and the cell sheet then replenished with a suspension of red blood cells. Infected cells will adsorb the red blood cells, because some viruses in the process of extrusion from the cells will react with them. This reaction is known as hemadsorption.

3. *Metabolic inhibition test*: This method is based on the principle that cell metabolism changes the pH of the medium. Cells infected and destroyed by virus will no longer metabolize and cease to alter the pH. Changes in pH, of course, can be read macroscopically by incorporating sensitive indicators in the culture medium.

4. *Plaque formation*: In this method, cell sheets are inoculated and the virus is allowed to penetrate the cells. The culture medium is then removed, and replaced by a similar medium supplemented with 1% agar; the agar medium settles as an overlay onto the cell sheet. When released from an infected cell, a virus will only be able to infect cells in its immediate proximity. Distinct "plaques," clear patches of areas where all cells have been destroyed, will thus develop and are visible macroscopically.

THE IDENTIFICATION OF VIRUSES

As we cannot study individual viruses, and as degenerative changes (CPE) are too vague a measure to identify viruses accurately, we depend largely on serologic methods in our attempts to identify viruses.

The following methods are listed in the order of frequency in which they are generally used:

a. *Neutralization*: Diluted virus suspensions are mixed with known concentrations of type-specific antisera, and these mixtures may then be inoculated into animals, eggs, or cell cultures. When type-specific antiserum reacts with the virus, an obvious neutralization of virus growth will be apparent.

b. *Hemagglutination or hemadsorption inhibition*: These methods are similar in principle to the preceding method, but hemagglutination inhibition in particular is advantageous over neutralization because hemagglutinating viruses can be identified by this method without the further use of cell cultures. Instead of virus growth, virus action on red blood cells is neutralized by specific antiserum.

c. *Complement-fixation*: Virus-suspensions may be employed and tested with specific sera, in a reverse manner to that used in the conventional CF test. However, because many cross-reactions occur by this method, complement fixation is best utilized as a tool to group different viruses rather than to type them (e.g., all adenoviruses have at least one CF antigen in common).

21-3 CLASSIFICATION

The main differences between viruses and bacteria are:
1. Metabolic activity. Viruses lack all metabolic enzymes and depend upon their host cells to supply them.
2. Size. Viruses measure only 20 to 350 nm in diameter. One micrometer is 1000 nanometers (nm), which means that only the largest viruses are visible under the light microscope.
3. Nucleic acid composition. Viruses possess either DNA or RNA, but never both.
4. Antibiotic susceptibility. All viruses are resistant to antibiotics.

Viruses differ from one another as follows:
1. Size and nucleic acid composition (see above).
2. Morphology, symmetry, and number of capsomeres. (Capsomeres are distinctive subunits of the capsid.)
3. Susceptibility to chemical and physical agents, in particular ether.
4. Molecular weight of nucleic acid of the virion. (A virion is an intact virus particle.)
5. Virion composition—enveloped, complex, or naked.
6. Site of capsid assembly in the host.

These characteristics have been used in the classification of viruses (see Table 21–1). Obviously, it would be difficult to routinely identify viruses isolated in the diagnostic laboratory by determining the characteristics outlined in Table 21–1. The determinations discussed in section 21–2 are much more practical for routine use. A more detailed diagnostic approach is discussed in the next section. Because of the extreme variety and multiplicity of viral diseases, we limit ourselves here to the outline presented in Table 21–2. For more detailed information, refer to the bibliography, and to citations 2 and 3 in particular.

Table 21–1. Major classification of human viruses

Virus or virus group	Nucleic acid	Capsid symmetry	Virion composition	Site of capsid assembly	No. of capsomeres	Ether sensitivity	Size in nm	Molecular weight
Mastadenovirus	DNA	Cubic	Naked	Nucleus	252	Resistant	70–90	23
Papovaviridea	"	"	"	"	72	"	43–53	3.5
Herpesviridea	"	Complex	Enveloped	"	162	Sensitive	100–150	54–92
Orthopoxvirus (Vaccinia)			Complex	Cytoplasm	?	Resistant	230–300	160
Picornaviridea (Entero-, Polio- and Rhinovirus)	RNA	Cubic	Naked	Cytoplasm	32	"	20–30	2–2.8
Reoviridea	"	"	"	"	92	"	75–80	15
Togaviridea (Yellow fever, Rubella)	"	"	Enveloped	"	32	Sensitive	40–70	3
Orthomyxoviridea (Influenza)	"	Helical	"	"	6–9	"	90–120	2–4
Paramyxoviridea (Mumps, Measles)	"	"	"	"	18	"	150–300	4–8
Lyssavirus (Rabies)	"	"	"	"	18	"	70–175	3–4

21-4 DIAGNOSTIC VIROLOGY

Many specimens sent to a virus laboratory are accompanied by a simple requisition or slip of paper with no more information than the patient's name and the proverbial "virus studies." These specimens are usually shelved. If you were to ask a biochemist or hematologist to do "biochemical" or "hematology" studies and were to wait for his reaction, you could understand why the virologist rejects such specimens.

Diagnostic virology, then, begins at the bedside, and laboratory tests can only be attempted when at least a fair history accompanies the specimen. The diagnostic approach may constitute one or a combination of the following.

CLINICAL OBSERVATION

A full clinical examination should provide data on:
a. Symptoms, signs and their duration.
b. Immunization status (artificial and natural).
c. Recent and past history of the patient and his family.
d. Epidemiology of the area and industrial hazards of the individual.
e. Laboratory findings, WBC, differential counts, other tests performed while the patient was under observation.

The clinical observations are most important as a guide to the laboratory approach. A reasonable case history must always accompany the first specimen sent to the virus laboratory of each individual. Only when this information is available will the virologist be able to decide on the course of action to be taken in the laboratory. The virologist should be able to answer the following questions from the information provided:
a. Which host will be most suited for isolation attempts? Obviously he could not start to inoculate each specimen into all the different animals and cell cultures at his disposal.
b. Which serologic test should be tried first?
c. Might not some other type of specimen be better suited for study of this particular case?

COLLECTION OF SPECIMENS

The decision regarding the type of specimen to be taken from the patient lies with the physician. In most instances, however, the technologist collects the specimen. They should both know which specimens are to be used for attempts at isolation, serologic studies, or direct examination.

Specimens for Isolation

a. *Skin scrapings and smears of lesions.* The physician should always take these specimens. Slides must be left to dry in air; do not fix by heat or alcohol; place face to face, after marking the side of the slide with the smear, separate the slides by a match or toothpick, and secure with tape or an elastic band.

b. *Vesicular or pustular fluids.* Collect these in capillary tubes and then seal with paraffin wax or Sealease, and place in a small test tube supported with cotton to prevent breakage.

c. *Tops of lesions and scabs*: Collect in a test tube, stopper, and secure the stopper with adhesive tape.

d. *Blood*: Separate serum from the clot, and send both serum and clot in two separate test tubes.

e. *Autopsy specimens*: Naturally, the pathologist collects these specimens.

f. *Throat swabs or washings*: As some reference centers prefer one over the other, check local preferences. Use sterile nutrient broth or saline as gargling fluid. Special outfits, complete with the preferred gargling fluid, may be supplied by your local health department or virus laboratory. Take swabs from the nasopharynx and throat; break the swabs in a test tube containing broth, saline or special medium as provided by the virus laboratory in your area, and secure with a stopper or cap.

g. *Feces*: Collect approximately 20 grams in a suitable wide-mouthed container.

h. *Cerebrospinal fluid*: Collection of this specimen is under the jurisdiction of the physician.

Specimens for Serology. Always collect two serum samples—one during the acute phase and the other during the convalescent phase of the disease. Separate the serum from the clot, keep cool but do not freeze. Freezing and thawing tend to decrease the antibody titer. Thus, when serum from the acute phase has undergone repeated freezing and thawing and then later tested in parallel with convalescent phase sera, a false difference in titer may be demonstrated.

PRESERVATION OF SPECIMENS

Because most viruses are highly labile with regard to changes in pH, temperature, drying, and storage, the following points must be strictly observed in order for the viruses to survive:

a. Always use sterile containers free from chemical matter.

   b. Submit the specimen as soon as possible to the virus laboratory.
   c. Never use containers in which disinfectants have been stored.
   d. Keep specimens at 4°C or freeze immediately and keep frozen (except blood).
   e. If possible, use transport media and containers supplied by the regional virus laboratory.

REQUISITIONS

The person shipping the specimens must ensure that each specimen is accompanied by a requisition slip that contains at least the following minimal information:
   a. Patient's name, age, and sex.
   b. Doctor's name and address or name of the referring hospital.
   c. Nature of the specimen and date obtained.
   d. Date of onset of the illness.
   e. Symptoms and signs (particularly dermatologic and neurologic).
   f. Presumptive diagnosis, progress, and prognosis. Possible source of infection; contact with animals, birds.
   g. Laboratory findings if available (cell counts, differentials).

TRANSPORT

Ensure that frozen specimens do not fill more than two-thirds of their containers. Stopper all containers securely. Send frozen specimens on dry ice in the special containers as provided by the department of health. Mark ALL parcels on the outside "Specimens for virus studies; pathologic material."

DIRECT LABORATORY EXAMINATION

Smears of lesions and tissues obtained by autopsy or biopsy may be stained by a variety of techniques and then examined under light, fluorescent, or electron microscopes. Direct examination, however, has rather limited applications in diagnostic virology. It is used to differentiate between poxviruses and herpesviruses (electron microscopy) and in the diagnosis of rabies (fluorescence microscopy). Recent developments in fluorescence microscopy technology have added to the armament of the virologist, allowing more rapid methods of clinical significance.

Table 21-2. Some common viruses, the diseases they may cause, and the general diagnostic laboratory approach

Virus	Disease that may be caused	Specimen for isolation	Host for isolation	Identification method	Serology
				Diagnostic approach	
Variola	Smallpox	Vesicle fluid	Eggs	Specific pocks	CF or HI
Herpes simplex	Cold sores	Ulcer swab,	TC	Specific pocks	CF
	Meningoen-cephalitis	CSF			
Influenza A	Asian flu	Throat swab	Eggs	HI	CF or HI
Mumps	Parotitis, orchitis, meningoen-cephalitis	Saliva, CSF	TC	HI or Neutralization	HI
Adenovirus and others	Atypical pneu-monia and other	Throat swab Feces	TC	Neutralization	CF
Poliovirus	Poliomyelitis	Throat swab Feces or CSF	TC	Neutralization	Neutralization CF
Coxsackie viruses ECHO virus	Aseptic menin-gitis and other	Feces or CSF	TC	Neutralization	Neutralization
Rhinoviruses	Common cold	Nasal secretions	TC	Neutralization	Neutralization

CF = Complement fixation; HI = Hemagglutination inhibition; TC = Tissue culture; CSF = Cerebrospinal fluid. (Reproduced from Can. J. Med. Techn., **31**: 80–87, 1969.)

VIRUS ISOLATION

A general approach to the isolation of virus proceeds as follows: specimens are treated to remove contaminants such as bacteria and yeasts, and are then inoculated into the most appropriate host or hosts. These hosts are then observed for detection of virus growth, and when growth is detected the isolate may be identified by some of the methods previously mentioned in Section 21–2.

SEROLOGIC EXAMINATION

Few serologic findings have any diagnostic value when a single specimen is examined. Only a considerable rise in antibody titer indicates an active infection. For serologic studies therefore, a serum specimen withdrawn during the acute phase should be sent to the laboratory as soon as the disease becomes apparent, preferably accompanied by a fitting clinical picture and the suspected identity of the causative agent. This must be followed by a second sample taken during the convalescent phase of the disease, or 10 to 14 days following the first specimen. It is from the serologic examination of both these specimens that some diagnostically significant results may be obtained. Obviously, these results usually have only a retrospective value to the clinician and the patient.

SUMMARY

Table 21-2 presents the more common human viruses, the diseases they may cause, and the diagnostic approach most suitable for their isolation and identification.

FURTHER READING

1. Andrewes, C., and Pereira, H. G.: *Viruses of Vertebrates*. 3rd ed. Baltimore, Williams & Wilkins Co., 1972.
2. Acton, J. D., et al.: *Fundamentals of Medical Virology*. Philadelphia, Lea & Febiger, 1974.
3. Lennette, E. H., et al.: *Manual of Clinical Microbiology*. 2d ed. Washington, D.C., American Society for Microbiology, 1974.

chapter 22

Fungi, Yeasts and Molds

22-1 BASIC MYCOLOGY

Fungi are composed of somatic or vegetative structures that may take the form of single cells or tubular strands of many cells. The true yeasts are the simplest forms and produce only somatic structures. They usually do so by budding, a process by which a single spore buds out from the parent cell, matures while still attached to the mother cell, separates, and finally forms budding

285

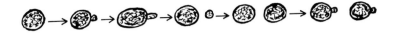

Fig. 22-1. Progressive budding.

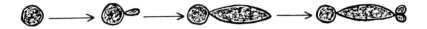

Fig. 22-2. Production of pseudomycelium.

spores itself (see Fig. 22-1). The yeastlike fungi produce a pseudomycelium, by elongating the original bud and subsequently producing a pair of terminal buds projecting from the elongated original bud (see Fig. 22-2). Other yeast cells produce numerous endospores and release these by rupture of the parent cell (see Fig. 22-3).

All true yeasts and some of the yeastlike fungi develop into colonies much as do the bacteria. Some yeastlike fungi produce bacterialike colonies at 37°C, but moldlike colonies at 25°C.

What are moldlike colonies? What is a mycelium? In the opening sentence of this chapter, we talked about tubular strands of many cells. These tubes are known as *hyphae* (singular, hypha). Hyphae may be fused (see Fig. 22-4) or individual hypha may be separated by septa (see Fig. 22-5). Hyphae eventually "weave" themselves into a feltlike mat, which is known as a *mycelium.*

A *moldlike colony* consists of two parts:
1. The *vegetative mycelium*, the part actually feeding and growing near or into the medium.
2. The *aerial mycelium*, the part protruding from the medium. The aerial mycelium of mold is particularly evident as the "furry" growth we often notice on bread and fruits. Spores develop from the aerial mycelium.

A *spore* is any structural unit which, when separating from the parent organism, is capable of developing into a new, individual organism. Fungal spores function as units of propagation; they are slightly more resistant to unfavorable environments than are the vegetative and other units. They are generally slightly less susceptible to heat and to disinfectants than are vegetative bacteria. Sterilization methods may therefore be modified accordingly when fungal spores constitute a hazard.

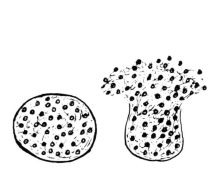 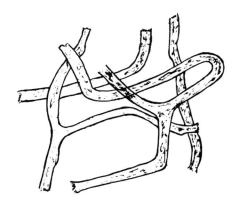

Fig. 22–3.   Eruption of endospores.   **Fig. 22–4.**   Nonseptate hyphae.

When deposited on or in a suitable medium or environment, fungal spores germinate, often by developing a tubelike projection called a germ tube. The germ tube further elongates and grows into hyphae (see Fig. 22–6).

Spores may be produced by sexual or asexual processes. Most medically important fungi sporulate asexually. Differentiation of the pathogenic fungi rests mainly on the type of spores produced or on the structures from which the spores originate. The remainder of this section, therefore, is devoted to the developmental processes and structures of fungal spores.

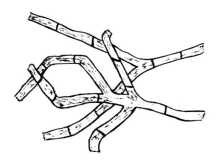 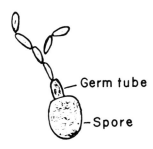

Fig. 22–5.   Septate hyphae.   **Fig. 22–6.**   Germ tube formation.

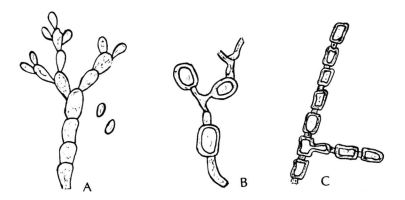

Fig. 22-7. A, Blastospores; B, Chlamydospores; C, Arthrospores.

ASEXUAL SPORULATION

The simplest form of true sporulation is that by which the spores form directly from vegetative mycelium. Spores so formed are collectively called *thallospores*. Three distinct types of thallospores are known:

1. *Blastospores* are produced by budding from the tips of the mycelium, either as single spores or as small clusters of spores (see Fig. 22-7A).
2. *Chlamydospores* are produced by rounding off and by enlargement of certain hyphae. They usually develop a thick wall around the spore, easily recognized in preparations stained with lactophenol cotton blue (see Fig. 22–7B).
3. *Arthrospores* are produced by division of individual hyphae, developing into strands of square or cylindrial thick-walled spores (see Fig. 22–7C).

A more complex form of sporulation occurs when spores are formed, singly or in groups, from specialized hyphae. Hyphae especially developed to produce spores are called *conidiophores*. The spores arising from the conidiophore are called *conidia*. When conidia are larger in diameter than the average hypha, they are referred to as macroconidia; when smaller, they are called microconidia.

Macroconidia may take many different shapes:

1. They may be septate or nonseptate.

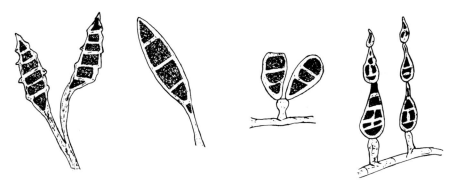

Fig. 22–8. Various macronidia.

2. They may have spindle, sausage, club, racket or nodular shapes.
3. They may originate from the conidiophore singly, in pairs, or in clusters (Fig. 22–8).

Microconidia generally have the same shape and size. However, the manner in which they "sprout" or arise from the conidiophores is characteristic:

1. Some arise directly from the hyphae. These are the sessile conidia (see Fig. 22–9).
2. Some develop a short pedicle from which the conidia arise—the pedunculate conidia (see Fig. 22–10).
3. Some arise from swollen conidiophores that have developed superstructures called sterigmata. The actual conidiophore may be branched or grossly swollen (see Fig. 22–11).

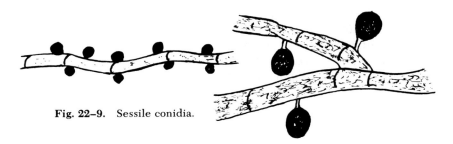

Fig. 22–9. Sessile conidia.

Fig. 22–10. Pedunculate conidia.

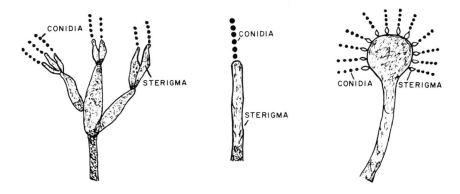

Fig. 22–11. Conidia production from swollen conidiophores.

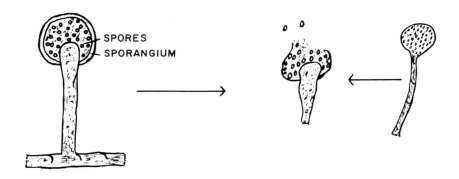

Fig. 22–12. Sporangiospore development.

4. Others develop in swollen structures on stalklike conidiophores. These conidiophores are better known as sporangiophores; the swollen structure as a sporangium, and the spores as sporangiospores. Sporangiospores are released by final rupture of the sporangium (see Fig. 22–12).

SEXUAL SPORULATION

Of the several modes of sexual sporulation, we shall limit ourselves to two:

1. The production of *ascospores*, whereby two specialized

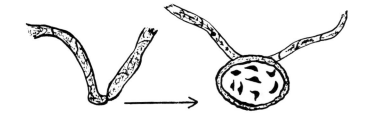

Fig. 22–13. Ascospore development.

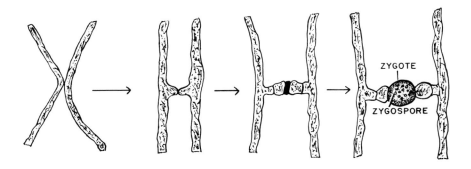

Fig. 22–14. Zygospore development.

hyphae fuse to form an ascus (or sac), in which the spores develop (see Fig. 22–13).

2. The production of *zygospores*, a different form of fusion or linkage of hyphae, and the formation of a zygote in which the spores develop (see Fig. 22–14).

22-2 CLASSIFICATION OF FUNGI

Few mycologists seem to agree on how to classify the fungi, and almost all textbooks on the subject disagree with one another. As members of the allied health professions, we are mainly interested in identifying those fungi that cause disease in man. Therefore, we are inclined to adopt a classification system that will allow us to differentiate the pathogenic fungi from one another and from the saprophytes. In doing so, we should not lose sight of the fact that such a classification system may deviate from a truly biologic classification. Thus, we briefly present a basic biologic classification and follow with a medical classification that is more workable for us.

BIOLOGIC CLASSIFICATION

Phylum Eumycophyta: This phylum of the plant kingdom is composed of the true fungi. In general, these form tubular filaments with definite cell walls. The phylum is divided into four classes:

Class 1. Phycomycetes
Class 2. Ascomycetes
Class 3. Basidiomycetes
Class 4. Deuteromycetes

Most pathogenic fungi belong to Class IV. Indeed, the Moniliales, Order III of this class, contains over 90% of all pathogenic fungi. We will define the Moniliales as having conidia borne on conidiphores. The order Moniliales contains well over 600 genera and some 10,000 species. Fortunately for us, most of these are nonpathogenic to man. The common pathogenic genera of the Moniliales:

Candida	*Aspergillus*
Sporotrichum	*Penicillium*
Trichophyton	*Geotrichum*
Microsporum	*Blastomyces**
Epidermophyton	*Histoplasma**

Order IV, the Pseudosaccharomycetales, contains most of the other pathogenic fungi. This order may simply be defined as the yeastlike fungi. The common pathogens are *Cryptococcus* and *Coccidioides*.

MEDICAL CLASSIFICATION

The biologic classification offers no guide to the diagnosis of mycotic diseases in man. A medical classification, based on the body sites most commonly affected by different fungi, is a more practical approach and therefore widely followed by diagnosticians. An example of such a classification divides the fungi in groups as:

   a. *Saprophytic fungi,* those most commonly found as ordinary saprophytes.
   b. *Superficial fungi* (dermatophytes), the most common causes of mycoses† of the outer layers of the skin, the hair shaft, and the nails.

---

*These are yeastlike at 37°C.
†A mycosis is a mycotic (fungal) infection.

c. *Mucous membrane invaders*, those fungi that chiefly cause infections of linings of the mouth and the respiratory and urinary tracts.

d. *Subcutaneous fungi*, which mainly affect the deeper skin tissues.

e. *Systemic fungi*, which usually cause infections of internal organs.

22-3 GROWTH CHARACTERISTICS OF FUNGI

Fungi require complex organic substances as nutrients. Most fungi are saprophytic in nature, while some demonstrate parasitism. Relatively little is known about the physiology and biochemistry of the various fungi; therefore, few diagnostic tests are based on these disciplines. Differentiation of the fungi still depends largely on cultural and microscopic morphology. Even more so than is the case with bacteria, slight variations in culture media or conditions affect the characteristics displayed by many fungi.

Plain peptone water will support the growth of most fungi. The addition of yeast extracts often enhances the production of the more typical hyphae and spores. Pigmentation is usually most characteristic when the cultures are grown on media containing dextrose, maltose, or both.*

Fungi grow best in moist environments at a pH ranging between 5.6 and 7.0 and at temperatures between 25° and 30°C. Some fungi may demonstrate dimorphism. When grown at 25°C they may produce a cottony, moldlike colony, and at 37°C they may produce waxy or butyrous, moist colonies.

When pigmented colonies show tiny patches of white, examine the pigmented areas for typical hyphae and spore formation. The white patches are usually "sterile" and are believed to develop from mutating cells.

22-4 SAPROPHYTIC FUNGI

Although few saprophytic fungi cause disease in man, they frequently contaminate media and specimens. Two genera, *Aspergillus* and *Penicillium*, are particularly interesting.

ASPERGILLUS

Species of this genus are numerous and ubiquitous. *A. fumigatus* is the cause of most cases of aspergilloses in man.

---

*Sabouraud's dextrose broth or agar is most commonly employed for culture of fungi and yeasts.

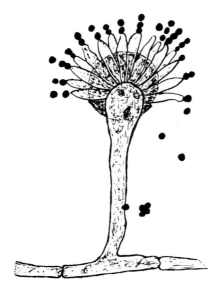

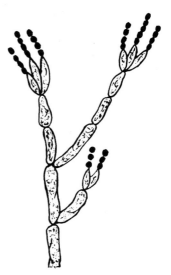

Fig. 22–15. *Aspergillus.*   **Fig. 22–16.** *Penicillium.*

Typical aspergillosis develops into a severe, invasive pulmonary infection. Aspergilli have septate hyphae and produce conidia from flask-shaped sterigmata on wide, vesiclelike, conidiophores (see Fig. 22–15). On Sabouraud-dextrose agar at 25°C, the growth of aspergilli is rapid. At first, they grow into a white fluff (48 hours). Later they develop into various shades of greenish-blue, yellowish-green, tan, or even black. Their surfaces are velvety to cottonlike, turning to powdery in older cultures.

PENICILLIUM

Although the products of certain *Penicillium* species are toxic to some individuals, their primary medical importance lies in their ability to produce potent antibacterial substances. *Penicillium* have septate hyphae and produce conidia from flasklike sterigmata on branching conidiophores (see Fig. 22–16). Their cultural characteristics are similar to those of *Aspergillus*.

22-5 SUPERFICIAL FUNGI

Only three organisms can logically be classified in this group. They infect the outer layers of the hair shaft or the skin.

MALASSEZIA FURFUR

These organisms cause the widespread disease, tinea versicolor. The name tinea has been in use since ancient times and refers to "ringworm disease." The characteristic spread of many fungal diseases—slowly expanding from a small central location to ringlike areas surrounding this center—led to the belief that mycoses were caused by a worm.

Tinea versicolor is characterized by the development of dark, scaly patches on various parts of the body, mainly the chest and the back. *M. furfur* has not been cultured and is known only from its appearance in clinical specimens. Under Wood's lamp, the scales show a pale yellow fluorescence in the dark.

CLADOSPORIUM WERNECKII (MANSONII)

C. werneckii causes the tropical disease tinea nigra, which is characterized by black blotches on the body and, more particularly, on the palms of the hand.

Skin scrapings reveal brown to dark green, septate branched hyphae, 1.5 to 3.0 μm thick, with chlamydospores and swollen epithelial cells.

TRICHOSPORON BEIGELII (CUTANEUM)

T. beigelii is the cause of piedra, a mild infection of the hair, demonstrable by soft, lightly to darkly pigmented nodules along the hair shaft.

22-6 CUTANEOUS FUNGI (THE DERMATOPHYTES)

Organisms of this group mainly cause infections of the skin, nails, and hair. They are usually referred to as "dermatophytes," and constitute the largest group within the pathogenic fungi. Three genera are recognized and may be differentiated by the diseases they cause or by their characteristic macroconidia.

MICROSPORUM

Organisms of this genus mainly cause mycoses of the skin and hair. Infected hairs fluoresce when examined under Wood's lamp. There are three major species, *M. audouinii*, *M. canis*, and *M. gypseum*, and several minor ones.

M. audouinii is the most common cause of tinea capitis, ringworm of the scalp. Members of this species are often referred to as being anthropophilic, since they seem to be limited to man.

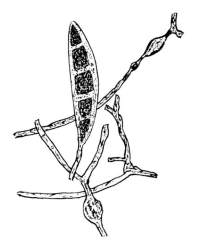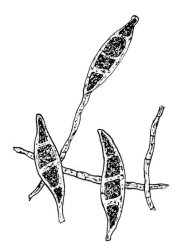

Fig. 22–17. *Microsporum audouinii.*   **Fig. 22–18.** *Microsporum canis.*

Microsporum produces spindle-shaped macroconidia from about 35 to 150 μm in length. *M. audouinii* produces pectinate hyphae with few macroconidia if any (see Fig. 22–17). On Sabouraud-dextrose agar at 25°C, *M. audouinii* grows slowly, producing flat, grayish to tan colonies with a thin aerial mycelium. The vegetative mycelium may be light to dark brown in color. Sporulation is somewhat enhanced by the addition of yeast extract.

M. canis is primarily an animal pathogen and therefore often called zoophilic (animal loving). It frequently causes "ringworm" in domestic animals such as dogs and cats, from which man may become infected.

Microscopically, *Microsporum canis* resembles *M. audouinii*, but there are no pectinate hyphae and macroconidia are more numerous (see Fig. 22–18). It grows rapidly, producing flat, disc-like colonies, with a thin aerial mycelium, brightly yellow at the periphery and white in the center. The vegetative mycelium is first yellow, turning into a deep orange.

Microsporum gypseum is really a soil saprophyte and is called geophilic (earth loving). On rare occasions, it may cause tinea capitis in man. In culture, it sporulates even more rapidly than *M. canis* and macroconidia are often seen in clusters or pairs (see Fig. 22–19). Colonies have a coarse, powdery surface, with deep yellow to orange or brown pigmentation.

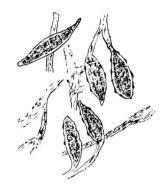 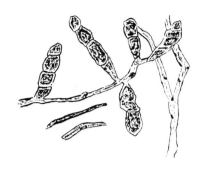

Fig. 22–19. *Microsporum gypseum.*   **Fig. 22–20.** *Epidermophyton floccosum.*

EPIDERMOPHYTON

This genus contains only one species, *E. floccosum*, the cause of tinea cruris, or ringworm of the areas surrounding the genitalia, especially the insides of the thighs. It may also invade the nails but not the hair.

Chains of arthrospores may be seen in skin scrapings. In culture they develop numerous sausage-shaped, septate (2 to 4) macroconidia (see Fig. 22–20). They grow slowly into flat or radially folded colonies, at first white and fluffy, later turning a tan or olive-green, with a velvety to powdery surface.

TRICHOPHYTON

Organisms of this genus may infect the skin, hair, and nails. In North America the most common diseases are tinea pedis (athlete's foot), and tinea unguium (nail infection), and less commonly, tinea barbae (ringworm of the skin of the face of bearded persons). Infected hairs usually do not fluoresce under Wood's lamp. The main species are: *T. mentagrophytes, T. rubrum, T. tonsurans, T. schoenleinii* and *T. violaceum.*

T. mentagrophytes is the most common cause of athlete's foot. It may also infect hair and then produce arthrospores outside the hair shaft. Microscopically, numerous small, slender, elongated microconidia are frequently seen alongside the hyphae. Depending on the strain, few or many, thin-walled, club- to spindle-shaped, septate (2–5) macroconidia will also develop (see Fig. 22–21). *T. mentagrophytes* grows rapidly, usually producing white cottony colonies, but coarse granular strains also occur, especially from

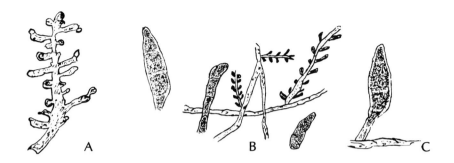

Fig. 22–21. *Trichophyton. A, T. mentagrophytes; B, T. rubrum; C, T. tonsurans.*

animal sources. The vegetative mycelium is usually light brown, but may be a pale orange to a deep red.

T. rubrum is a less common cause of mycoses of the skin. Although it rarely invades hair, it remains ectothrix (outside the hair) when it does. Microconidia may be seen along the hyphae, but peculiarly club-shaped, blunt-ended macroconidia are more characteristic (see Fig. 22–21). They grow slowly, into flat or heaped up colonies, with a white, fluffy surface and a vegetative mycelium that ranges in color from pinkish-brown to a deep red or deep purple.

T. tonsurans frequently infects hair and is of the endothrix (within the hair) type. Numerous microconidia form in a manner similar to *T. rubrum.* The macroconidia, however, are usually few and of a bent-spindle shape (see Fig. 22–21). They grow slowly, producing a fine, powdery growth, which is at first flat and later builds up to a more velvety colony. The color of the aerial mycelium ranges between a creamy white to tan, the vegetative mycelium, between yellow and dark brown.

T. schoenleinii invades the hair and frequently produces hyphae and even mycelium throughout the hair shaft. The mycelium is very irregular of the so-called "antler type." *T. schoenleinii* grows slowly, into irregular, tough, folded colonies, with a white to tan colored surface, and a much darker vegetative mycelium.

T. violaceum also invades the inside of the hair shaft. Microscopically, it is much like *T. schoenleinii* but spores form anywhere along the hyphae, instead of mainly at the ends, changing their appearance from "antlerlike" to nodular throughout.

22-7 MUCOUS MEMBRANE INVADERS

These are often referred to as the yeastlike fungi, because morphologically as well as physiologically they are more similar to the true yeasts than to the fungi or molds. Two genera, which have each been placed in different families by different workers, are important here—*Cryptococcus* and *Candida*.

CRYPTOCOCCUS

C. neoformans is almost like a true yeast. These organisms are simple, unicellular, round or oval, and reproduce only by budding (blastospores). They lack all further morphologic development, although a large capsule can usually be seen when the cells are examined in India ink preparations (see Fig. 22–22).

Cryptococcoses are mainly infections of the respiratory tract, but they may develop into chronic infections or even meningitis.

On Sabouraud-dextrose agar, the organisms grow quite well at 25°C, producing moist, butyrous colonies of a creamy color. They also grow at 37°C.

CANDIDA

These organisms reproduce by blastospore formation either from pseudomycelium (see Fig. 22–2) or from budding yeast cells.

Diseases caused by *Candida* species are collectively referred to as candidiases. In older textbooks, they may be found under moniliases, as the most frequent pathogen—*C. albicans*—was previously classified as *Monilia albicans*. *C. albicans* causes a variety of disease patterns, ranging from the more common mucous membrane infections to deep systemic infections. Common diseases caused by this organism are:

a. *Thrush*, which appears as small white patches on the mucous membrane of the mouth. When stripped off, the patches leave inflamed, red membranes.

b. *Vulvovaginitis*, which may be caused by a number of organisms. In diabetic patients, pregnant women, and in women on prolonged antibiotic treatment, vulvovaginitis is caused most commonly by *C. albicans*.

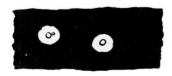

Fig. 22–22. *Cryptococcus* capsules.

c. *"Black hairy tongue infections,"* which occur most frequently in heavy smokers and in patients on prolonged antibiotic treatment.

d. *Pulmonary pneumonitis.*

e. Disseminated forms, which often occur following prolonged treatment with antibiotics or immunosuppressive drugs, and in individuals who have immunodeficiencies.

Antimycotic drugs, such as nystatin, amphotericin, and griseofulvin, may be used in the treatment of these diseases.

Laboratory Diagnosis. Since these are the most common mycotic infections, their diagnosis by laboratory means is described in more detail:

Collection and submission of specimen. In most instances this is a clinical rather than a laboratory responsibility. Care should be taken that specimens are placed in clean, sterile containers. No special precautions are required in storage or transport, as the organisms survive quite well. Some regional reference laboratories prefer to have specimens submitted already planted on Sabouraud-dextrose agar.

Direct examination. Budding cells and different types of mycelium may be apparent in wet preparations. When mycelium is absent, check for capsulation by the India ink method to rule out *Cryptococcus neoformans*, especially when the clinical diagnosis is pulmonary infection.

Isolation. Inoculate specimens directly on Sabouraud-dextrose agar, incubate at 25°C, and examine daily for evidence of growth. *Candida* species grow well and appear as white, soft colonies that later develop into feathery outgrowths into the medium.

Identification. C. albicans may be readily differentiated from other *Candida* species by recognition of their ability to produce chlamydospores. The best medium for such production is chlamydospore agar. This medium should be plated, and the agar inoculated by inserting a needle, with inoculum, at a 45° angle into the medium. A coverslip should be placed over the inoculation site, and following a few days at 25°C the plate may be examined directly under the microscope for chlamydospores (Fig. 22–23).

Candida species may be further differentiated by their ability to ferment different carbohydrates. Fermentation studies, however, are not quite as simple as those discussed for the bacteria.

22-8 SUBCUTANEOUS FUNGI

The subcutaneous fungi mainly invade the skin, particularly subcutaneous tissues. Several saprophytes may rarely invade sub-

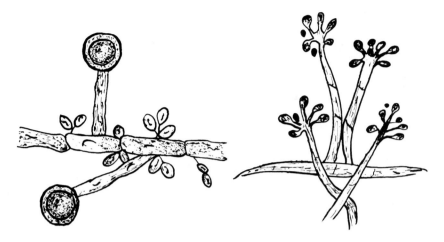

Fig. 22–23. *Candida albicans*   Fig. 22–24. *Sporotrichum schenckii.*
     chlamydospores.

cutaneous tissues. The most frequent invader is *Sporotrichum schenckii*, which produces a disease known as sporotrichosis. In this disease, subacute or chronic lesions affect the skin and subcutaneous tissues.

In tissue scrapings, the organisms appear as small, oval, yeastlike budding cells. On Sabouraud-dextrose agar at 25°C, the organisms form small moist colonies in two to three days, and wrinkled, membranous colonies after five days. Clusters of microconidia may be borne on conidiophores from septate hyphae (Fig. 22–24).

Actinomyces and *Nocardia* species are often grouped with the subcutaneous fungi, even though they belong to a different form of life altogether, the Actinomycetales. They are discussed in that section (see p. 251).

22-9 SYSTEMIC FUNGI

The systemic fungi mainly invade internal organs of the body, including bone and subcutaneous tissues. Again, we limit ourselves to a brief discussion of organisms that cause serious diseases in man only.

BLASTOMYCES DERMATITIDIS

This organism is the cause of North American blastomycosis, an often fatal pulmonary infection. A similar disease occurs in

South America but appears to be spread by a different organism, *Paracoccidioides brasiliensis*. Both North American and South American diseases are usually chronic, and progress from a mild infection of the mucous membranes to the lungs.

B. dermatitidis organisms may be recognized in infected tissues or sputa as typical budding cells; the parent cell has a double wall, and the bud, a single wall. *P. brasiliensis* produces multiple buds, each attached to the parent cell by constricted tubes. Both species are difficult to grow, requiring blood-enriched media.

A complement fixation test has been developed which serves as the main tool for diagnosis.

HISTOPLASMA CAPSULATUM

Once considered rare, histoplasmosis is believed to be widespread in North America. Serology tests have produced evidence to conclude that on this continent alone some 30 million people have come in contact with *H. capsulatum*.

Histoplasmosis is usually benign; when symptomatic, it is primarily a respiratory disease of a lasting nature. The symptoms resemble those of tuberculosis and the disease is often fatal. The organisms grow with difficulty in culture. Tuberculate chlamydospores were once believed to be diagnostic for this organism, but since they may also be produced by some other fungi, they are only suggestive evidence of histoplasmosis. Cultures are yeastlike at 25°C and moldlike at 37°C.

COCCIDIOIDES IMMITIS

These organisms also cause severe pulmonary infections. They are found predominantly in the western United States, particularly the San Joaquin Valley of California and have been reported as far south as northern Argentina and to the east in Texas. Coccidiodomycosis is also known as San Joaquin Valley Fever.

In tissue and body fluids, the organisms produce characteristic spherules, which are large structures (5 to 200 μm in diameter), which contain numerous endospores.

22-10 LABORATORY DIAGNOSIS OF MYCOSES

SPECIMENS

Hairs and scales from lesions can be removed with sterile forceps and placed between two microscope slides. Flame the slides at the inner surfaces, secure them with an elastic band, wrap them in Kraft paper and identify the specimen. Nonscaling lesions should first be cleansed with 70% ethanol. The specimen may then be taken by gently scraping the outer rim of the lesion with a scalpel and collecting the scrapings onto a flamed slide or sterile Petri dish. Infected nails should be scraped at the affected areas. Other specimens may be collected in the usual manner (see Chapter 24).

DIRECT EXAMINATION

Fungal spores are easily disseminated into the environment. Thus, before embarking on any mycology studies, special precautions must be taken:

a. Use a fan-operated, filter-equipped fume hood, especially when dealing with possible systemic pathogens.
b. Manipulate cultures only over towels that have been soaked in disinfectant.
c. Remove stoppers or lids slowly and move loop slowly and with extreme care.
d. If a culture is spilled in a room, sterilize with formalin vapors or ethylene oxide; better yet, engage a professional fumigator.

Make a preparation by placing the specimen in a drop of 10 to 40% potassium hydroxide (KOH) on a clean glass slide. Add a cover slip, and heat the preparation gently over a flame. The purpose of the hydroxide is to digest the tissue and make the fungal elements more readily visible. If the specimen has not cleared sufficiently on first examination, reheat and, if necessary, add more hydroxide to prevent it from drying out. Examine the preparation under the low power objective, with the condenser lowered or the diaphragm slightly closed. Direct examination may help to determine whether or not a fungus is present in the specimen. It rarely allows immediate identification of the species.

When examining infected hairs, the position of spores and their arrangement may indicate whether the fungus belongs to the genus *Microsporum* or the genus *Trichophyton*. However, in nails and skin specimens, species of *Microsporum, Trichophyton* and *Epidermophyton* all present a similar picture. Artifacts such as oil droplets, air bubbles, pollen grains, and fibers of wool or cotton may be mistaken for spores or hyphae. Identification of the infecting fungus is attempted only after culture and isolation.

Infected hairs may also be exposed to Wood's lamp, which is a simple ultraviolet light used in the dark. Hairs infected with *Microsporum* usually fluoresce, while those infected with *Trichophyton* do not.

ISOLATION

Infected material may be cultured directly on Sabouraud-dextrose agar, to which 20 units of penicillin and 40 units of streptomycin per milliliter of medium have been added to prevent overgrowth by bacterial contaminants. Keep the cultures at room temperature and examine daily for evidence of growth. When this occurs, examine microscopically and search for morphologic structures characteristic of the different genera and species.

In order to perform such examinations, it is often necessary to cut a small piece off the tougher colonies. This must be done with great care, to disturb the structures the least. The tougher pieces may be gently teased out in a drop of 10% KOH or lactophenol cotton blue on a glass slide.

IDENTIFICATION

Laboratorians of a medium-sized hospital must be able to differentiate *Candida* from *Cryptococcus*, and *C. albicans* from other *Candida* species and yeasts. They must also learn to identify *Microsporum*, *Epidermophyton*, and *Trichophyton*, and the major species of *Microsporum* and *Trichophyton*, from one another.

Further, *Aspergillus*, *Penicillium*, *Coccidioides*, *Blastomyces*, and *Histoplasma* should be recognized. If it is accepted that no organism is ever guaranteed to be nonpathogenic and if consultation from reference laboratories is sought when necessary, mycology need not be the frightening discipline it is so often projected to be.

FURTHER READING

1. Hazen, E. L. et al.: *Laboratory Identification of Pathogenic Fungi Simplified*. 3rd ed. Springfield, Illinois, Charles C Thomas, 1970.
2. Beneke, E. D., and Rogers, A. L.: *Medical Mycology Manual*. 3rd ed. Minneapolis, Burgess Publishing Co., 1971.
3. Missett, P. A.: Identification of yeastlike fungi. Canad. J. Med. Techn., *34*: 63–79, 1972.
4. Emmons, C. W., Binford, C. H., Utz, J. P. and Kwon-Chung, K. J.: *Medical Mycology*. 3rd ed. Philadelphia, Lea & Febiger, 1977.
5. Huppert, M. et al.: Rapid methods for identification of yeasts. J. Clin. Microbiol., 2: 21–34, 1975.

chapter 23

Parasitic Animals

23-1 BASIC PARASITOLOGY

Parasitology covers the area of biology that considers the phenomena associated with the dependence of one living organism on another. In the general sense, a *parasite* is any organism that lives at the expense of a host. A *host* is usually a larger organism that provides physical protection, nourishment, or both. As such, parasitology would cover much of bacteriology and mycology, all of virology, the study of the protista, metazoa, many arthropods and some of the annelida. Since we have already discussed the bacteria, viruses, fungi, and yeasts, we shall limit ourselves to the other groups of organisms listed, and of these we shall consider only those parasitic animals that commonly cause disease in man.

In order to obtain a better understanding of parasitism, however, let us digress a little. One of the most important concerns of any organism centers around its search for food. To have this basic need satisfied, the energies of other living things, whether they be animal or vegetable, must be exploited. In the broad sense, therefore, all animals are parasitic and become parasitized at one stage or another.

We must differentiate among various forms of association between different animals, such as symbiosis, commensalism, mutualism, and parasitism. Symbiosis simply means the living together of two different species; the associates are called symbionts. In commensalism, one of the species benefits from the other without causing harm to its benefactor; the benefactor is usually the larger organism and is commonly called the host. In mutualism, both species derive benefits from their association. In parasitism, only one of the species benefits at the expense of the other species.

Relatively few parasites can reproduce, mature, and reproduce again within the confines of one host. Some parasites have become so dependent on a particular host that they seem able to live only within or on that host. Examples of these are *Giardia lamblia*, an intestinal flagellate restricted to man, and *Pediculus humanus*, the human body louse. Parasites so restricted, of course, can be eradicated theoretically by treating all humans affected by them. Most parasites, however, are not as restrictive as that, and they occur in various animals as well as in man. In fact, man is often only an incidental host while domestic or wild animals serve as the main reservoirs.

Parasites that cannot survive outside their host are called *obligate parasites*; those that can live outside the host are called *facultative parasites*. Some parasites have rather intricate life cycles and may depend on more than one host to reach maturity. Good examples of these are the cestodes, of which *Dibothriocephalus latus*, the fish tapeworm, needs to develop in four stages in three different hosts. When bacteria invade certain areas of the body, we speak of an infection. We also speak of infections when larger parasites enter the body. Certain parasites, however, do not enter the body but feed on the body; such invasions are referred to as *infestations* (ticks and leeches).

Man may become infected or infested by parasites from a number of sources:

a. *Soil or water* may be contaminated with excreta containing viable worms, intermediate larvae, eggs, or cysts.
b. *Food* often contains parasites in immature infective stages (ova, cysts, and larvae) or adult worms (beef, pork, and fish tapeworms, trichinae).

    c. *Blood sucking or biting insects* may transmit or transfer malaria parasites, viruses, rickettsiae, and trypanosomes.

    d. *Other individuals*, either directly or indirectly, may transmit parasites (lice).

    e. Some parasites lay eggs in the perianal region, and infected individuals frequently reinfect themselves from this source. Such infections are called *autoinfections*.

The most common portals of entry, in descending order, are the mouth, the skin, and percutaneously from biting insects, the blood.

It is obviously difficult for allied health professionals to learn much about parasitology. Their course of study is usually far too comprehensive to dwell in detail on many issues that would be of interest if not of importance. However, it is also difficult to recognize and differentiate the various pathogenic parasites without having some basic understanding of their structure and function. The remainder of this chapter is devoted to a general classification of the parasites and a comparison of the common pathogens within each major group. We shall mainly discuss structures that aid in diagnosis, and will not necessarily relate these structures to their function. Thus, the reader must realize that in most instances descriptions of individual organisms and their importance to medicine is far from complete. For further information, one may consult the bibliography.

23-2 CLASSIFICATION OF PARASITIC ANIMALS

In the following abridged classification, only organisms commonly associated with man are represented.

Kingdom Protista. Comprised of all unicellular organisms, including bacteria, algae, slime molds, fungi, protozoa, and ciliates.

    Phylum Protozoa. Comprised of all unicellular animals, except Ciliophora.

      Superclass Sarcodina. Move by means of pseudopods, includes the amebas

Genera:	*Entamoeba*	Species:	*histolytica*
			coli
	Endolimax		*nana*
	Iodamoeba		*bütschlii*

      Superclass Mastigophora. Move by means of flagella.

Genera:	*Trichomonas*	Species:	*vaginalis*
			tenax
	Pentatrichomonas		*hominis*
	Dientamoeba		*fragilis*
	Giardia		*lamblia*

Chilomastix	*mesnili*
Trypanosoma	*gambienese*
	rhodesiense
	cruzi
Leishmania	*donovani*
	tropica
	braziliensis
	mexicana

Class Sporozoa. Lack specific means of locomotion.

Genera: *Plasmodium*   Species: *vivax*

falciparum

malariae

ovale

Toxoplasma   *gondii*

Isospora   *hominis*

Phylum Ciliophora. Move by means of cilia.

Genera: *Balantidium*   Species: *coli*

Kingdom Metazoa. Comprised of all multicellular animals.

Phylum Platyhelminthes. The flat worms.

Subclass Cestoda. The tapeworms. (Consist of a scolex, "neck," and a chain of body units called proglottids. No body cavity or digestive tract; hermaphrodites.)

Genera: *Dibothriocephalus*   Species: *latus*

Taenia   *solium*

Taeniarhynchus   *saginatus*

Hymenolepis   *nana*

Echinococcus   *granulosus*

Class Trematoda. The flukes. (No body cavity; incomplete digestive tract; hermaphroditic or diecious.)

Genera: *Schistosoma*   Species: *japonicum*

mansoni

haematobium

Paragonimus   *westermani*

Opisthorchis   *sinensis*

Fasciola   *hepatica*

Phylum Nematoda. The round worms. (Elongated, with a cylindrical body; a complete digestive tract, and a hollow body cavity.)

Genera: *Ascaris*   Species: *lumbricoides*

Enterobius   *vermicularis*

Necator   *americanus*

Ancylostoma   *duodenale*

Wuchereria   *bancrofti*

Strongyloides	*stercoralis*
Trichinella	*spiralis*
Trichuris	*trichiura*

Phylum Annelida. The segmented worms.

   Hirudinea; the leeches. These are the only parasites of this phylum.

Phylum Arthropoda; the bilaterally symmetrical, segmented invertebrates. These are more commonly known as the insects. Insects play a large part in the transmission of infectious diseases, in which case they are known as *vectors*. Some insects parasitize man or animals: mites— *Sarcoptes scabiei*—are the cause of scabies; lice— *Pediculus humanus* var. *capitis*, the head louse, *Pediculus humanus* var. *corporis*, the body louse, and *Phthirus pubis*, the crab louse; fleas—*Pulex irritans*, the human flea; bedbugs—*Cimex lectularius*—which are not true parasites.

23-3 PROTOZOA AND CILIOPHORA

When speaking of these organisms, we shall refer to the group in general as protozoa, except in those instances in which the ciliophora differ significantly.

The human parasites of this group vary in size from 5 μm *(Entamoeba histolytica)* to 150 μm *(Balantidium coli)* in diameter. Their shape depends on whether or not the surface layer is firm. When it is not they may take different shapes. The cytoplasm may be divided into ectoplasm and endoplasm. *Ectoplasm* is any conspicuously differentiated outer layer of cytoplasm. The *endoplasm* is the usually more fluid cytoplasm surrounding the nucleus.

The nucleus may be compact, in which case the dense chromatin fills the entire nucleus (see Fig. 23–1), or vesicular, with the chromatin appearing as beads or clumps along the nuclear membrane. In the latter type of nucleus, the endosome, or karyosome (denser nuclear material), may be located centrally (see Fig. 23–2), or eccentrically (see Fig. 23–3).

The protozoa move by pseudopods, flagella, or undulating membranes; the ciliophora move by means of cilia. The flagella originate from a blepharoblast, a basal granule visible at the "root" of the flagella. An undulating membrane may also allow some mobility and is responsible for the rotating motion of some *Trichomonas* species (see Fig. 23–4).

Protozoa may ingest food by phagocytosis, by diffusion, or through a cytostome—a primitive mouthlike structure (see Fig.

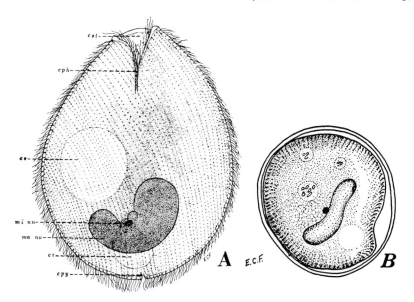

Fig. 23–1. *Balantidium coli.* A, trophozoite; *B*, cyst. × 750. *cph*, cytopharynx, within cytostome; *cpy*, cytopyge; *cst*, cytostome; *cv*, contractile or pulsating vacuole; *ma nu*, macronucleus; *mi nu*, micronucleus. *A*, *B*, from Faust, E. C., Beaver, P. C., and Jung, R.: *Animal Agents and Vectors of Human Disease.* ed. 4. Philadelphia, Lea & Febiger, 1975.

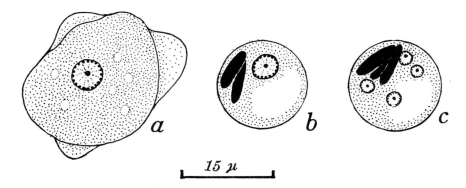

Fig. 23–2. *Entamoeba histolytica:* *a*, trophozoite; *b*, immature cyst; *c*, ripe cyst. × 1600. (From Faust, E. C., Beaver, P. C., and Jung, R.: *Animal Agents and Vectors of Human Disease.* ed. 4. Philadelphia, Lea & Febiger, 1975.)

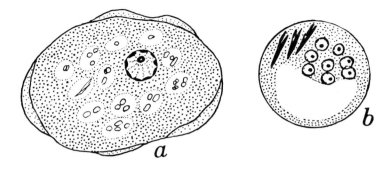

Fig. 23–3. *Entamoeba coli. a,* trophozoite, *b,* ripe cyst. × 1600. (From Faust, E. C., Beaver, P. C., and Jung, R.: *Animal Agents and Vectors of Human Disease.* ed. 4. Philadelphia, Lea & Febiger, 1975.)

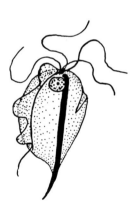

Fig. 23–4. *Trichomonas hominis* from a diarrheic stool. × 1600. (From Faust, E. C., Beaver, P. C., and Jung, R.: *Animal Agents and Vectors of Human Disease.* ed. 4. Philadelphia, Lea & Febiger, 1975.)

23–1). Excretion may also be accomplished by diffusion, by expulsion from contractile vacuoles, or even by expulsion from a cytopyge, which is a primitive anus (see Fig. 23–1).

In keeping with the nature of parasites, protozoan nutrient requirements are complex, requiring highly organized organic compounds, such as amino acids, vitamins, and carbohydrates, as well as the array of inorganic and organic substances required by most cells. Protozoa may ingest bacteria, red blood cells, tissue elements, and the like.

Most protozoa are able to transform into cysts from trophozoites. *Trophozoites* are the true motile and feeding forms. Under adverse conditions, the trophozoites enter into a precystic

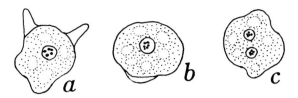

Fig. 23–5. *Dientamoeba fragilis, a, b, c,* trophozoites. × 1600. (From Faust, E. C., Beaver, P. C., and Jung, R.: *Animal Agents and Vectors of Human Disease.* ed. 4. Philadelphia, Lea & Febiger, 1975.)

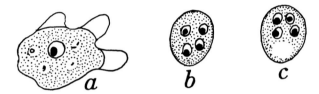

Fig. 23–6. *Endolimax nana. a,* trophozoite; *b, c,* ripe cysts. × 1600. (From Faust, E. C., Beaver, P. C., and Jung, R.: *Animal Agents and Vectors of Human Disease.* ed. 4. Philadelphia, Lea & Febiger, 1975.)

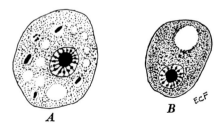

Fig. 23–7. *Iodamoeba buetschlii. A,* trophozoite; *B,* cyst. In the nucleus the distinctive pattern of the chromatin granules radiating out from the karyosome is characteristic in both stages of this ameba. The dense glycogen vacuole shown in the cyst may also be sometimes observed in the trophozoite. × 1500. Iron-hematoxylin stain of Schaudinn-fixed fecal film. (From Faust, E. C., Beaver, P. C., and Jung, R.: *Animal Agents and Vectors of Human Disease.* ed. 4. Philadelphia, Lea & Febiger, 1975.)

form and develop into nonmotile cysts. The *cysts* are protected by a cyst wall much the same as are bacterial spores. The process of cyst formation is called *encystation*. The ultimate "hatching" of a motile metacystic trophozoite from a cyst is called excystation.

Depending on the organism and on the specimen under study, the laboratorian may identify protozoan infections by finding either the trophozoites or the cysts. Some protozoa encyst as a necessary function of the life cycle *(Entamoeba)*. Specimens from patients infected with these organisms usually reveal both trophozoite and cyst forms.

Trophozoites are more sensitive to the environment outside the host than are most bacteria, and will survive for only short periods of time outside a suitable host. The cystic forms likewise are not as resistant to heat as bacterial spores. Concentrations of phenol, formalin and chlorine that kill vegetative bacteria will also kill cysts, but more time is required. Many types of protozoa (sporozoa excluded) have been cultured on artificial media. Irregular trials at culturing clinical material should not be attempted, since the techniques involved are very exacting. Table 23–1 and Figures 23–1 to 23–11 should allow the student to become familiar with the more common pathogenic protozoa. One should realize, however, that many specimens, particularly stool specimens, may contain artifacts that might be mistaken for cysts, trophozoites, ova or even worms. Several such artifacts are presented in Fig. 23–12.

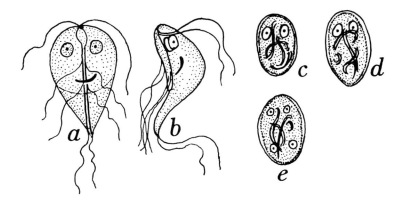

Fig. 23–8. *Giardia lamblia. a*, trophozoite, ventral view, and *b*, profile view; *c, d*, immature cysts; *e*, mature cyst. × 1600. (From Faust, E. C., Beaver, P. C., and Jung, R.: *Animal Agents and Vectors of Human Disease.* ed. 4. Philadelphia, Lea & Febiger, 1975.)

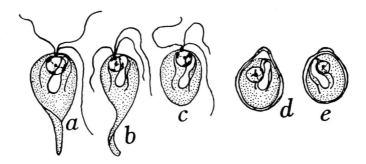

Fig. 23–9. *Chilomastix mesnili, a, b, c,* trophozoites; *d, e,* cysts. × 1600. (From Faust, E. C., Beaver, P. C., and Jung, R.: *Animal Agents and Vectors of Human Disease.* ed. 4. Philadelphia, Lea & Febiger, 1975.)

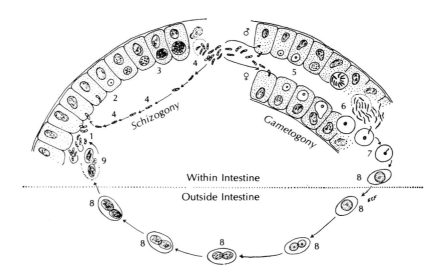

Fig. 23–10. Diagram illustrating the life cycle of *Isospora belli,* coccidian parasite of man. *1,* sporozoites entering intestinal mucosa; *2,* young trophozoite in mucosal cell; *3,* development of schizont; *4,* merozoites freed of parent membrane; *5,* gametocytes, male (above) and female (below), developed from merozoites; *6,* gametes; *7,* union of gametes to form zygote; *8,* maturing stages of oocyst; *9,* sporocysts freed of oocyst wall. (From Faust, E. C., Beaver, P. C., and Jung, R.: *Animal Agents and Vectors of Human Disease.* ed. 4. Philadelphia, Lea & Febiger, 1975.)

Entamoeba histolytica and *Giardia lamblia* are the most clinically important intestinal protozoa; they are found frequently in liquid stools. *Entamoeba coli, Dientamoeba, Endolimax, Balantidium coli, Iodamoeba, Chilomastix* and *Isospora* are detected less frequently, and may be found in formed and liquid stools. *Trichomonas vaginalis* is often associated with vaginitis or urethritis and it may be found in vaginal or urethral secretions. *T. hominis* is nonpathogenic. *Isospora* and *Giardia* may be present in smaller numbers and concentration methods may be necessary (see zinc-sulfate flotation and formalin-ether centrifugation tests, p. 324).

Trypanosoma may be seen in peripheral blood smears or in the cerebral spinal fluid of patients suffering from "sleeping sickness" or other syndromes. Most trypanosomiases are almost exclusively restricted to some area of central Africa. *Trypanosoma cruzi* is the cause of Chagas' disease, which is found in tropical and subtropical regions of continental America. Chronic Chagas' disease frequently causes fatal damage to heart muscle.

Evidence of *Leishmania* may be found cutaneously, or in spleen and liver biopsies. *L. donovani* has been cultured from the blood. *Leishmania* is transmitted by the "sandfly," and therefore it is restricted geographically.

Plasmodium species cause malaria; they are transmitted to their hosts by mosquitoes. Malaria results from plasmodial infection of the parenchymal and red blood cells. Diagnosis may be made from bloodsmears stained by Giemsa's method.

Toxoplasma gondii causes toxoplasmosis, a disease that is particularly destructive to parenchymal and reticuloendothelial cells. Toxoplasms are frequently found in cats and they spread as oospores from fecal litter in soils or other media. The infection can be transmitted transplacentally, which may result in serious abnormalities of the newborn. Blood smears stained by Giemsa's method may reveal the organisms. Two serologic tests, the passive hemagglutination test and the indirect fluorescence antibody test, are commonly employed in the diagnosis and control of toxoplasmosis.

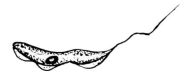

Fig. 23–11. Trypanosome.

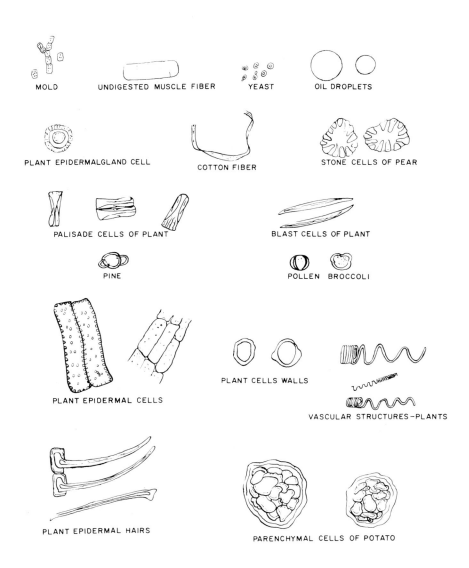

Fig. 23–12. Some common artifacts found in feces.

Table 23–1. Characteristics of some common Protozoa

		Entamoeba histolytica	Entamoeba coli	Endolimax nana	Iodamoeba bütschlii	Dientamoeba fragilis
T R O P H O Z O I T E S	Size (in μm)	20–40 average 25	15–50 average 35	6–15 average 8	8–20 average 10	5–15 average 12
	Inclusions	Erythrocytes	Bacteria	Bacteria	Bacteria	Bacteria
	Karyosome	Small, central	Large, eccentric	Large, central or eccentric	Large and granular, central or eccentric	4–8 chromatin granules
	Motility	Very active	Sluggish	Sluggish	Sluggish	Active
C Y S T S	Size (in μm)	5–20 average 10	10–30 average 15	6–15 average 8	6–20 average 10	No cysts
	Shape	Rounded	Rounded	Rounded, oval or ellipsoid	Odd-shaped	No cysts
	Nuclei	1–4	1–8	1–4	1	No cysts

23-4 TREMATODA

The parasitic flukes have the most complex life cycles of all the helminths. Some members change into six different forms between the ovum stage and maturity.

The schistosomes are known as the blood flukes, but the ova of *Schistosoma japonicum* and *S. mansoni* are usually found in the feces. Ova of *S. haematobium* are found more frequently in the urine, but may also appear in the feces. The ova are distinct from one another. *S. mansoni* ova bear a prominent lateral spine; those of *S. haematobium*, a distinct terminal spine; and the ova of *S. japonicum*, a small terminal spine. Size and shape are additional diagnostic features (see Fig. 23–13).

Paragonimus westermani, the lung fluke, has typical ova, which may be coughed up in the sputum (see Fig. 23–13).

The liver flukes, *Opisthorchis (Clonorchis) sinensis* and *Fasciola hepatica*, are known as the Chinese and sheep liver flukes respectively. Their distribution, however, does extend to other species and geographic areas. Their ova are quite distinct and may be found in feces (see Fig. 23–13).

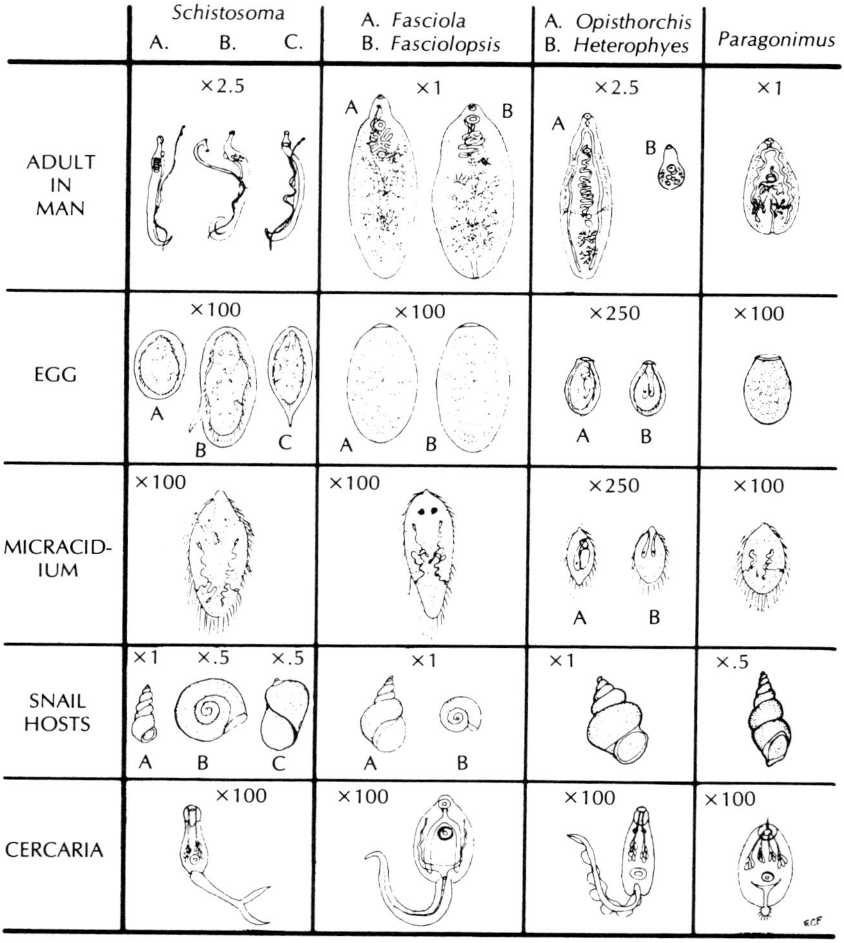

	Schistosoma A. B. C.	A. Fasciola B. Fasciolopsis	A. Opisthorchis B. Heterophyes	Paragonimus
ADULT IN MAN	×2.5	×1	×2.5	×1
EGG	×100	×100	×250	×100
MICRACID-IUM	×100	×100	×250	×100
SNAIL HOSTS	×1 ×.5 ×.5	×1	×1	×.5
CERCARIA	×100	×100	×100	×100

Fig. 23–13. Important stages and differential characteristics of the common digenetic trematodes that parasitize man. Under Schistosoma, A represents *Schistosoma japonicum;* B, *S. mansoni* and C, *S. haematobium.* (From Faust, E. C., Beaver, P. C., and Jung, R.: *Animal Agents and Vectors of Human Disease.* ed. 4. Philadelphia, Lea & Febiger, 1975.)

23-5 CESTODA

The tapeworms are composed of a definite head, the scolex, and a body, the strobila. The body is divided into segments called proglottids. The scolex is small, measuring about 2 mm or less. New proglottids are produced immediately below the scolex, and as they form they displace the previously formed segments. As the segments move down the strobila, they mature until they become filled with eggs (gravid) and are shed intact or disintegrate. (Proglottids of *Dibothriocephalus latus* shed eggs by way of a uterine pore.) So, in one complete worm, all stages of proglottid development are present.

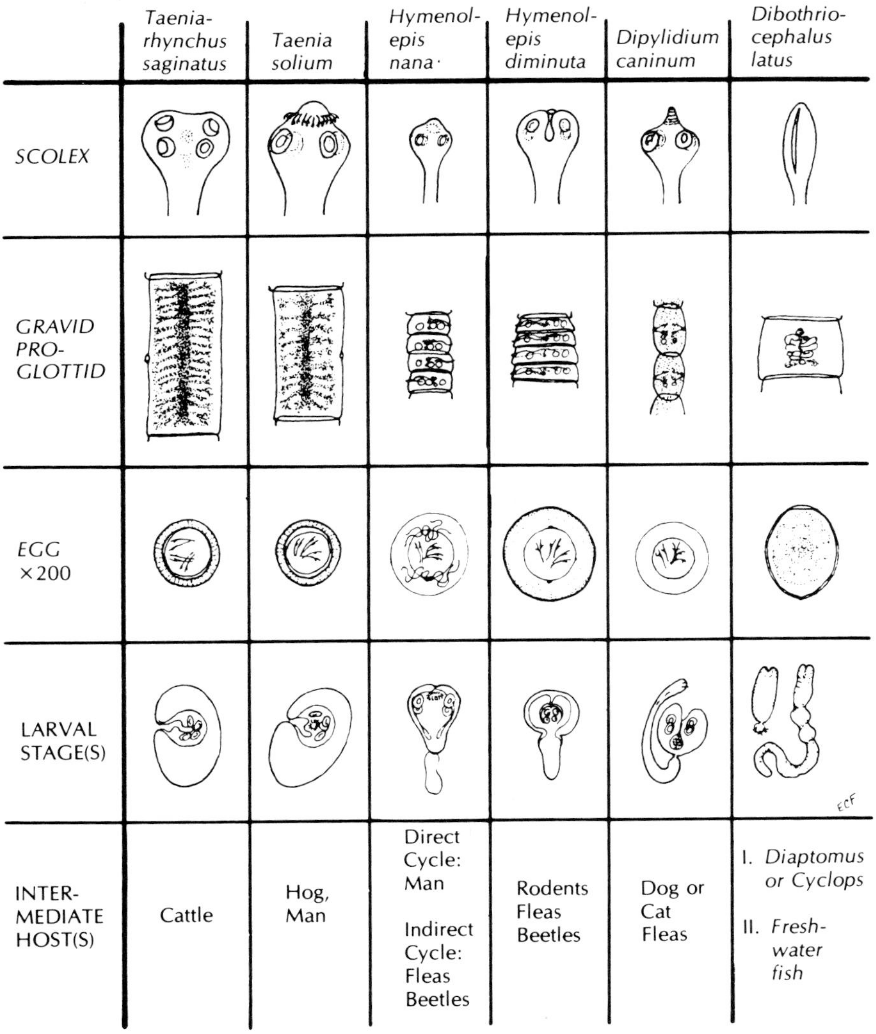

	Taenia-rhynchus saginatus	Taenia solium	Hymenol-epis nana·	Hymenol-epis diminuta	Dipylidium caninum	Dibothrio-cephalus latus
SCOLEX						
GRAVID PRO-GLOTTID						
EGG ×200						
LARVAL STAGE(S)						
INTER-MEDIATE HOST(S)	Cattle	Hog, Man	Direct Cycle: Man Indirect Cycle: Fleas Beetles	Rodents Fleas Beetles	Dog or Cat Fleas	I. *Diaptomus or Cyclops* II. *Fresh-water fish*

Fig. 23–14. Important stages and diagnostic characteristics of the tapeworms that commonly parasitize man. (From Faust, E. C., Beaver, P. C., and Jung, R.: *Animal Agents and Vectors of Human Disease.* ed. 4. Philadelphia, Lea & Febiger, 1975.)

Each segment is covered by an elastic cuticle and each segment has a muscular system that allows the segment to move in a bowlike manner. Two nerve trunks commence in the scolex and run over the entire length of the worm.

The main activity of the tapeworm is the production of numerous eggs. For this purpose, each proglottid is endowed with male and female reproductive organs. Following fertilization, all reproductive organs, except the uterus, degenerate in all tapeworms except *D. latus*. This fact is useful in diagnosis, because by examining the lower proglottids, we can differentiate species of tapeworms on the basis of the shape of the uterus (see Fig. 23–14).

The life cycles of the cestodes are complex. As many as four different hosts may be required to complete a full cycle. Man may serve as a definitive or an intermediate host, or as both. To control diseases caused by cestodes, use can be made of their complex life cycles. The more complex the cycle, the greater the options available for control measures.

Most humans who carry tapeworms tolerate them reasonably well. Symptoms may range from mild to severe nutrional deficiencies to intestinal obstruction, which occurs rarely. Anthelmintic drugs are available for therapy, and are indicated when an infection has been diagnosed. Diagnosis is based on detection of ova or segments (see Fig. 23–14).

23-6 NEMATODA

Nematodes are cylindrical, threadlike, nonsegmented roundworms. They have a digestive tract complete with "mouth" and "anus." They are also bisexual. None of the nematode worms have a uniform thickness. They taper at the head or the tail. When at rest, some are straight and others have a natural curve, spiral, or hook. The males of most species have a pronounced curve at the posterior end, near the copulatory organ, the spicule.

The body covering is a tough, noncellular cuticle, usually marked by transverse striations. Some intestinal roundworms attach themselves to the villi with their "mouth" and ingest blood and mucosal cells *(Ancylostoma* and *Necator)*. Others penetrate the intestinal wall *(Strongyloides)* or "weave" themselves into the mucosa of the intestinal wall *(Trichuris)*. Infection by *Enterobius*, *Trichuris* and *Ascaris* usually occurs by ingesting infective ova. *Enterobius* is often sustained by autoinfection. This organism deposits eggs at night in the perianal or perineal regions, which become itchy. Scratching may result in transferring eggs to the mouth. *Enterobius* is quite common in North American children.

Trichuris trichiura, whipworms, live primarily in the cecum and may remain there for years. Symptoms may range from mild discomfort and weight loss to bloody diarrhea and emaciation. Ova are produced in large numbers, shed in feces, and hatched in moist, warm environments. Infection is by ingestion of mature eggs.

The ova of *Ascaris* hatch intestinally, but the larvae must enter the circulation through the mucosal wall in order to reach the lungs, where they develop further. They then break into the alveolar spaces, move up the bronchial tree, and are finally swallowed to develop into adult worms in the alimentary canal. It is not uncommon for adult *Ascaris* worms to be brought up in vomit.

Trichinella spiralis is transmitted by ingestion of larvae encysted in the skeletal muscles of uncooked, infected meat (pork and bear meat). Diagnosis is based on detection of the encysted larvae or serologic tests.

The two hookworms, *Ancylostoma duodenale* and *Necator americanus* cannot be differentiated by their ova. Both enter the body through the skin, but the ova require some time in the soil before maturation can occur.

Strongyloides stercoralis is similar to the hookworms in that it enters the body by way of the skin. The larvae reach the lungs through the circulatory system, move through the alveolae to the bronchial tree, are swallowed, and mature in the small intestine. Eggs are deposited into the mucosa and develop rapidly. The larvae are passed in the feces, so that ova in stools are rare. Figure 23–15 presents the chief identification features of commonly found intestinal nematodes.

23-7 LABORATORY DIAGNOSIS

Generally, two types of laboratories examine specimens for parasites: the clinical laboratory in a hospital or doctor's clinic, and the public health laboratory. In the clinical laboratory, fresh samples may be examined for trophozoites, ova, and cysts. Public health laboratories are usually located at a distance from the patient, and samples to be sent there are usually unsuitable for examination of trophozoites by the time they arrive. To preserve larvae, ova, and cysts and to render the specimen less hazardous in transport, specimens to be mailed to a distant laboratory may be preserved in 10% formalin. Specimens may be collected in any sterile, clean, widemouthed container. A disposable waxed cardboard container with an overlapping, tight-fitting lid is most suitable. These not only ensure a container that never has been used before but also permit handling and simple decontamination

Name	Enterobius vermicularis (pinworm)	Trichuris trichiura (whipworm)	Ascaris lumbricoides (large roundworm)	Trichinella spiralis (trichina worm)	Necator, Ancylostoma (hookworm)	Strongyloides stercoralis (threadworm)	Wuchereria, Brugia, Loa, Onchocerca et al. (Filariae)
Adults, size ♂	2–5 × 0.1–0.2 mm.	30–45 mm. long	15–31 cm × 2–4 mm.	1.4–1.6 mm. × 40–60 μm	7–11 × 0.3–0.5 mm.	lacking	19–45 mm. × 60–350 μm
♀	8–12 × 0.3–0.5 mm.	35–50 mm. long	20–35 cm. × 3–6 mm.	3.0–3.5 mm. × 60–90 μm	9–13 × 0.4–0.6 mm.	2.2 mm. × 30–74 μm	33–100 mm. × 120–500 μm
Usual location	Free or superficially attached to mucosa of cecum, appendix and colon	Attached to mucosa of cecum, appendix, colon and rectum	Free in small intestine	Females in mucosa of small intestine	Attached to mucosa of small intestine	Females in mucosa of small and large intestines	Lymph channels and intercellular spaces of visceral and somatic tissues
Stage of progeny leaving human host	Almost fully embryonated egg	Unembryonated egg	Unembryonated egg	None; larva in muscles	Egg in early stage of cleavage	Rhabditoid larva	Microfilaria (pre-larva)

Required development to stage infective for man	Few hours at anus or on clothing, larva in egg	2–3 weeks minimum in soil, larva in egg	2–3 weeks in soil, 2nd larval stage in egg	3 weeks in muscles of pig or other host, advanced larva in fibrous capsule	6 days or more in soil, free 3rd-stage (filariform) larva	One day in feces or soil, free 3rd-stage (filariform) larva	1–2 weeks in blood-sucking arthropod, 3rd-stage (filariform) larva
Usual method of human exposure	Taken into mouth and swallowed	Taken into mouth and swallowed	Taken into mouth and swallowed	Ingested in inadequately processed meat	Penetration of skin or by ingestion (*Ancylostoma*)	Penetration of skin	Skin invasion when infected arthropod takes blood meal
Migration in human body and development to adult stage	Egg hatches in intestine; larva migrates to cecum and matures in 15–28 days	Egg hatches in intestine; larva migrates to cecum, attaches to mucosa and matures in 10–12 weeks	Egg hatches in intestine; larva migrates to lungs, develops 1–2 weeks, molts, returns to intestine and matures in 8 to 10 weeks	Excysted larvae invade mucosa of upper small intestine and mature in 5–7 days	Larva in skin migrates via blood vessels to lungs, develops 1–2 weeks, molts, then migrates to small intestine via trachea, becomes attached and matures in 6 or 7 weeks (*Necator*), or without development in lungs matures in 5–6 weeks (*Ancylostoma*)	Larvae in skin enter blood vessels, migrate to small intestine via lungs; enter mucosa and mature in 4 weeks or less	Larvae in skin migrate to sites of adult predilection; mature in several months to 1 year

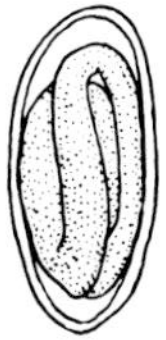

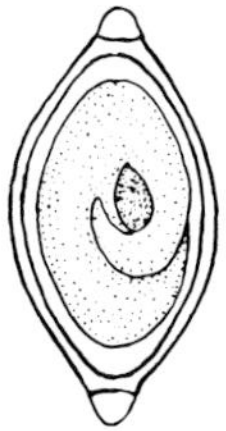

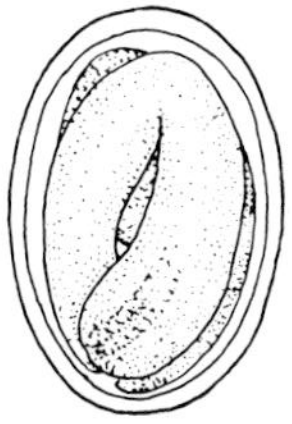

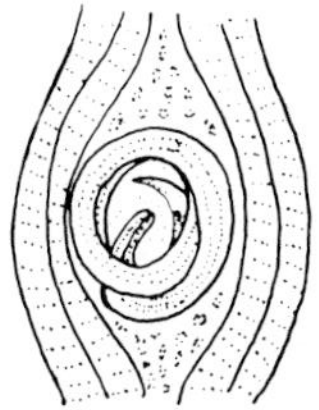

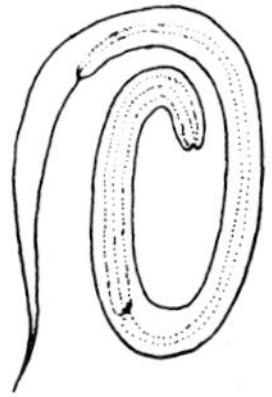

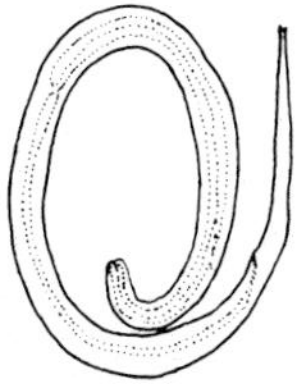

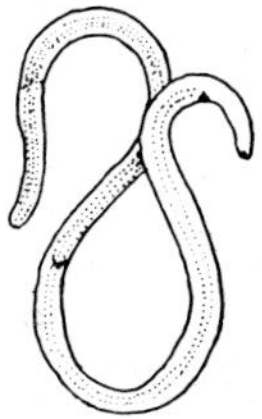

Fig. 23–15. Stages in the life cycles of the common roundworms of man. (From Faust, E.C., Beaver, P.C., and Jung, R.: Animal Agents and Vectors of Human Disease. ed. 4. Philadelphia, Lea & Febiger, 1975.)

323

by incineration. For mailing specimens, a better choice is a screw-capped glass container filled one-third with feces.

For simple, direct examination of stool specimens, use an applicator stick to emulsify enough stool in saline or water to obtain a murky suspension. Drop a coverglass over this preparation, ensure that the slide is dry at the bottom, and examine under low and hi dry magnifications.

Cysts and eggs can often be seen best if D'Antoni's iodine is used instead of saline or water. Three preparations of three different areas of the specimen should be examined and all the slides screened carefully before reporting that no trophozoites, ova or cysts have been seen.

Several methods of concentrating the ova and cysts present in a specimen have been developed. The zinc-sulfate flotation test and the formalin-ether centrifugation test are probably the most widely used tests. The latter is the only method recommended to diagnose schistosome eggs, but remember that ether is potentially dangerous, and requires a well-vented area removed from sparks or open flames.

FORMALIN-ETHER CENTRIFUGATION TEST

1. Fill a conical-tipped 15-ml centrifuge tube half-full with tap water.
2. Place at least 2 ml of feces in the water and mix well using a wooden applicator. Fill the tube to ½ inch of the rim with additional water and mix well again.
3. Centrifuge at 1500 rpm for 2 mintues. Decant the supernatant fluid.
4. Add 10 percent formalin to the sediment until the tube is one-half full, mix thoroughly, and allow to stand for five minutes.
5. Add about 3 ml of ether (until tube is three-fourths full); stopper the tube (or use thumb or Parafilm) and shake vigorously; remove the stopper or thumb carefully to prevent spraying of material due to pressure within the tube.
6. Centrifuge at 1500 rpm for about two minutes. Four layers should result: a small amount of sediment containing most of the parasites; a layer of formalin; a plug of fecal debris on top of the formalin; and a topmost layer of ether.
7. Free the top plug of debris from the sides of the tube by ringing with an applicator stock and carefully decant the top three layers.

8. Mix the remaining sediment with the small amount of fluid that drains back from the sides of the tube. Drag sediment from tube onto a fecal slide by means of applicators. Prepare iodine mount of the sediment for microscopic examination.

ZINC-SULFATE FLOTATION TEST

1. Mix one part of formed stool with ten parts warm water in a conical-tipped 15-ml centrifuge tube.
2. Strain 10 ml of this mixture through one layer of wet cheesecloth into a paper cup; crimp the cup and pour the suspension back into the same centrifuge tube. Fill with tap water.
3. Centrifuge this filtrate for 45 to 60 seconds at 2500 rpm.
4. Pour off the supernatant into a disinfectant, resuspend the sediment in tap water, and centrifuge again; repeat until the supernatant is clear.
5. To the final sediment add 3 to 4 ml of 33% zinc sulfate solution (specific gravity 1.180). Mix thoroughly and then fill the tube to within ½ inch of the rim with the same solution.
6. Centrifuge again for at least 90 seconds.
7. Transfer material from the surface of the liquid to a glass slide by means of a loop, stir in a drop of dilute iodine solution, add a cover glass, and examine.

FURTHER READING

1. Beck, J. W., and Davies, J. E.: *Medical Parasitology*. St. Louis, C. V. Mosby Company, 1976.
2. Spencer, F. M. and Monroe, L. S.: *The Color Atlas of Intestinal Parasites*. 2nd ed. Springfield, Ill., Charles C Thomas, 1975.
3. Faust, E. C., Beaver, P. C., and Jung, R. C.: *Animal Agents and Vectors of Human Disease*. 4th ed. Philadelphia, Lea & Febiger, 1975.
4. Noble, E. R., and Noble, G. A.: *Parasitology*. 4th ed. Philadelphia, Lea & Febiger, 1976.

Part III
DIAGNOSTIC
MICROBIOLOGY

chapter 24

Specimen Collection
and Processing

24-1 GENERAL POINTS OF NOTE

The findings of any analytic laboratory can only be as good as the specimens referred to it. Microbiologic analysis, particularly, depends largely on the quality of the specimens analyzed. When specimens are improperly collected, some organisms may be introduced to the specimens other than those originally present at the site of collection. These extraneous organisms, or contaminants, cannot be distinguished from those that were present initially. Therefore, the introduced organisms (contaminants) also form part of the analytic material and, hence, part of the final report. Moreover, contaminants usually grow better on most routine media, and consequently outgrow, mask, or even completely obliterate the few pathogens that may have been present in the specimen before contamination.

From the foregoing it should be obvious that much care must be taken in the collection, transport, and handling of specimens. In this chapter we discuss the more common types of specimen referred for microbial analysis, their proper collection, transport and storage, and their initial processing in the laboratory.

PROPER COLLECTION OF SPECIMENS

The specimen must be collected from the proper site at the proper time. This warrants some knowledge of anatomy, but more importantly, it entails a common sense approach and some tact. The proper time usually means before antibiotic treatment is initiated, although in some instances, it refers to a specific stage of the disease when isolation from a particular area may be most promising.

Tact and care should be exercised during specimen collection to prevent embarrassment or discomfort to the patient. The quality of the specimen improves considerably when the laboratory worker seeks the cooperation of both the patient and the nursing staff. The patient and the staff should be informed of any potential danger to themselves and to the specimen. When the patient or the nursing staff collects the specimen, emphasize the necessity for prompt submission.

The procedures used for collection must also prevent contamination. Specimens for microbiologic assay may be contaminated in two general ways:
a. biologically, by the introduction of extraneous organisms,
b. chemically, by the introduction of harmful or interfering chemicals.

As already mentioned, the specimen can be contaminated easily from on-lying areas (such as sputum contaminated with saliva). More often, however, the source of contamination is the specimen container. Containers for all specimens to be submitted for microbiologic analysis must be chemically and biologically sterile.

Chemical contamination may range from detergents and other cleansing products left in bedpans or urine bottles, to spices and vinegars remaining in an assorted array of bottles and jars used for specimen containers by ill-informed patients. Chemical contamination often results in destruction of the pathogens long before the specimen reaches the laboratory.

Extraneous organisms may be introduced to the specimen by anyone who handles it improperly. They may also be present in poorly cleaned, inadequately sterilized, or haphazardly stored specimen containers.

TRANSPORTATION OF SPECIMENS

Specimens should be submitted to the laboratory without delay and should be safeguarded during transport from heat, extreme cold and other damaging factors. If the specimen is to be transported over any distance, the mail is often the fastest means of transport. Postal regulations vary from country to country. In most countries, pathologic specimens must be identified by label as "pathologic specimens." In any event, the specimen must be safeguarded against breakage and leakage. Glass tubes should be securely stoppered, the stopper taped down with adhesive tape, the tube protected by cotton (to absorb moisture in the event that the tube breaks), the cotton-wrapped tube placed in a metal container, and the metal container placed in a cardboard mailing box. Complete sets of mailing containers are commercially available* and are usually supplied by regional public health laboratories. To ship delicate specimens over great distances, special containers that can control the temperature at 4°C or 37°C are commercially available.† These containers have an energy pack that can be activated by either freezing or heating; this energy pack will regulate the temperature within the container in which it is placed after activation. For relatively short distances (across town or within a hospital complex), a reliable, speedy dispatch service is particularly important.

Specimens kept for any great length of time may be unsatisfactory for two main reasons:

A. The pathogens that were initially present may no longer be viable and thus can no longer be isolated.

B. Fewer pathogens than nonpathogens may be present. Because most nonpathogens outgrow pathogens, delay will decrease the chances of isolating pathogens from increasing numbers of nonpathogens.

When quantitative measures are to be undertaken, any delay interferes with accurate counts that represent the flora present in the specimen at the time of collection.

IDENTIFICATION OF SPECIMENS

The specimen must be readily identifiable from an attached label and accompanied by a suitable requisition. The label should identify the specimen by the patient's name and the source of the

---

* Arthur H. Thomas Co., Philadelphia, Pa.
†Royal Industries, Santa Ana, California.

specimen (throat, wound or rectal swab). In addition, the requisition should give the doctor's name and address, the date and time of collection, and the examination requested. Many laboratories design their own requisitions. A well-designed requisition form can serve as a laboratory worksheet, a final report, a file report and, of course, a request for a single or a series of test procedures.

24-2 DIFFERENT TYPES OF SPECIMENS

Each particular type of specimen requires specific care in collection, handling and processing. In this section, we discuss some pertinent points for each of the more common types of specimen.

BLOOD

The blood is probably the single most important specimen to be submitted for microbiologic assay. Organisms isolated from blood are always significant. Therefore, extreme care must be taken not to introduce any organisms either by venipuncture or by manipulation of the specimen afterwards.

To obtain a blood specimen, carefully cleanse the skin and then treat it with a 3.5% tincture of iodine or a 70% solution of ethanol. Allow the alcohol to dry well, so as not to introduce any into the needle and hence into the specimen. Furthermore, some workers often forget that once the skin is disinfected, the area from which the blood is to be taken should be kept "sterile." Some technologists dutifully cleanse and disinfect the skin, only to "feel" the vein before inserting the needle.

The best chances for isolation are obtained when about 10 ml of blood are collected directly into a blood culture bottle that contains a suitable medium.*

Some anticoagulants have a bactericidal or bacteristatic effect. When whole blood is collected, either 3 ml of a 2% sodium citrate solution or 1 mg of heparin per 10 ml of blood is recommended. The enzyme EDTA is definitely disqualified as an anticoagulant for blood to be cultured.

Because whole blood breaks down rapidly and then becomes even more effective as an antibacterial agent, prompt transport to the laboratory and immediate inoculation into trypticase soy, thio-

---

* Satisfactory blood collecting kits are available from: Difco Laboratories, Detroit, Mich.; Bioquest, B.B.L. Division, Cockeysville, Md.; Hyland Laboratories, Costa Mesa, California; and others.

glycolate broths, or other suitable media is absolutely essential. More recently, the addition of sodium polyanethol-sulfonate (Liquoid) or sodium fluoride to the blood culture medium has been advocated. These agents act as anticoagulants as well as neutralize the antibacterial activity of the blood.

CEREBROSPINAL FLUID

Like blood, the spinal fluid is normally sterile. Once collected, the spinal fluid must be cultured immediately unless it is to be examined for viruses, in which case it may be frozen and kept at −20°C. The collection of cerebrospinal fluid is obviously a medical task.

URINE

From male patients, a clean-catch midstream urine specimen collected in a sterile bottle is usually satisfactory. From female patients, it is recommended that specimens be obtained by catheterization.

Since urine is a reasonably good growth medium for many bacteria found in the urinary tract, prompt submission and processing are again mandatory. If the specimen cannot be processed immediately, it must be kept between 4° and 10°C.

If urine specimens cannot be processed immediately, or if the laboratory has only limited facilities for culturing specimens, urine culture systems are recommended. Urine culture systems are slides that have been coated with two or more kinds of media. After the slides have been dipped into the urine sample, they are placed in the tube provided with the system and the entire system is incubated. The slide is examined for growth after 18 hours. Several satisfactory systems are available,* and because each differs slightly from the other, package inserts must be consulted for interpretation of results.

THROAT SWABS

It is often forgotten that areas from which swabs are taken are inflamed and therefore irritable to the patient. In particular, the throat is sensitive, and a dry swab should never be used. The cotton tip on an applicator stick should be firm and cover the stick well.

---

*Bactercult, Wampole Laboratories, Stamford, Conn.; Bacteriuria, Bioquest, BBL Division, Cockeysville, Md.; Bactube, Roche Diagnostics, Nutley, N.J.; Dipinoc, Royal Scientific, Inc., Buffalo, N.Y.; Dipslide, Oxoid, Ltd., Basingstoke, Hants, England; Uricult, Orion Diagnostica, Helsinki, Finland (distributed by I.C.N. Life Sciences Group. Cleveland, Ohio); Uridip, Ortho Diagnostics, Raritan, N.J.

Flexible stick swabs* are better yet. Prior to using it, the swab should have been placed in a cotton-plugged tube and both tube and swab sterilized together. Remove the swab from its tube and moisten it slightly by dipping it into trypticase or another suitable broth.

Inform the patient beforehand about what you are trying to accomplish and make him comfortable. Ask the patient to open his mouth, and hold the tongue in place with a sterile tongue depressor. Without touching the buccal cavity, firmly insert the swab into the throat, ensuring good contact with the inflamed area. Withdraw the swab immediately, again being careful not to touch the inside of the mouth. Place the swab back into its original tube, label, and relay to the laboratory. If the swab cannot be plated out immediately, store at 4° to 10°C.

When diphtheria is suspected, collect two swabs, and inoculate one on Loeffler's medium at the bedside (see Chapter 12).

EAR SWABS

An infected ear is exquisitely painful. Ear swabs must be taken with the greatest of care. A flexible swab stick should always be used. My best advice is to let the physician do it.

WOUND SWABS

Wounds, too, can be rather painful. The best chances of isolation exist when specimens are obtained by swabbing the outer ridges as well as the deeper folds. The outer ridges usually yield such aerobes as *Staphylococcus, Escherichia coli* or *Pseudomonas*; the deeper folds might reveal anaerobes. The swabs from the deeper folds should immediately be placed into a tube of blood culture broth or a tube of prereduced medium,† which is best to preserve anaerobic bacteria.

GENITAL SWABS

From male patients, a swab may be taken from the inflamed urethra. For this purpose, a thin wire loop with a swab attached, the Calgiswab,* may be used.

From females, several different locations may be chosen, depending on the area of greatest inflammation. An experienced gynecologist is best prepared to obtain specimens from females. All genital swabs should be planted on warm (37°C) chocolate agar

---

*Calgiswabs and Calgitubes, available from Colab Laboratories, Inc., Chicago Heights, Ill. are ready-made, disposable tubes containing flexible alginate swabs.
†Scott Laboratories, Fiskeville, Rhode Island.

plates immediately. When this is impossible, the swab should be submerged in a suitable transport medium such as Stuart's or Amies. Vials containing these media can be obtained commercially,‡ and the rather messy process of filling small containers to capacity can be eliminated. The swab, when plunged into the vials, can simply be broken off, and the cap tightly resecured. Even the highly sensitive gonococcus has survived in Stuart's medium for up to 48 hours.

FECES OR RECTAL SWABS

The stool is not the most difficult specimen to collect, store or process. Collection, however, is usually a task of the patient, who must be informed on how to proceed to obtain a satisfactory specimen.

Never should the feces be "fished" from the toilet bowl. The easiest means of collection is provided when the patient can be instructed to defecate directly into a sterile, waxed cardboard container. When feces are not obtainable, a rectal swab is the next best specimen. A sterile swab is inserted well into the anus and then placed in a cotton-plugged sterile tube for transport.

SPUTUM

The patient himself is the only one who can provide a proper specimen of sputum. It is most important that the patient be informed of the necessity of his cooperation and the need for deep sputum rather than for a throat wash by saliva. A suitable container must be left with the patient so he or she can cough up sputum as it becomes available. Such a container should not be an unsightly jar or a dangerous Petri dish.

An excellent collection system has been developed* that is not only neat looking but also safe in handling. It provides a permanent fixture that can remain at the bedside at all times, fitted with a replaceable centrifuge tube, handy for transport and processing. The unit is leakproof and shatterproof, and can be discarded by incineration when the patient is discharged. A properly collected specimen should be treated as described in Chapter 25, or as in Chapter 17, if it is to be examined for tubercle bacilli.

FURTHER READING

Stokes, E. J.: *Clinical Bacteriology*, 4th Ed. London: Edward Arnold, Publ., 1976.

---

‡Difco Laboratories, Detroit, Mich.; and Baltimore Biological Laboratories, Cockeysville, Md.
*Available from Falcon Plastics, B. D. Laboratories, Inc. Baltimore, Md.

chapter 25
The Analytic Approach

In the microbiology laboratory, we assay some specimens for microbial content, others for specific or nonspecific antibody content, and still others for drug content. In previous chapters, we have already discussed the specific approaches to be taken in order to diagnose various infectious diseases. In ensuing chapters we also discuss various methods of antibody detection and of antibiotic susceptibility testing in detail. In this chapter, we intend to clarify a more general approach to bacterial analysis. Bacterial analysis consists of two distinctly separate steps: isolation of bacteria from mixtures in a specimen, and identification of such isolates.

25-1 ISOLATION OF BACTERIA FROM CLINICAL SPECIMENS

To be clinically useful, a microbiologic report need not necessarily reflect the total microbial content of a submitted specimen. In fact, it would be economically unfeasible and practically impossible to isolate and identify each and every type of bacterium contained in a clinical specimen. It would also make little sense, because it would confuse rather than assist the majority of physicians in their attempt to correctly diagnose and treat a patient. What is required of a microbial report is that it lists all clinically significant organisms found to be present in the submitted sample. In order to determine such facts, the microbiologist must be able to differentiate between findings that are clinically significant in each specimen and those that are irrelevant. In most instances, the clinically significant findings are limited to a listing of potential pathogens. In some instances, all that is required is a determination of whether or not a specific pathogen is present, for example: "*Salmonella* or *Shigella* not isolated from feces," "No *Staphylococcus aureus* or *Streptococcus pyogenes* isolated from throat swabs," "No *Neisseria gonorrhoeae* isolated from genital swabs," and "No acid-fast bacilli seen." In other instances, a listing of total findings may be valuable.

To isolate all pathogens from any specimen, the specimen must be planted on a suitable medium. The choice of media to use is almost unlimited, and must be determined with much forethought. If the objective is to isolate one particular pathogen, a single selective medium could be chosen that would allow isolation of that pathogen and at the same time prevent interference of its growth by other organisms present in the specimen. On the other hand, if the objective is to isolate any or all possible pathogens, as is usually the case, then the technologist should choose all those different media that would provide the growth requirements for all potential pathogens. To select the best media, the technologist must know the normal flora of a specific specimen as well as its potential pathogens.

In this section, we consider the organisms commonly found in various specimens, the pathogens that are commonly isolated from these specimens, and a choice of media that would allow isolation of all such pathogens. The choices of media are mine, and by no means the only choices possible. A small laboratory may find it difficult to keep some of the suggested media in routine stock, whereas a large laboratory could widen the choice considerably.

BLOOD

Blood is collected in a blood culture broth, which is incubated at 35°C and subcultured after 24 hours and 48 hours, and then again every 48 hours for at least 14 days. Care must be exercised to prevent contamination while subculturing.

Any bacteria present in the blood are clinically significant. Those more commonly found are: *Neisseria meningitidis, Streptococcus pneumoniae* and *Haemophilus* species. Less frequently one may find *Staphylococcus aureus, Streptococcus* species, *En-*

terobacter, Brucella, Francisella, Clostridium and other anaerobes. Except for *Brucella* and *Francisella*, all of these grow reasonably well on blood agar when the original blood culture is subcultured. Of course, each time a subculture is made, at least two blood agar plates must be inoculated: one for anaerobic culture, the other for culture under 10 percent CO_2. A staphylococcal streak should also be applied to allow growth of *Haemophilus*.

CEREBROSPINAL FLUID

The cerebrospinal fluid (CSF) should be spun at 1500 rpm for ten minutes, the supernatant collected in a sterile test tube for biochemical analysis, and the sediment planted on chocolate agar plates. Any bacteria isolated from the CSF are clinically significant. *Neisseria meningitidis, Haemophilus influenzae* and *Streptococcus pneumoniae* are most commonly isolated from CSF. *Staphylococcus aureus* and *Pseudomonas* are probably next in frequency, and other bacteria occur rarely.

URINE

The urine can contain a variety of different bacteria. When more than three different types of bacteria are found, each in fairly equal proportion, the urine specimen has probably been contaminated. In urinary tract infections, one type of bacteria usually predominates.

Contaminants may consist of *Staphylococcus albus, Proteus, Escherichia coli, Enterobacter, Bacillus,* diphtheroids, yeasts and streptococci. Of these, *E. coli, Enterobacter,* and *Proteus* species are often pathogenic, and should be considered as such when they occur in large numbers or by themselves. *Staphylococcus aureus, Streptococcus faecalis, Pseudomonas,* and any others isolated in large numbers should be considered pathogenic.

Many laboratories perform quantitative or semiquantitative analysis on urine. For this purpose, several different techniques have been developed. I recommend Hoeprich's method, which uses a calibrated loop, because it is simple, fast, and reasonably accurate. Reasonable accuracy is all that is required because the diagnostic significance of the number of bacteria found in the urine is based on a scale of 1000 per ml, 10,000 per ml, 100,000 per ml, or more than 100,000 per ml. The calibrated loop method allows quantitation well within these ranges. A loop calibrated to contain 0.01 ml of liquid specimen is used. One loopful each of a well-mixed, uncentrifuged urine sample is added to a blood agar plate and a MacConkey agar plate. The urine should be spread out as evenly as possible over the entire surface of the plate. This may be facilitated by the use of a sterile, bent glass rod. The plates are incubated at 37°C for 18 hours and the total number of colonies of each plate is counted. This count should be multiplied by 100 (0.01 ml inoculum) to arrive at the number of viable bacteria per ml of the original urine specimen.

The total number of colonies on MacConkey medium might be smaller than that on blood agar, because the latter allows growth of both gram-positive and gram-negative bacteria, whereas gram-positive bacteria are largely inhibited on MacConkey medium.

It is also wise to inoculate one tube of thioglycolate broth with about 0.5 ml of urine. If both plates fail to show growth, and the thioglycolate appears cloudy, some anaerobes may have grown in the thioglycolate broth, which then should be investigated. The presence of anaerobes should also be suspected when a Gram's stain from a thioglycolate culture displays organisms that cannot be accounted for on either MacConkey or blood agar.

THROAT SWABS

The normal flora of the throat might contain: *Streptococcus viridans, Streptococcus faecalis, Staphylococcus albus, Neisseria,* diphtheroids, *Escherichia coli, Bacillus, Clostridium,* yeasts and even *Mycobacterium* species. The more common pathogens of the throat are: *Streptococcus pneumoniae, Streptococcus pyogenes, Staphylococcus aureus, Haemophilus influenzae, Corynebacterium diphtheriae, Klebsiella* and *Candida.* A throat swab should routinely be planted on one blood agar plate furnished with a *Staphylococcus* streak and incubated under CO_2; one MacConkey agar plate or similar medium; and one broth composed of either cooked meat or thioglycolate. When diphtheria is suspected, a Loeffler's slant and a tellurite plate should also be inoculated. If a *Staphylococcus* survey is the main objective, a simple salt mannitol agar could suffice. *Streptococcus pyogenes* (beta hemolytic) and *Staphylococcus aureus* are significant even if isolated in relatively small numbers. Other pathogenic organisms are usually predominant.

EAR SWABS

The middle ear is most commonly infected by the following: *Pseudomonas aeruginosa, Staphylococcus aureus, Proteus, Escherichia coli* and less commonly with any of the organisms that may be found in the throat. Ear swabs should be processed in a manner similar to throat swabs.

WOUND SWABS

Organisms most frequently isolated from wound swabs are *Staphylococcus aureus, Escherichia coli, Proteus, Pseudomonas, Bacteroides, Clostridium,* and *Streptococcus.* On rare occasions, one may find *Pasteurella, Corynebacterium, Bacillus, Nocardia, Erysipelothrix* and *Mycobacterium.*

Wound swabs may be processed in the same way as throat swabs, with care exercised when some of the more unusual bacteria are suspected, as will be evident from direct examination of a smear under Gram's stain. In addition, one blood agar plate is inoculated and incubated anaerobically.

GENITAL SWABS

The main pathogens isolated from these specimens are *Neisseria gonorrhoeae* and *Trichomonas vaginalis.* Other organisms frequently found are *Haemophilus, Escherichia coli, Bacteroides, Candida,* and *Mycobacterium.* The isolation of *N. gonorrhoeae* has already been discussed in Chapter 13. For isolation of the other organisms, steps as discussed under wound swabs may be followed. *Trichomonas* infections are discussed in Chapter 23.

FECES

The feces may contain almost any type of bacteria. The main pathogens isolated from the feces are *Salmonella, Shigella, Staphylococcus aureus* and enteropathogenic *Escherichia coli* (e *E. coli*). Because the pathogens are usually present in relatively small numbers, as compared to nonpathogens, the use of highly selective and enrichment media is recommended. A suitable combination of media would be Salmonella-Shigella agar (SS), MacConkey agar (MacC), and selenite broth (Sel). If either e *E.coli* or *Staphylococcus aureus* is suspected, a blood agar or salt mannitol agar respectively could be added. The combination SS, MacC and Sel will allow isolation of *Salmonella* and *Shigella* in most instances, and at the same time permit isolation of other Enterobacteriaceae if such would be required.

If *Salmonella* or *Shigella* are present in fairly large numbers, they will be detectable within 18 hours on the SS and perhaps even on MacC. If they are present only in very small numbers, and fail to appear on either MacC or SS within 18 hours, they may be recovered from the selenite broth by subculture on SS. The selenite should have been inoculated with a pea-sized portion of feces at the

same time the first SS and MacC plates were inoculated. If no
Salmonella or *Shigella*-like colonies are evident on the second SS
plate following 18-hour incubation, it may be assumed that no such
organisms were present in the specimen (see also Chapter 29 for
these media).

SPUTUM

Bacterial pneumonia may be caused by *Klebsiella, Staphylococcus aureus, Haemophilus influenzae, Streptococcus pneumoniae, Pseudomonas* and *Mycoplasma.* Isolation of *Mycoplasma*
is hardly a routine procedure. However, most of the other types of
bacteria can be isolated by planting the sputum on a battery of
media similar to those outlined under throat swabs.

When the sputum is viscid and difficult to handle, a few
milliliters of sterile saline may be carefully added to the specimen.
Slightly stirring the sputum in this saline will release enough
bacteria to allow their isolation by planting a loopful of the saline.
Vigorous agitation must be avoided, less the technologist create
dangerous aerosols.

For the isolation of *Mycobacterium tuberculosis,* the reader is
referred to Chapter 17.

ANAEROBIC CULTURE

When attempting to isolate strict anaerobes, certain precautions must be taken to ensure any degree of success:

1. All media must be prepared without the formation of
   oxidized substances.
2. All media must be stored at a low oxidation-reduction
   potential until inoculated.
3. Oxidation of the specimen during collection, transportation
   and storage must be prevented.
4. Oxidation of either the specimen or the medium must be
   prevented during inoculation.
5. An efficient anaerobic environment must be provided during incubation.
6. Oxidation of the isolate must be prevented during subsequent subculture procedures.

The isolation and culture of anaerobic bacteria often require
expertise and equipment that might not be available in small
laboratories. Refer to Chapters 6 and 16 for further comments on the
isolation of anaerobes.

25-2 IDENTIFICATION OF ISOLATED BACTERIA

Once bacteria have been isolated in pure culture, the main tasks remaining are the establishment of antibiotic susceptibility patterns (Chapter 27) and the identification of the organisms. In this section, we shall discuss the main criteria governing the identification of unknown isolates.

In essence, identification is similar to classification. To identify an unknown bacterial culture, however, it is not usually necessary, nor is it at all practical, to ascertain all the characteristics of an isolate. Remember that classification, and hence identification, is always a subjective exercise. Each worker must adopt for classification and identification those characteristics that best suit his or her particular requirements. In adopting any system that utilizes relatively few characteristics, it is inevitable that more importance will be placed on some characteristics than on others. To be consistent, however, each worker should determine at the onset which characteristics are more and which are less important in the system to be adopted. Once that choice has been made, it should not be altered unless the entire system is revised. The final system adopted should conform to some acceptable classification system (see Chapter 7).

The first and foremost requirement for identifying an unknown culture is that the culture be pure (i.e., consists of only one type of bacterium). Most difficulties in identification result from a failure to realize that often one is testing a mixed culture. Whenever undue difficulties arise, it is wise to inoculate the culture under study on a suitable medium and to check whether it is in fact pure. Even colonies picked from highly selective media may not be pure, as the selective medium may inhibit but not kill bacteria of a different type. Subculture of such colonies on other types of media may result in the growth of the underlying bacteria as well as the bacteria constituting the primary colony.

Once a pure culture has been obtained, identification is a relatively simple procedure and should be based on a system of determinative elimination of the most easily ascertainable characteristics. The number of characteristics to be determined will vary with each isolate, but should include only those characteristics that will aid the effective differentiation of the isolate. The most basic characteristics should be determined first, followed in logical sequence by the more difficult, more cumbersome, or less significant characteristics. In some instances an organism can be placed in its appropriate genus on the basis of only four basic determinations (e.g., a gram-negative rod that has polar flagella, is oxidative, and produces a greenish pigment is obviously a *Pseudomonas* species and most likely *P. aeruginosa*). In most cases, however, the process of differentiation is far more complicated, and many more characteristics must be known before the identity of the isolate can be determined with any degree of certainty. The most logical general sequence of characterization is listed below:

1. Determine gross cellular morphology (such as coccus, rod, branching, spore formation and location, and capsule formation). This is best done under phase contrast by studying live suspensions to eliminate distortions due to drying. Determine motility.
2. Determine routine staining reactions, such as Gram's reaction (which is most useful when done on fresh cultures), acid-fastness, and fluorescence microscopy.
3. Determine cultural characteristics. (Is the organism aerobic or anaerobic? Is it fastidious? What are its growth patterns on selective media? If hemolytic, what type of hemolysis? Does it produce pigment?)
4. Determine biochemical characteristics. These studies can become exhaustive and are easily overutilized even by experienced microbiologists. Use only those tests that would further differentiate the organism within the group to which it has been assigned on the basis of other characteristics. The primary biochemical characteristics are catalase and oxidase production and fermentative or oxidative activity. The need to determine other biochemical characteristics should be based on data already gathered; these tests are listed in the appropriate chapters in Part II.
5. Determine serologic identity. Only in a few instances is it worthwhile to perform serologic procedures at the beginning of the investigation; these circumstances have been identified in Part II. In most cases, serologic procedures are required only when data obtained by the previous four steps have not identified the organism.
6. Determine animal pathogenicity. The modern microbiologist utilizes animal pathogenicity tests only as a last resort.

More specific testing sequences applicable to partially characterized isolates are outlined in Charts 25–1 and 25–2. In most instances, an accurate identification can be made without much difficulty within 48 hours following receipt of the specimen.

Chart 25–1. Primary identification of aerobes

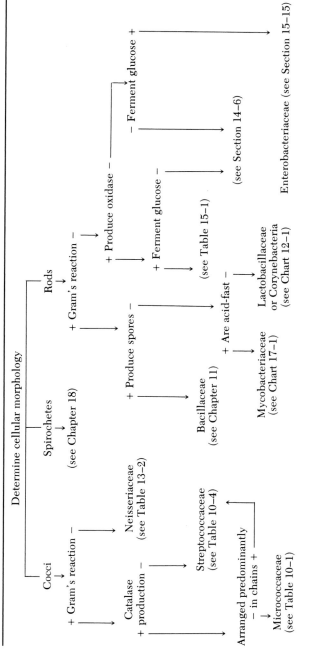

Guide to Chart 25–1: Determine only those characteristics required to reach a reference point, then refer to the respective chart, table or section.

Chart 25–2. Primary identification of anaerobes*

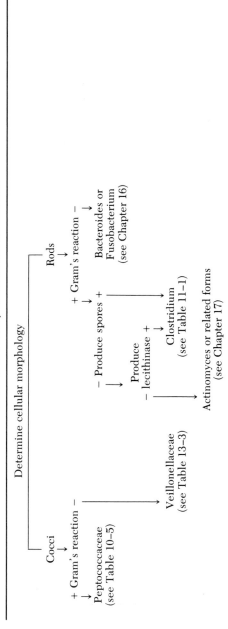

Guide to Chart 25–2: Determine only those characteristics required to reach a reference point, then refer to the respective chapter or table.

* Anaerobes, for the purpose of primary identification, are defined as those isolates that grow exclusively or considerably better in the absence of oxygen.

FURTHER READING

1. Bailey, W. R., and Scott, E. G.: *Diagnostic Microbiology*. 4th ed. St. Louis, C. V. Mosby Co., 1975.
2. Cowan, S. T., and Steel, K. J.: *Manual for the Identification of Medical Bacteria*. 2nd ed. Cambridge, England, Cambridge University Press, 1974.
3. Stokes, E. J.: *Clinical Bacteriology*. 4th ed., London, Edward Arnold, Publishers, 1976.
4. Hoeprich, P. D.: Culture of the urine. J. Lab. Clin. Med., **56**: 899-907, 1960.
5. Bartlett, R. C.: *Medical Microbiology, Quality, Cost and Clinical Relevance*. New York, John Wiley & Sons, 1974.
6. Smith, L. D.: *The Pathogenic Anaerobic Bacteria*. 2nd ed. Springfield, Ill., Charles C Thomas, 1975.

chapter 26

Quality Control

26-1 DEFINING QUALITY CONTROL

In the past decade, much has been written regarding quality control in the clinical laboratory. Great efforts have been made to place quality control programs on a sound mathematical or statistical basis. These efforts have met with reasonable success in disciplines such as biochemistry and hematology. In other disciplines, the mathematical or statistical approach is not readily applicable. Particularly in microbiology, such treatment of quality control would be virtually impossible, for several reasons:

a. Most microbiologic determinations cannot be placed within the broadest limits of variations allowed in mathematics.

b. During almost every step of microbiologic analysis, the analyst exercises critical judgement and is not governed by precisely defined steps to be taken next.

c. Results obtained by microbiologic analyses vary not only because of the techniques and approaches chosen by different analysts, but also because of the multiplicity of variations that different cultures may produce.

349

Thus, quality control in the microbiology laboratory cannot be defined by the usual terms applicable in other disciplines.

26-2 THE OBJECTIVES OF QUALITY CONTROL

The ultimate objective of any quality control program is perfection of all work results. In the laboratory, perfection of work results can be obtained only when all aspects of work performance are executed perfectly. All aspects of work performance involve not only the methods and equipment used, but also the manpower employed. The cooperation of the entire laboratory staff—administrative, secretarial, technical, as well as maintenance—is necessary for a successful quality control program. The main objective, therefore, can only be achieved when all the individuals responsible for a work result operate as a well-coordinated unit. Some more specific objectives are:

a. Isolation of all pathogens from all specimens submitted.
b. Correct identification of all isolates.
c. Correct and meaningful assay of susceptibility of pathogens to antimicrobial agents.
d. Accurate determination of serum antibody levels.
e. Prompt submission of interpretative reports.

Let us analyze these specific objectives more closely.

ISOLATION OF PATHOGENS

In order to isolate all pathogens from all specimens, it is absolutely necessary that specimens be properly collected, transported, stored, and treated when required (see Chapter 24). Also, each specimen should be processed without delay and planted on a set of media that permit isolation of all possible pathogens. It follows that all media must be prepared and kept according to strict specifications (see p. 351).

Strictly speaking, none of the foregoing can be considered a quality control on the performance of a microbiology laboratory. In that sense, a true quality control would consist of the submission of known specimens for analysis and comparison of results. The analyst should not know which specimens constitute the controls. If specimens are submitted in duplicate as a means of quality control, one should be entered under a fictitious name, so that the analyst is kept unaware of the duplication. In both instances, the results are preferably monitored and collated by an outside agency. Of course, the results of all known specimens should coincide with the standard findings; duplicate specimen analyses should be identical.

Only when the results of these quality control tests have been consistently accurate under routine conditions can a microbiology laboratory be relied upon to perform acceptable analyses on routine specimens. Of course, this criterion represents the ideal, which encounters obvious difficulties when applied to actual conditions.

CORRECT IDENTIFICATION OF ISOLATES

In order to identify an isolate correctly, a number of criteria must be met:

1. The isolate must be in pure culture (see Chapter 6 or 25).
2. A recognized procedure must be adopted. A general approach is discussed in Chapter 25; specific methods, reagents and media are listed in Chapters 29 to 31. Each laboratory should prepare and follow its own specific procedures manual, which should be updated continuously.
3. Satisfactory media and reagents must be employed. Quality control of these are discussed further in this section.
4. Equipment must be adequate. Some details for ensuring that equipment is performing satisfactorily are discussed under "Internal Monitoring," p. 355.

Quality Control of Media and Reagents. All media and reagents must be subjected to some sort of routine testing before they may be used in the laboratory. Ideally, a few samples of each batch of medium and each batch of reagent should be tested with two known cultures. One culture should be known to display whatever characteristic(s) one expects to find with the medium or reagent under test (e.g., produces hemolysis on blood agar). The other culture should be known to be unable to produce that characteristic on the particular medium or with the particular reagent (e.g., fails to produce hemolysis on blood agar). Of course, it would be impractical to test the ability of each batch of blood agar to produce all possible colonial variations that different bacteria might display. On the other hand, the value of checking media and reagents only "once in a while" is limited. A practical, middle-of-the-road approach must be adopted to ensure that all media and reagents are as reliable as one may reasonably expect. Some factors that might lead to the production of unsatisfactory media or reagents follow:

a. *Improper storage.* Improperly stored dehydrated media may deteriorate. If exposed to air, the dried material will absorb moisture, which may cause the product to break down, or may result in an unknown dilution factor when the medium is prepared for use. Heat also destroys many ingredients in dehydrated media.

All dried media should be stored in a dry, cool place.

Avoid stockpiling, so that media are stored no longer than six to twelve months. Media stored beyond such periods should not be expected to yield satisfactory results.

b. *Weighing and dilution factors.* Simple errors in weighing or in calculating dilution factors may lead to improper preparation of dehydrated media and improper results. These considerations are often overlooked.

c. *Tapwater.* The use of improperly distilled tapwater or distilled water contaminated by algae to reconstitute dehydrated media may also result in an unsuitable product. How often is the distilled water reservoir in your laboratory cleaned?

d. *Dirty glassware.* Dirty glassware or glassware improperly rinsed of detergents provides another source of constant error.

e. *Improper homogenizing or mixing.* Improperly homogenizing media or improperly mixing reagents will create products that are too concentrated or too dilute.

f. *Overheating or oversterilizing.* Either factor will cause many ingredients to break down, resulting in softening, destruction of the agar, caramelization, destruction of carbohydrates, change of pH, destruction of buffers, or other effects.

Most media in use in the bacteriology laboratory are obtained in dehydrated form from reliable supply houses, where they have already undergone rigid quality-control testing. These products are generally of high quality and perform satisfactorily when prepared according to the manufacturer's specifications. Nevertheless, to detect errors that may have occurred during preparation of the product, as just discussed, it is good practice to subject each batch of media to some form of quality control. For some routine media, this control procedure may simply consist of logging results that are routinely observed without any extra effort; for example, MacConkey agar will display typical lactose positive and lactose negative colonies in any laboratory that processes more than 20 specimens a day. For other media, the control procedure consists of inoculating two or more samples of the batch with known cultures, then incubating and processing each sample as required (such as adding ferric chloride to a phenylalanine slant), reading the results, and comparing the results with standard norms.

The choice of known cultures for quality control tests is limited only by their suitability and availability. Special batches of known cultures that have a wide scope of different reaction patterns are

Table 26–1. Determinations and respective cultures that yield positive and negative results in control procedures

Determination	Positive culture	Negative culture
Catalase reaction	Staphylococcus epidermidis	Streptococcus faecalis
Oxidase reaction	Pseudomonas aeruginosa	Escherichia coli
Esculin hydrolysis	Streptococcus faecalis	Streptococcus pyogenes
Citrate utilization	Enterobacter aerogenes	Escherichia coli
Coagulase production	Staphylococcus aureus	Staphylococcus epidermidis
Lysine or ornithine decarboxylation, and Arginine dihydrolysis	Salmonella newport	Proteus vulgaris
Gelatin hydrolysis	Proteus mirabilis	Escherichia coli
Hydrogen sulfide production	Proteus vulgaris	Escherichia coli
Indole production (check both the medium and Kovac's reagent)	Escherichia coli	Proteus mirabilis
Malonate utilization	Enterobacter aerogenes	Escherichia coli
Methyl-red test	Escherichia coli	Enterobacter aerogenes
Voges-Proskauer reaction	Enterobacter aerogenes	Escherichia coli
Niacin test	Mycobacterium tuberculosis	Any nonchromogen
Nitrate reduction	Escherichia coli	Pseudomonas aeruginosa
ONPG reaction	Escherichia coli	Proteus morganii
Phenylalanine deamination	Proteus vulgaris	Escherichia coli
Urease production	Proteus vulgaris	Escherichia coli
Motility	Proteus vulgaris	Klebsiella pneumoniae
Fermentation of:		
Glucose		
Adonitol		
Arabinose		
Inositol		
Lactose	Escherichia coli	Pseudomonas aeruginosa
Mannitol		
Raffinose		
Rhamnose	Enterobacter aerogenes	Proteus morganii
Salicin		
Sorbitol		
Sucrose		
DNase production	Serratia marcescens	Staphylococcus epidermidis
Glucose O/F:		
Oxidation	Pseudomonas aeruginosa	Acinetobacter lwoffi
Fermentation	Escherichia coli	Pseudomonas aeruginosa

commercially available* and a boon to the smaller laboratory, where maintaining adequate stock cultures has always been the major problem limiting quality control efforts. A list of routine tests and appropriate organisms that yield positive and negative reactions in each case is presented in Table 26–1. Media or reagents should be tested when prepared, and again each month thereafter if stored for long-term use.

Staining reagents are best monitored by preparing a mixture of appropriate organisms on a microscope slide and processing the slide with the new batch of reagents. A good control mixture for Gram's stain would be a mixed broth culture of *Staphylococcus* and *Escherichia coli*. For control of acid-fast reagents, a liquefied sputum specimen could be lightly seeded with mycobacteria, autoclaved at 126°C for 30 minutes, and stored at 4°C for continuous weekly use.

QUALITY CONTROL OF SUSCEPTIBILITY TESTS

Susceptibility testing is fully discussed in Chapter 27. Quality control of susceptibility tests should at least involve the incorporation of standard strains of *Staphylococcus aureus* and *Escherichia coli*.* Such strains should be assayed at least once a week against all commercially prepared antibiotic discs employed in susceptibility tests. Although the antibiotic discs purchased from commercial sources are subject to rigid quality control by the manufacturers, who are also under constant scrutiny by government inspectors, each laboratory should again check whether these discs conform to standards when used with their media by their personnel. Standard zones of inhibition are listed in Table 27–1.

QUALITY CONTROL OF SEROLOGIC TESTS

Quality control in the clinical laboratories had its origin in the serology lab. For decades, serologic tests have been subjected to reasonably rigid controls, and results obtained in one laboratory could, more often than not, be corroborated by others. (Serology is considered in greater detail in Chapter 28.)

The titers reported on many sera subjected to antibody studies are usually the result of rather exact quantitative analyses. Often, however, the titers obtained by one method, or even by the same method employed in different laboratories, do not always agree with those obtained by other methods or by other workers. Much can still be done to make serologic analyses more accurate. It is

---

*Bactrol Disks, Difco Laboratories, Detroit, Mich.

here that a quality control program based on mathematics and statistics could find its way into the clinical microbiology laboratory.

REPORT WRITING AND DISPATCHING

No quality control program is complete without an efficient means of report writing and report dispatching.

The report writing is usually the function of the technologist in charge. Reports should be concise, clearly written and in plain, easy to understand language. Duplication of reports should be avoided as much as possible, unless a photocopier is available, to eliminate possible errors in the duplicate copies. The laboratory must, at all times, keep a legible copy on file for future reference. If a photocopier is not available, a double requisition-report, fitted with a carbon between, could reduce the workload as well as the errors. Finally, reports must be released soon after they are written. This demands an efficient and conscientious office staff.

26-3 INTERNAL MONITORING

As you have undoubtedly observed, the evaluation of laboratory performances should be an integral part of daily laboratory procedures. Throughout this text, we have discussed means of control for various tests and procedures. However, more specific quality control monitoring should become a daily routine.

Besides the measures already discussed in the previous section, quality control should include the monitoring of all equipment in use. This important aspect of quality control is often overlooked, even though it is frequently the cause of trouble, difficulty or error. Some equipment checks may be listed as follows:

1. Microscopes must be cleaned frequently and optics checked for dirt spots that could be responsible for erroneous reports.
2. Temperature charts or logs should be maintained on all thermal equipment, such as autoclaves, ovens, waterbaths, incubators, refrigerators, and freezers.
3. Thermometers should be calibrated at least every six months.
4. pH meters should be calibrated weekly.
5. Balances should be checked once a year.
6. Centrifuges should be monitored routinely by tachometers, and the tachometers checked once a year.

7. Glassware must be checked for cleanliness and wear. Chipped glassware must be discarded. Glass used for measuring must be calibrated periodically.
8. Gaspak jars must always contain an indicator strip.
9. CO_2 levels in incubators should be checked daily on the supply tank as well as on the instrument panel. Actual CO_2 levels should be measured at least every six months.
10. Autoclaves should be monitored by the use of test spore strips* or other reliable indicators of sterility.

Internal monitoring may be extended by the introduction of known specimens. To be effective, such specimens should be submitted along with the routine specimens and should be unidentifiable to the analysts who process them (see also page 350).

Another approach is the exchange of clinical specimens by two or more local laboratories for the purpose of simultaneous testing. Followed by a comparison of results, this is a simple, effective means of quality control. Such exchanges should not be a source of embarrassment for any of the participating laboratories. The results could simply be exchanged between chiefs or coordinators, who could then check them with their own results and institute correctional procedures where necessary. Those who are embarrassed to learn that their performance can be improved have no place in the clinical laboratory. Only by constant and rigid evaluation of test procedures, followed by correction when necessary, will a laboratory be able to achieve the highest standards.

26-4 EXTERNAL MONITORING

Several other monitoring programs are available:
a. The College of American Pathologists† provides specimens and cultures at quarterly intervals. Every three months, a new set of different specimens is prepared and made available for widespread distribution.
b. Several state, provincial or regional laboratories provide similar sets at different intervals.
c. Some commercial concerns‡ have various monitoring sets available which they change at regular intervals.

Because these specimens would be difficult to conceal as "routine specimens," their value as true quality control programs,

---

* Available from Baltimore Biological Laboratory, Cockeysville, Md.
† 230 North Michigan Ave., Chicago, Ill., 60601.
‡ Hyland Laboratories, Costa Mesa, California; Difco Laboratories, Detroit, Mich.

is questionable. However, as a means of monitoring the proficiency of the participant, they are a definite aid in overall control of standards. When properly used, they also assist in the continuing education of laboratory staff.

FURTHER READING

1. Tonks, D. B.: *Quality Control in Clinical Laboratories.* 2nd ed. Toronto, Warner-Chilcott Laboratories, 1972.
2. Griffin, O. F., and Greeban, L. B.: Practical charting technics in quality assurance programs. Dade Monograph No. 2, Miami, Florida, 1971.
3. Prier, J. E., Bartok, J. T., and Friedman, H.: *Quality Control in Microbiology.* Baltimore, University Park Press, 1975.
4. Ellis, R.J.: *Manual of Quality Control Procedures for Microbiological Laboratories.* 2d ed. Atlanta, Center for Disease Control, 1976.

chapter 27
Susceptibility Testing

27-1 INTRODUCTION

The most significant reports produced in the clinical microbiology laboratory are those that guide the treatment of patients receiving antimicrobial agents. The student would do well to review briefly the discussion on antimicrobial agents beginning on page 114.

For susceptibility testing, a pathogen should preferably be isolated in pure culture. Only in a few instances can susceptibility tests be performed directly on the isolation media (cerebrospinal fluid culture). Pure cultures should be tested against an appropriate variety of different antibiotics in order to obtain an antibiogram of the isolate. An antibiogram lists the relative susceptibilities of a given isolate to a number of different antibiotics. As seen in Table 9–1, many antibiotics usually affect either gram-positive or gram-negative bacilli, and sometimes both. Therefore, one can use common sense in selecting which antibiotics to test on a particular isolate. The ultimate choice will depend on the isolate, the investigator, and the service that a particular laboratory can afford to give.

Various methods can be used to test susceptibility patterns of bacteria. We will consider only two methods here: the disc diffusion (Kirby-Bauer) test, and the tube diffusion test.

27-2 THE KIRBY-BAUER METHOD

This is the most commonly used method for determining the susceptibility of bacteria to antibiotics. It is a single disc diffusion test. Disc diffusion tests utilize paper discs that have been soaked in a specific concentration of antibiotic solutions and subsequently allowed to dry. When an agar plate is seeded evenly with a particular culture of bacteria, and antibiotic discs are placed on the surface of the plate, the antibiotic diffuses from the disc into the medium. If the culture is susceptible to an antibiotic, a zone of growth inhibition surrounds the disc containing that antibiotic. If the culture is resistant to an antibiotic, growth occurs up to and even underneath the disc.

Although the zone size depends mainly on the strength of the antibiotic and the susceptibility of the culture under study, it is also affected by a number of other factors.

Type of Medium Used. A medium that supports rapid and heavy bacterial growth yet does not inhibit or interfere with antibiotic diffusion should be used. The most suitable medium appears to be Mueller-Hinton agar. This medium permits good growth of most pathogens, and may be supplemented with 5% blood for the more fastidious isolates. The pH of the medium should lie between 7.2 and 7.4, as tested at 20°C.

Environmental Factors. Streptomycin is inactivated under anaerobic conditions. The potency of other antibiotics is altered under 10% CO_2 and varies also with pH changes. These factors should be taken into account when testing cultures that require CO_2 or anaerobiasis, and those that produce predominantly acid end-products.

The Depth of the Medium. Since the test is based on the diffusion of the antibiotic away from the disc, more or less antibiotic will be present in smaller or larger zones depending on the depth of the medium. Therefore, a depth of 40 mm has been established as a standard. This can be attained by pouring exactly 25 ml of medium into a plate with a 90-mm diameter, or 60 ml into a plate with a diameter of 150 mm.

The Size of the Inoculum. Results will vary if different concentrations of viable organisms are subjected to the same concentrations of antibiotics on discs. A standard inoculum may be obtained by "picking" three to ten colonies of the culture under study and growing these for two to five hours in tryptose phosphate broth. The culture should then be diluted, if necessary, with sterile water or saline, so that the turbidity of the culture medium will be the same as that of a standard solution composed of 0.5 ml of 1% $BaCl_2$ in 99.5 ml of 1% H_2SO_4. The standard and the culture should be in similar tubes and compared with each other under a good light source against a white background with a heavy black line. New standards must be prepared monthly. Broth cultures that have been allowed to stand overnight should not be used for standardization, because they may contain large numbers of dead organisms.

The Application of the Inoculum. The inoculum should be spread evenly over the entire surface of a relatively dry agar plate. This should be done with a sterile swab dipped into the standard inoculum. The swab should not be too wet and should leave no marks on the agar surface.

The Application of the Discs. The discs should be applied no later than 15 minutes after the inoculum has been seeded. Delay will result in a growth period of the organisms before the antibiotics have a chance to diffuse into the medium. Discs must be applied aseptically, with flamed forceps or special disc dispensers.* The discs should be spaced at least 24 mm apart from center to center, and 15 mm away from the edge of the plate.

The Choice of Discs. In the United States and Canada, commercially available discs are reliable. The Food and Drug Administration in the United States and the Canadian Centre for Disease Control have set rigid standards that are forcefully controlled. The technologist should also enforce these standards. Never use outdated discs, and avoid deterioration by improper storage.

The technologist decides which discs to place on which isolates. For gram-negative bacteria, the following could be chosen: ampicillin, colistin, cephalothin, nitrofurantoin, chloramphenicol, tetracycline, kanamycin, carbenicillin, gentamicin, and cotrimoxazole. For the assay of gram-positive bacteria, the choice would involve ampicillin, cephalothin, streptomycin, erythromycin, tetracycline, penicillin, methicillin, clindamycin, gentamicin,

---

*Difco Laboratories, Detroit, Mich. and Baltimore Biological Laboratories, Cockeysville, Md.

nitrofurantoin, and cotrimoxazole. In all cases, the disc potencies should be those listed in Table 27–1. Upon special request, the choice of discs can be easily altered.

The Time of Incubation. Plates should be incubated soon after the discs have been applied. Delay may result in zones of inhibition that are larger than usual because the antibiotic diffuses before bacterial growth has begun.

The Incubation Period. This should be no longer than 24 hours at 37°C. The standards vary considerably for cultures that require longer growth periods.

OUTLINE OF KIRBY-BAUER TEST

All of the foregoing factors should be considered when antibiotic susceptibility tests are performed. With these factors in mind, the Kirby-Bauer test proper may be outlined as follows:

a. Pick three to ten colonies of the culture under study and place in 4 ml of tryptose phosphate broth.

b. Incubate the broth for two to five hours and standardize the culture.

c. Inoculate the standardized culture evenly on Mueller-Hinton plates.

d. Apply the antibiotic discs to the plates.

e. Incubate the plates under the required conditions.

f. Measure the zones of inhibition surrounding the discs. These measurements are recorded in millimeters of the diameter of the zone, including the disc. Take these measurements within 24 hours of inoculation, and include only areas of complete inhibition. Measurement may be facilitated by the use of a caliper or a transparent overlay.

g. Compare the zone diameters with a chart, such as Table 27–1, and record the results as susceptible, intermediate, or resistant. If a transparent overlay is used, compare the zones of specific antibiotics that are printed on the overlay with the test plates.

h. Sulfonamides allow bacterial growth for several generations before inhibition becomes evident. When testing these agents, disregard the slight growth surrounding the disc and measure the zone from the edge of the heavy growth. Also, when testing *Proteus* species with sulfonamides, ignore a thin veil of swarming organisms.

i. Some technical errors are worth mentioning: Sliding the disc over the surface of the medium will cause oval zones;

Table 27–1. Interpretation of results of the Kirby-Bauer test

Antimicrobial Agent	Disc Potency in Micrograms or Units	Inhibition Zone Diameter in mm		
		Resistant	Intermediate	Susceptible
Amikacin	10	8 or less	9–13	13 or more
Ampicillin:				
with *Staphylococcus aureus*	10	20 or less	21–28	29 or more
with any other	10	11 or less	12–13	14 or more
Bacitracin	10	8 or less	9–12	13 or more
Carbenicillin				
with *Pseudomonas aeruginosa*	50	12 or less	13–14	15 or more
with *Escherichia coli* and *Proteus*	50	17 or less	18–22	23 or more
Chloramphenicol	30	12 or less	13–17	18 or more
Clindamycin	2	14 or less	15–16	17 or more
Colistin	10	8 or less	9–10	11 or more
Co-trimoxazole	25	10 or less	10–15	16 or more
Erythromycin	15	13 or less	14–17	18 or more
Gentamicin	10	12 or less	—	13 or more
Kanamycin	30	13 or less	14–17	18 or more
Lincomycin	2	9 or less	10–14	15 or more
Methicillin	5	9 or less	10–13	14 or more
Neomycin	30	12 or less	13–16	17 or more
Nitrofurantoin	300	14 or less	15–16	17 or more
Novobiocin:				
without blood in the medium	30	17 or less	18–21	22 or more
Oleandomycin	15	11 or less	12–16	17 or more
Oxacillin	1	10 or less	11–12	13 or more
Penicillin G:				
with *Staphylococcus aureus*	10	20 or less	21–28	29 or more
with any other	10	11 or less	12–21	22 or more
Polymyxin B	300	8 or less	9–11	12 or more
Streptomycin	10	11 or less	12–14	15 or more
Sulfonamides	250	12 or less	13–16	17 or more
Tetracycline	30	14 or less	15–18	19 or more
Tobramycin	10	11 or less	12–13	14 or more
Vancomycin	30	9 or less	10–11	12 or more

placing the disc too near to the edge of the plate will cause eccentric zones. In either case, measure the size of the zone from the smallest diameter. In the first instance, some of the antibiotic is wiped onto a wider surface of the plate and therefore diffuses further. In the second instance, the antibiotic diffuses sideways once the edge of the medium has been reached.

27-3 THE TUBE DILUTION METHOD

Serial dilutions of a particular antibiotic or a number of different antibiotics are mixed with standard inocula of a culture under investigation. By this method, it is possible to ascertain the minimal inhibitory concentration of a particular antibiotic to a particular culture. This may be achieved by incubating the antibiotic dilutions and culture inocula for a predetermined time, and determining the presence or absence of growth. The tube dilution method is useful for testing the susceptibility of organisms that require CO_2, anaerobic atmospheres, or special enriched media that cannot be tested by the agar diffusion method.

Keep in mind that the minimal inhibitory concentration (MIC) is not necessarily the minimal lethal concentration (MLC). Also note that many of the factors discussed under the Kirby-Bauer method also play a role in the tube dilution test.

The test itself is time-consuming and therefore not recommended as a routine method. The test may be performed as follows:

a. Dilute frozen stock solutions of the required antibiotics in sterile water to contain 200 μg or units/ml.

b. Dilute this solution further for each concentration of antibiotic to be tested. Use aseptic technique and 10 plugged or capped sterile test tubes. The test tubes should be small, 13 by 100 mm; the dilutions must be serial and in volumes of 0.5 ml, so that the range will be 100, 50, 25, 12.5, 6.25, 3.1, 1.5, 0.75 and 0.37. The last tube should not contain any antibiotic and will serve as a growth control.

c. To each tube, add 0.5 ml of the test culture, diluted to contain approximately 10^5 viable organisms per milliliter. For most cultures, this concentration can be obtained by diluting an overnight broth culture to 1:1000 in fresh broth.

d. Incubate at 37°C for 18 hours, or until the last tube demonstrates growth.

e. The results are reported as the least amount of antibiotic required to inhibit the growth of the culture. For example, if the sixth tube is the first one to show growth, the minimum inhibitory concentration for that antibiotic will be at the previous tube, which is 6.25 μg/0.5 ml or 3.1 μg/ml.

27-4 SERUM LEVEL ASSAY

In some instances it is clinically valuable to determine the actual levels of antibiotics attained in the serum. Table 9–1 lists the common levels of some frequently used antibiotics that may be found in the serum. The assay of these serum levels is a relatively simple method, somewhat similar to the tube dilution method. Instead of known quantities of antibiotics in suspension, the patient's serum is serially diluted and mixed with fixed suspensions of the incriminated isolate. The serum level is then expressed as the reciprocal of the highest serum dilution that inhibits the growth of the organism. In general, the serum bactericidal level of an antibiotic should be at least 1:8 to be effective in difficult infectious cases.

The serum assay may be performed as follows:

a. Collect a blood sample before therapy has been initiated and use serum from that specimen as a control.
b. Collect blood samples after at least 24 hours of therapy, and aseptically collect the serum from those samples.
c. Test this serum within three hours, or freeze it at −20°C until testing can be done.
d. Aseptically, prepare eight serial dilutions of serum in Mueller-Hinton broth in 1.0-ml volumes. Dilutions should range from 1:1 to 1:128. Tubes should have stoppers.
e. Add 0.05 ml of a 1:1000-dilution of a six-hour broth culture of the test organism.
f. Incubate all tubes at 35°C for 18 hours.
g. Determine the bactericidal endpoint. This is done by subculturing 0.05 ml of each tube that shows no growth (no turbidity) to a fresh tube of broth and repeating the incubation. Subcultures that remain clear indicate bactericidal action in the tube from which the subculture was made.
h. Express the serum level as the highest dilution factor that resulted in bactericidal action.

27-5 QUALITY CONTROL

Practical quality control methods have not been developed yet for monitoring the tube dilution or serum level assay methods. The disc diffusion test (Kirby-Bauer method) has been in such widespread use that it has prompted the development of practical quality control measures. The most commonly used measures employ two standard cultures to monitor the minimum zone size a particular disc should display in order to rate as satisfactory. These cultures are the Seattle strains of *Staphylococcus aureus* and *Escherichia coli* (American Type Culture Collection numbers 25923 and 25922 respectively*). Maximal acceptable standard de-

*These cultures are available in easily dispensable and stable pellet form, Bactrol Disks, Difco Laboratories, Detroit, Mich.

viations and mean zone diameters using these cultures have been determined for most available antibiotic discs. Detailed descriptions of control procedures are inserted with the Bactrol Disks, or may be obtained free of charge. Regrettably, when deviations are registered, laboratory workers frequently blame the susceptibility discs and often fail to investigate other shortcomings that may be responsible for the error.

FURTHER READING

1. Bauer, A. W., et al.: Antibiotic susceptibility testing by a standardized single disk method. Am. J. Clin. Path., 45:493-496, 1966.
2. Blazevic, D. J., et al.: Quality control testing with the disk antibiotic susceptibility test of Bauer-Kirby-Sherris-Turck. Am. J. Clin. Path., 57:592-597, 1972.
3. Bartlett, R. C., and Mazens, M.: Analytical variability in single disk antimicrobial susceptibility test. Am. J. Clin. Path., 59:376–383, 1973.
4. Ericsson, H. M., and Sherris, J. C.: Antibiotic sensitivity testing: report of an international collaborative study. Acta Pathol. Microbiol. Scan., Section B, (Supplement 21), 1–90, 1971.
5. Barry, A. L.: *The Antimicrobic Susceptibility Test: Principles and Practice.* Philadelphia, Lea & Febiger, 1976.

chapter 28
Serology

28-1 BASIC PRINCIPLES OF SEROLOGY

The student would do well to review the immunology section of Chapter 9 before embarking on this chapter. *Immunology* is the study of antibody production and of antibody-antigen reactions in vivo (within the body). *Serology* is the study of antibody-antigen reactions in vitro, which means under artificial conditions or by laboratory methods. More precisely, serology is the study of phenomena whereby antibodies react in vitro with their corresponding antigens, and the development and control of the most sensitive, most specific, and simplest methods whereby each antibody-antigen reaction may be demonstrated. This section aims to explain the general principles underlying serologic methods. The following sections of this chapter discuss some commonly used serologic methods in more detail.

Each antibody-antigen reaction requires rather exact conditions. The exactness of these conditions varies, of course, with the complexity of the test. Electrolyte balance, temperature, and time are crucial factors in most tests; osmotic pressure, pH, and other factors are important in many others. Most antibody-antigen reactions occur in two distinct stages: (1) the specific combination of the antibody with its corresponding antigen; (2) the observable reaction, such as agglutination, precipitation, lysis, or other phenomena. Each stage may differ with regard to such factors as time, temperature, electrolyte balance, or other requirements. Furthermore, these two stages do not always follow one another clearly, but often overlap.

Terms used to describe antibodies and antigens are often named after the method by which they can be detected, or after the effect they have on one another. Hence, the terms precipitin and precipitinogen refer to the antibody and the antigen respectively that form precipitates when they combine. Agglutinins are antibodies that clump cells together in large aggregates; lysins, antibodies that can promote the breakdown or lysis of cells containing their antigen. There are many other reactions and terms.

How specific are antibody-antigen reactions? Any substance can be an antigen, and each antigen stimulates the production of an antibody specific to itself. This means that there are as many different antibodies as there are different antigens. However, not all of these millions of antigens can stimulate antibody production in every individual. As discussed in Section 9-2, only antigens foreign to an individual normally stimulate antibody production in that individual.

Let us suppose that capital letters from A to Z represent all antigens, and that lower-case letters from a to z represent all antibodies. Let us further suppose that an immunologically normal person would possess *only* those antigens represented by the letters in his name. If we have two individuals named Mr. Saul and Mr. Zeus, Mr. Saul could produce all antibodies except a, l, s, and u; Mr. Zeus could produce all antibodies except e, s, u, and z. If both Mr. Saul and Mr. Zeus were challenged with antigens B and C, both would produce antibodies b and c. However, if both were challenged with antigens A and E, only Mr. Saul would produce antibody e, and only Mr. Zeus would produce antibody a.

Although antibody-antigen reactions are specific—that is, each particular antibody reacts only with its particular antigen—some situations arise in which the reaction appears to be nonspecific. *Cross-reactions* comprise one situation in which the antibodies

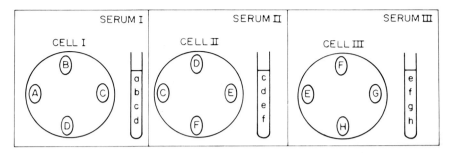

Fig. 28–1. Cross reactions of three different antisera. Serum I will react with cells I and II. Serum II will react with cells I, II, and III. Serum III will react with cells II and III.

appear to react with unrelated antigens. Refer to Figure 28-1. In that figure, cell I is composed of antigens A, B, C, D; if a susceptible individual is challenged with cell I, his serum will contain antibodies a, b, c, and d. Cell II has antigens C, D, E, and F; a susceptible individual stimulated with this cell will produce antibodies c, d, e, and f in his serum. Similarly, a third individual challenged with cell III, which has antigens E, F, G, and H, will have antibodies e, f, g, and h in his serum. Each antiserum (serum containing antibodies) will react not only with the cell used for its production, but also with any cell that carries an antigen corresponding to an antibody in that antiserum. Serum I will react with cells I and II; serum II, with cells I, II, and III; serum III, with cells II and III. These are known as cross-reactions.

The *prozone phenomenon* is another factor that sometimes upsets serologic results. This occurs when too much antibody is mixed with too little antigen, or vice versa. Figure 28–2 demonstrates the possible results in either case.

To be able to form aggregates for precipitation or agglutination, antibodies and antigens must be present in relatively equivalent amounts. In Figure 28–2, antibodies are represented by the symbol –0–, which indicates two available combining sites. Antigens are represented by the plus sign, +, which indicates four available combining sites. The equivalent zone, in which antibodies and antigens have combined to form aggregates, comprises the middle panel of Figure 28–2. In panel I, antibody is far in excess; although it combines with the antigen, it saturates all antigen sites, eliminating the possibility of aggregation. Likewise, when the antigen is in

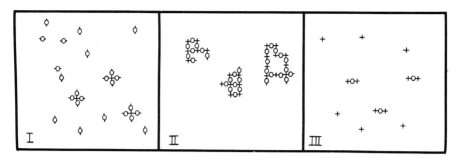

Fig. 28–2. Illustration of the prozone phenomenon and the equivalent zone. ⊙ = antibody; + = antigen. I shows the prozone phenomenon of excess antibody; II, the equivalent zone; and III, excess of antigen.

excess (panel III), all antibody sites are saturated before aggregates can be formed.

When we test sera containing high concentrations of antibody, a positive result may not be observed because of this prozone phenomenon. By diluting such sera and adding known amounts of antigen to each dilution, the equivalent zone may be achieved. Such a test would show a negative result in the first dilutions, followed by a positive result in subsequent dilutions, until a dilution is reached at which antigen is in excess.

In this section, only some basic principles of serology have been considered. The interested reader is directed to reading reference 2 for more detail.

28-2 C-REACTIVE PROTEIN (CRP)

CRP is a substance that is not found in normal sera but occurs frequently in sera of patients with inflammatory or other tissue-damaging syndromes. Thus, the demonstration of CRP in the serum is a nonspecific measure for the presence of infection or tissue injury.

In the CRP test, the CRP is the antigen, and the reagent ACRP (or CRPA) is the antibody. The CRP test is therefore one of the many so-called reverse serology tests, by which one attempts to identify unknown antigens by using known antibody.

The test itself is simple. Excellent CRPA-sera are commercially available.* The test serum, which has been heat inactivated

---

*Difco Laboratories, Detroit, Mich.; Hyland Laboratories, Costa Mesa, Calif.; Behring Diagnostics, Montreal, Canada.

at 56°C for 30 minutes, is drawn up into one half of a regular capillary tube. CRPA-serum is then drawn following the test serum, ensuring that no air separates the two reagents. When the tube is nearly filled, half and half with each, the capillary tube is inverted and placed in an upright position. If the test serum contains CRP, a precipitate appears at the interphase between serum and CRPA. In this type of test, the possibility of a prozone phenomenon is largely eliminated because antigen and antibody (serum and CRPA) slowly diffuse into one another, finding the equivalent zone naturally.

A quantitative CRP test is possible by diluting the test serum before it is drawn into capillary tubes, and testing various dilutions with the CRPA. The highest dilution at which the test would still be positive is then taken as a factor expressing the "titer" of CRP in the test serum. For example, if test serum is diluted from 1:1 to 1:64 by serial doubling dilutions, and the first four tubes are positive, the CRP titer of the test serum would be 1:8.

28-3 FEBRILE ANTIBODY TESTS

A number of febrile diseases such as brucellosis, typhoid fever, typhus, Rocky Mountain spotted fever, and several others may be serologically diagnosed by employing suspensions of certain bacteria. To be effective, these bacteria must be either responsible for causing the febrile disease, or carry an antigen identical to one carried by the agent responsible for the febrile disease.

All febrile antibody tests are basically the same, although some, named after the people who developed them, are known more widely. Of these, the Widal and the Weil-Felix tests are best known and serve as examples of other febrile antibody tests.

THE WIDAL TEST

Salmonella typhi and *S.paratyphi* A, B, and C are the most common causes of typhoid and paratyphoid fever. Suspensions of cultures of these organisms are subsequently used most commonly as antigens in the Widal test to detect antibodies against these diseases. Satisfactory antigens are commercially available.* The test procedure is fairly straightforward:

Preparation of the Specimen
   a. Obtain 5 to 10 ml of blood to be tested in a clean, dry test tube.

---

*Difco Laboratories, Detroit, Mich.; Lederle Laboratories, Pearl River, N.Y.

    b. Allow the blood to clot. Clot retraction may be facilitated by "ringing" a clean applicator stick around the clot, along the inside wall of the test tube.

    c. Separate the serum from the clot by centrifugation. Collect the clear serum.

    d. Do not heat the serum prior to examination. Significant antibodies are thermolabile and such treatment may destroy or lower the antibody titer.

Rapid Slide Test Procedure

    a. Pipette 0.08, 0.04, 0.02, 0.01 and 0.005 ml of serum onto a row of squares on a ruled glass plate using a 0.2-ml serologic pipette.

    b. Place a drop of the appropriate antigen for the slide test on each drop of serum.

    c. Mix each serum-antigen with an applicator stick, starting with the 0.005-ml serum dilution and working toward the 0.08-ml dilution. The final dilutions are approximately 1:20, 1:40, 1:80, 1:160 and 1:320, respectively.

    d. Rotate the glass plate by hand 15 to 20 times.

    e. Observe agglutination over a suitable light source and record:

        4+   Complete agglutination
        3+   Approximately 75 percent of the cells are clumped
        2+   Approximately 50 percent of the cells are clumped
        1+   Approximately 25 percent of the cells are clumped
        ±   Traces of agglutination only
        −   No agglutination

The titer is expressed as the reciprocal of the highest dilution that yields a 4+ reaction.

Controls. The use of both positive and negative controls in parallel with the test sera serves two purposes: first, it assures proper reactivity of the antigen, and second, it indicates agglutination results to be expected in both negative and positive sera. Both positive and negative sera are available from the same sources as the antigens; they should be diluted in the same proportions as the patient's serum and processed in exactly the same manner.

THE WEIL-FELIX TEST

Developed by Weil and Felix in 1916, this test employs suspensions of cultures of the OX19, OX2 and OXK strains of *Proteus*. Organisms of these strains share antigens with some of the agents responsible for several febrile diseases and can thus be used to detect antibodies against the various agents or diseases. Table

Table 28–1. Scope of diagnostic utility of febrile antibody tests

Antigen Employed	Disease to Which Antibodies Are Detectable	Time in Weeks of Appearance of Maximum Titer	Significant Titer
Salmonella "O" Group D	Typhoid fever	3–5	1:80*
Salmonella "H" Group D	Typhoid fever	4–5	1:80
Salmonella "O" Group A	Paratyphoid A	3–5	1:80*
Salmonella "O" Group B	Paratyphoid B	3–5	1:80*
Proteus OX 19	Typhus, or Rocky Mountain spotted fever	2–3	1:160
Proteus OX 2 and OX 19	Spotted fever	2–3	1:160
Proteus OXK	Scrub typhus	2–3	1:160
Brucella abortus	Brucellosis	3–5	1:80
Pasteurella tularensis	Tularemia	4–8	1:160
Leptospira	Leptospirosis	1–2	1:80

*These titers are significant only when found in the serum of nonvaccinated individuals.

28–1 lists the various antigens employable in febrile antibody tests and the diseases that each antigen may diagnose by reacting with antibodies in patient serum.

Tests similar to the Widal and Weil-Felix reactions may be carried out for brucellosis, tularemia and leptospirosis, utilizing suitable antigens. From a diagnostic point of view, it is important to realize some possible cross-reactions:

    a. Typhoid fever antibodies may cross-react with *Salmonella* "O" Group B.

    b. Apparently normal sera could contain *Proteus* antibodies.

    c. Tularemia antibodies may cross-react with both *Brucella abortus* and *B. melitensis* antigens.

    d. Recently vaccinated individuals may demonstrate an array of different high titers.

28-4 HETEROPHIL ANTIBODY TESTS

Infectious mononucleosis is an acute, generalized infectious disease of viral etiology. It predominantly attacks young adults, among whom nurses and interns seem to be either more susceptible or possibly most exposed individuals. Isolated cases in infants and the aged have been reported. The disease is self-limiting and seldom fatal.

The symptoms of infectious mononucleosis are extremely diverse, and may simulate those of several more important diseases.

Characteristic clinical, hematologic, pathologic, and serologic changes must be studied together in order to diagnose a case as infectious mononucleosis. Of course, here we are interested in the serology.

The serology of infectious mononucleosis warrants a brief introduction. In 1911, Forssman demonstrated that if a rabbit were injected with guinea pig tissue, the antibodies produced by that rabbit would agglutinate sheep red blood cells. The antibody responsible for this reaction was named Forssman antibody, and the antigen it reacted with, the Forssman antigen.

Soon after, others discovered that the Forssman antigen was widely distributed in nature. It has been found, among other sources, in various tissues of the guinea pig, cat, dog, mouse, and horse, in the red blood cells of sheep, as well as in various species of bacteria such as *Escherichia, Shigella,* and *Streptococcus pneumoniae.* The antigen is not present in the organs of cattle, rats, rabbits, pig, sheep, or man. In 1932, Paul and Bunnell discovered that the serum of patients suffering from glandular fever (infectious mononucleosis) also agglutinated the red blood cells of sheep.

The term *heterophil antibody* was introduced to designate an antibody that would react with an apparently unrelated antigen. We have already seen that cells are composed of many antigens, and that some antigens may be shared by different cells (see Section 28–1). The terms "apparently unrelated antigen" and "heterophil antibody" are therefore unfortunately chosen and should be abolished. The so-called heterophil antibodies react specifically with their antigen, just as any other antibody does. The antigen responsible for their production, however, is distributed more widely than most other antigens. Besides the Forssman and the infectious mononucleosis antibodies, the antibodies produced in response to serum sickness also agglutinate the red blood cells of sheep.

If we employ sheep red blood cells to detect agglutinating antibodies in a patient's serum, as we do in the Paul-Bunnell test, a positive result could indicate the presence of one or a combination of three types of antibodies:

    a. Infectious mononucleosis antibodies (IM)

    b. Forssman antibodies (FO)

    c. Serum sickness antibodies (SS)

This is because the sheep red blood cell carries all three corresponding antigens, IM, FO, and SS. The Paul-Bunnell test, therefore, is a presumptive test for infectious mononucleosis and will only reveal whether a serum contains sheep red cell agglutinins or

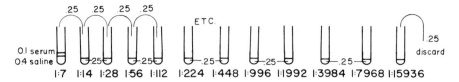

Fig. 28–3. Serial dilution of serum sample for the Paul-Bunnell test (the dilution factor of the 0.1-ml RBC is accounted for).

not. The test itself is fairly simple:

a. Inactivate test serum at 56°C for 30 minutes.

b. Make serial, twofold dilutions in saline in 0.25-ml volumes (see Fig. 28–3).

c. Add 0.1 ml of a 2% suspension of sheep red blood cells to each tube.

d. Leave the tubes at room temperature for two hours.

e. Read the titer as the highest dilution that will indicate agglutination of the red cells upon gentle tapping of the tube.

To diagnose a case of infectious mononucleosis by serologic methods, then, we need to differentiate between the three types of heterophil antibodies. This we may do by the Davidsohn differential test, which will differentiate the three types from one another.

The *Davidsohn differential test* makes use of the facts that guinea pig kidney cells carry both Forssman and serum sickness

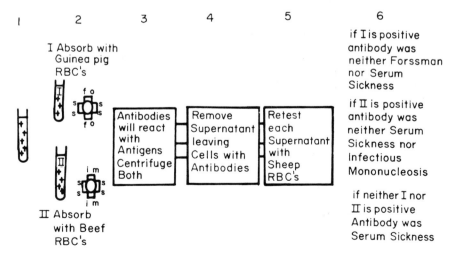

Fig. 28–4. Steps in the Davidsohn differential test.

Table 28–2. Selective absorption of heterophil antibodies

Type of Antibody	Cells Used for Absorptions	
	Guinea Pig Kidney	Beef Red Cells
Forssman	Absorbed	Not absorbed
Serum sickness	Absorbed	Absorbed
Infectious mononucleosis	Not absorbed	Absorbed

antigens (FO and SS), and beef red blood cells carry both serum sickness and infectious mononucleosis antigens (SS and IM). If we subject a portion of a serum positive in the Paul-Bunnell test to guinea pig kidney cells and another portion to beef red blood cells, the heterophil antibodies will selectively adhere to their antigens and may be removed by centrifugation and subsequent separation of the supernatant (Fig. 28–4). By retesting this supernatant with sheep red blood cells, we can tell which antibodies have been removed by which antigens, and hence which antibodies were present in the serum before absorption (see Table 28–2).

A number of companies supply reagents to be used in this test.* Detailed methodology varies with different products. Simplified screening tests have been developed that offer rapid provisional diagnosis of infectious mononucleosis.†

28-5 ANTISTREPTOLYSIN O

Todd discovered in 1928 that a broth culture of certain species of *Streptococcus* would hemolyze red blood cells. He attributed the lytic activity to a toxin, and called the toxin streptolysin. It was discovered later that some *Streptococcus* cultures produced two types of hemolytic toxins, subsequently called streptolysin O and streptolysin S. Streptolysin O is produced by most members of *Streptococcus* Group A, by human strains of *Streptococcus* Group C and by some strains of *Streptococcus* Group G. Streptolysin O is fairly antigenic and, hence, patients suffering infections by any of these organisms could produce antibodies to streptolysin O. Streptolysin O is oxygen-labile, lysing red blood cells only when in the reduced state. Once oxidized, it may be reactivated by reduction.

---

*Baltimore Biological Laboratories, Cockeysville, Md.; Difco Laboratories, Detroit, Mich.; Ortho Diagnostics, Raritan, N.J.
†*Hetrol Slide Test*, Difco Laboratories, Detroit, Mich.; *Mono check*, Hyland Laboratories, Costa Mesa, Calif.; *Monospot Test*, Ortho Diagnostics, Inc., Raritan, N.J.; *Monosticon Test*, Organon, Inc., West Orange, N.J.

The hemolytic activity is further inhibited by the presence of cholesterol. Streptolysin S is produced by some strains of *Streptococcus* Group A and is oxygen-stable. It is poorly antigenic, and is not believed to play a role in the production of antibodies in infected individuals. The antibody, antistreptolysin O or ASO, and its measurement, is the topic of discussion in this section.

The antigen, streptolysin O, can play a dual role in the final reaction: it may react with the antibody, antistreptolysin O, or it may react with the red blood cells. If it reacts with the antibody, it can no longer lyse red blood cells and is thus said to be neutralized. Obviously, it is possible to mix small amounts of antibody with large amounts of antigen. A subsequent addition of red cells to such a mixture would result in lysis of the red cells by excess antigen. Therefore, streptolysin O must be carefully standardized so that known amounts can be used in the test. This is accomplished by carefully measuring the antigen and expressing its strength in specific units; the unit system for this antigen was devised by Todd. For this purpose, the antigen is first measured in minimum hemolytic doses. One *minimum hemolytic dose (MHD)* is that amount of streptolysin O that will completely lyse 0.5 ml of a 5% suspension of rabbit red blood cells.

The method of measurement could be a simple titration as explained in Figure 28–3, using streptolysin instead of serum, and adding 0.5 ml of a 5% rabbit red blood cell suspension instead of sheep cells. The last dilution permitting complete lysis would then contain one MHD. If one Todd unit is 2.5 MHD, a simple calculation should be all that is required to express the results of the streptolysin titration in Todd units per milliliter.

THE ASO TITRATION

The antibody antistreptolysin O, or simply ASO, is also measured in Todd units. One unit of antibody, or ASO, is that amount that neutralizes one Todd unit of streptolysin O. The following reagents are required for this test:

    a. Streptolysin O buffer,* used as a diluent throughout the test.
    b. Red cells; a 5% suspension of rabbit red blood cells* suspended in streptolysin O buffer.
    c. Streptolysin O reagent,* the antigen, standardized to contain one Todd unit per 0.5 ml.
    d. Positive and negative serum controls.*
    e. Test serum, inactivated by heating to 56°C for 30 minutes.

---

*Available from Difco Laboratories, Detroit, Mich., Baltimore Biological Laboratories, Cockeysville, Md.

Table 28–3. Antistreptolysin O titration

Tube No.	Serum Dilution	Diluted Serum, ml	Streptolysin O Buffer, ml	Streptolysin O Reagent, ml		Rabbit Cells 3%, ml		Titer in Todd Units	Tube No.
1	1:10	1.0	0.0	0.5		0.5		10	1
2	1:10	0.2	0.8	0.5		0.5		50	2
3	1:100	1.0	0.0	0.5		0.5		100	3
4	1:100	0.66	0.34	0.5	INCUBATION	0.5	INCUBATION & CENTRIFUGATION	150	4
5	1:100	0.5	0.5	0.5		0.5		200	5
6	1:100	0.4	0.6	0.5		0.5		250	6
7	1:100	0.3	0.7	0.5		0.5		333	7
8	1:500	1.0	0.0	0.5		0.5		500	8
9	1:500	0.8	0.2	0.5		0.5		625	9
10	1:500	0.6	0.4	0.5		0.5		833	10
11	1:500	0.4	0.6	0.5		0.5		1250	11
12	1:500	0.2	0.8	0.5		0.5		2500	12
13	Streptolysin Control		1.0	0.5		0.5		Hemolysis	13
14	Red Cell Control		1.5	0.0		0.5		No Hemolysis	14

In the test proper, three dilutions of test serum are prepared:

A. 0.5 ml of serum plus 4.5 ml of buffer = 1:10

B. 1.0 ml of A plus 9.0 ml of buffer = 1:100

C. 2.0 ml of B plus 8.0 of buffer = 1:500

Portions of these dilutions plus further diluent, antigen, and red cells are distributed in a row of 14 test tubes and processed as outlined in Table 28–3.

To read, examine each tube carefully for signs of hemolysis. The streptolysin control should show complete hemolysis; the red cell control, no hemolysis. The normal range of ASO titers runs up to 100 Todd units/ml. Following acute streptococcal infections, the titer will rise to a maximum in about four to six weeks. Titers of 2500 units/ml or higher are quite common and may persist for up to six months, when they begin a slow decline. For this reason, high titers on single serum samples are no guarantee of a recent infection.

28-6 SYPHILIS SEROLOGY

Under Section 18–2, much has already been said about the different antigens involved in syphilis serology and about the diagnostic significance of various tests. Here, we shall concern ourselves with the mechanics of some of the more common tests and the principles involved in some others.

THE VDRL TEST

This test utilizes a carefully balanced mixture of cardiolipin, lecithin and cholesterol as a flocculating antigen in a simple slide test. The entire procedure consists of three major steps.

  1. **Preparation of Antigen Emulsion**
     a. Pipette 0.4 ml of buffered saline solution* to the bottom of a 30-ml round bottle or vessel.
     b. Add 0.5 ml of antigen* directly onto the saline while continuously but gently rotating the bottle or vessel on a flat surface.

     Caution: Temperature of both saline and antigen should be between 23° and 29°C. Antigen must be added drop by drop, but rapidly, so that all the 0.5 ml is added in about six seconds.

     Keep the pipette well away from the surface of the saline, and rotate the vessel rapidly but not too vigorously, so that no saline will splash onto the pipette. Proper speed of rotation is obtained when a circle about two inches in diameter is circumscribed about three times per second.

     c. Continue rotation for about ten seconds after all the antigen has been added.
     d. Add 4.1 ml of buffered saline.
     e. Stopper the vessel and shake 30 times in a period of no more than ten seconds.
     f. The antigen is now ready for use and may be used for a period of 24 hours.
  2. **Qualitative Test with Serum**
     a. Pipette 0.05 ml of inactivated serum into a ring on a special slide.
     b. Add one drop (1/60 ml) of antigen emulsion onto each serum.
     c. Rotate slides for four minutes. With mechanical rotation, circumscribe a ¾-inch diameter at 180 rpm; manually 2-inch diameter at 120 rpm.
     d. Read tests immediately after rotation.

Note: Serum controls of graded reactivity (reactive, weakly reactive, nonreactive) must always be included to ensure reliability of the results obtained.

  3. **Readings**

Read test microscopically with the low-power objective. The antigen will appear as short rod forms. Aggregation of those

---

*Available from Difco Laboratories, Detroit, Mich. and Lederle Laboratories, Pearl River, N.Y. Both saline and antigen should be obtained from the same firm.

particles into large or small clumps is interpreted as reactive or weakly reactive respectively. Zonal reactions result in loosely bound or irregular clumping.

THE RAPID PLASMA REAGIN CARD TEST

This test is rapidly replacing the VDRL test in popularity. The test is much less cumbersome than the VDRL, more sensitive, and probably more specific. In this test, unheated serum or plasma may be used. The antigen is ready-made* and quite stable. The antigen is coated on carbon particles, which are sized to allow easy reading when aggregated by antibody. The RPR test has been adapted successfully for use with the AutoAnalyzer.

THE REITER PROTEIN COMPLEMENT FIXATION TEST

This test uses a nonpathogenic treponemal strain as its antigen and is therefore more specific than either the VDRL or RPR card test. The complement fixation test is rather complex and beyond the scope of this text. Therefore, we shall limit ourselves to a general discussion of its principles.

Complement is a thermolabile substance present in the serum of normal individuals. In fact, it is a rather involved group of substances, but for the sake of this discussion we may consider it a single substance. Complement reacts nonspecifically with most antibody-antigen complexes. In doing so, it will be fixed or bound, and will no longer be able to react with other antibody-antigen complexes. If the antibody-antigen complex happens to be a cell with its antibody attached (a sensitized cell), the cell will be lysed by complement activity. In the complement fixation (CF) test, certain unobservable antibody-antigen complexes are mixed with

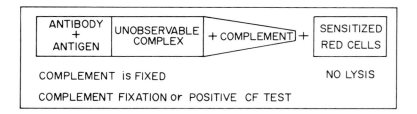

Fig. 28–5. Complement fixation or positive CF test.

---

*Hynson, Westcott and Dunning, Inc., Baltimore, Md.; the manufacturer supplies a 16-page brochure, fully outlining this test, free of charge.

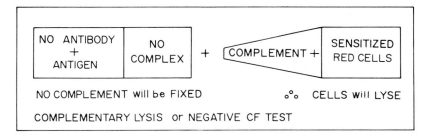

Fig. 28–6. Complementary lysis or negative CF test.

certain amounts of complement (Fig. 28–5). In such mixtures, complement will be fixed, and subsequent addition of sensitized cells (another antibody-antigen complex) will find no complement to react with, and the cells will remain intact. If antibody would be absent in the first instance, no unobservable antibody-antigen complexes would form, no complement would be fixed, and upon addition of sensitized cells, the cells would lyse (Fig. 28–6).

You can appreciate the complexity of the CF test procedure if you consider the possible results of the following:

    a. Too much complement is used.

    b. Antigen reacts with complement.

    c. Serum reacts with complement.

    d. Serum contains complement.

    e. Serum or antigen contains lysins.

THE FLUORESCENT TREPONEMA ANTIBODY TEST

This is the most specific test for syphilis. We have already discussed the basic principles of fluorescence microscopy in Chapter 3. Fluorescent antibodies have been labelled with a fluorescent dye. When the antibody is allowed to react with its antigen on a glass slide and the slide examined under the fluorescence microscope, the antigen appears as an illuminous object against a dark background.

The principle is so simple that the first fluorescent antibody techniques produced many nonspecific results. In order to produce effective fluorescent antibody tests, highly specific and pure reagents are an utmost necessity.

28-7 OTHER SEROLOGIC TESTS

Many more serologic tests could be described. The ones discussed here were chosen because they are either in common use in routine laboratories, or are particularly beneficial in explaining the principles of serology. Several relatively simple procedures have gained prominence during the last decade. Most of these employ latex particles coated with specific antigens. Such latex particles are rapidly aggregated by specific antibody; aggregates are easily visualized when the antigen-coated particles are mixed with serum containing antibodies on a glass slide.

Test kits for the rheumatoid factor, thyroid antibodies, ASO, infectious mononucleosis, CRP and many others are available from various sources.

FURTHER READING

1. Carpenter, P. L.: *Immunology and Serology.* 3rd ed. Philadelphia, W. B. Saunders Co., 1975.
2. Delaat, A. N. C.: *Primer of Serology.* Hagerstown, Harper & Row, 1976.

Part IV
SPECIFIC
METHODOLOGY

chapter 29

Culture Media: Their Preparation and Usefulness

29-1 CULTURE MEDIA

Any substance that can be used for the cultivation of microorganisms may be called a medium (plural, media) or, more precisely, culture medium.

PURPOSES OF MEDIA

Media serve one of two main purposes:
a. They promote microbial growth so that cultural characteristics can be ascertained.
b. They facilitate some biochemical reaction that is discernible either directly, by observation, or indirectly, by further reaction with additional reagents.

Of course, all these reactions, cultural as well as biochemical, depend upon the composition of the medium and the nature of the culture under study. We classify culture media as four different types:

    a. Basic media
    b. Enriched media
    c. Selective, differential and enrichment media
    d. Special media

29-2 BASIC MEDIA

These are the simplest media, containing only some meat extract or other simple infusion, peptone, salt, and water. The meat extract or infusion supplies the organisms with amino acids, vitamins, salts, and traces of carbon, nitrogen, hydrogen, and other elements. Salts, usually NaCl, serve to obtain the required isotonicity for the maintenance of constant osmotic pressures. Water serves as a solvent, a transport medium, or both. Because most water supplies contain a large amount of assorted minerals, of which copper is particularly harmful to many bacteria, one should always use carefully distilled water to prepare culture media. Vessels used to store distilled water should be cleaned periodically, as algae and other microbes may contaminate such supplies and produce substances toxic to many other microbes.

Media that contain only meat infusion, peptone, salt and water are in the liquid state; to study colonial characteristics, we must culture organisms on solid media. Solidification may be achieved by adding agar, gelatin, serum or egg albumin to the other ingredients. Agar, which is a polysaccharide obtainable from seaweed, is usually preferred. At a concentration of 2%, few bacteria can hydrolyze agar, and it has a melting point at approximately 92°C and a solidification point about 42°C.

At a concentration of 1.5% to 3.0%, agar provides a solid medium that will not disintegrate through physical means employed in the culture of most microorganisms. The wide range between its melting and solidification points is also beneficial, because it allows us to supplement basic media with additional nutrients required for growth. Blood and proteins may be added to a basic medium containing agar provided that the medium has been cooled to below 56°C; of course, the medium must be poured into plates before it cools to 45°C.

When large batches are to be prepared, the hazard of burning the media to the bottom of a flask may be reduced by preboiling about three quarters of the total volume of water required for the complete medium. This boiling hot water may then be added to the rest of the ingredients suspended in the remaining one quarter volume of water. The total length of time required to boil the entire mixture is thus drastically reduced and the chances of burning or charring are minimized.

NUTRIENT BROTH

Beef extract	3	g
Peptone	5	g
Distilled water	1000	ml

Dissolve the ingredients in the water over heat. Adjust the pH to 7.4. Dispense in suitable containers. Sterilize by autoclaving at 121°C for 15 minutes. Cool, incubate at 37°C for 18 hours, discard contaminated tubes, and store the remainder at 4°C.

Nutrient broth provides a medium that will support growth of a wide variety of microorganisms except the more fastidious ones.

NUTRIENT AGAR

Beef extract	3	g
Peptone	5	g
Sodium chloride	8	g
Agar	1000	ml

Dissolve ingredients by slow boiling; adjust the pH to 7.4; autoclave at 121°C for 15 minutes. Cool to approximately 60°C; pour approximately 15 ml aseptically into sterile, standard-size Petri dishes. Leave for about one hour to permit the mixture to solidify fully, then store the plates in the dark, medium uppermost to prevent water of condensation from collecting over its surface. Plated medium should be used within a week or so, as evaporation alters the concentration of the ingredients rather rapidly.

Alternately, this medium may be dispensed into suitable culture tubes before sterilization, following which the tubes may be slanted to obtain maximal slopes. Properly capped tubes may be stored at 4°C almost indefinitely.

TRYPTIC SOY BROTH

Tryptone	17	g
Soytone	3	g
Dextrose	2.5	g
Sodium chloride	5	g
Dipotassium phosphate	2.5	g
Distilled water	1000	ml

Prepare as you would nutrient broth. This mixture provides a richer medium than nutrient broth and supports the growth of a wider range of bacteria. The dextrose provides a ready source of energy but is rapidly converted into acid end-products. These end-products are partially buffered by the phosphate.

TRYPTIC SOY AGAR

Tryptone	15	g
Soytone	5	g
Sodium chloride	5	g
Agar	15	g
Distilled water	1000	ml

Prepare as nutrient agar. The advantages of adding dextrose, as in tryptic soy broth, are lost because buffers are less effective in solid media.

BRAIN-HEART INFUSION BROTH

Calf brain infusion from	200	g of brain
Beef heart infusion from	250	g of heart
Peptone	10	g
Sodium chloride	5	g
Disodium phosphate	2.5	g
Dextrose	2	g
Distilled water	1000	ml

Prepare as nutrient broth.

BRAIN-HEART INFUSION AGAR

Add 15 grams of agar to brain-heart infusion broth. Prepare as nutrient agar.

HEART INFUSION BROTH

Beef heart infusion from	500	g of heart
Tryptone	10	g
Sodium chloride	5	g
Distilled water	1000	ml

Prepare as nutrient broth.

HEART INFUSION AGAR

Add 15 grams of agar to heart infusion broth. Prepare as nutrient agar.

LIVER INFUSION AGAR

Beef liver infusion from	500	g of liver
Proteose peptone	10	g
Sodium chloride	5	g
Agar	20	g
Distilled water	1000	ml

Prepare as nutrient agar, adjusting the pH to 6.9. When sloped in tubes, this medium allows detection of H_2S production by *Brucella*. Hydrogen sulfide is detected by hanging a strip of filter paper, which has been dipped into a 10% solution of lead acetate and dried, from the lip of the tube.

The last five media described here are richer than the preceding ones because various amounts of different vitamins and amino acids are supplied directly by the infusions.

SABOURAUD'S DEXTROSE AGAR

Peptone	10	g
Dextrose	40	g
Agar	25	g
Distilled water	1000	ml

Dissolve by boiling, adjust to pH 7.6, dispense in 20-ml tubes, plug with cotton wool and autoclave at 121° for 15 minutes. Cool the tubes to permit maximal slant formation and store at 4°C.

Sabouraud's medium is particularly suited for the culture of yeasts and dermatophytes. Without agar it provides a broth suited for mass culture of yeasts.

29-3 ENRICHED MEDIA

You may argue that some of the aforementioned media are enriched media. However, if we define basic media as those that contain only meat extracts or infusions, peptone, salts and water, we may now define enriched media as basic media that are supplemented with body fluids, specific vitamins, amino acids, proteins, or any other nutrients.

BLOOD AGAR

Blood agar is one of the most commonly used media in a medical microbiology laboratory. It may be prepared by adding 5% to 10% defibrinated sterile blood to any basic agar medium. Be sure that the medium is cooled to just below 56°C before adding the blood (red blood cells hemolyze at 56°C, and proteins precipitate at 65°C). Pour into plates immediately, as described for nutrient agar.

Nutrient agar is often used as a blood agar base, but I recommend heart infusion agar. The NaCl level of the base should be a minimum of 0.5%; the optimal isotonicity is 0.9%.

Many hospitals use outdated human blood from their blood banks to prepare this medium. This is not recommended because such products may contain unknown antibodies, antibiotics, high dextrose levels, and the like. These substances could inhibit the growth of organisms one may wish to isolate.*

Sheep's blood appears to be best, especially when one can depend upon a known donor or reliable source. Remember, however, that sheep's blood inhibits the growth of *Haemophilus influenzae*. Rabbit or horse blood is satisfactory but difficult to obtain. Either enhances the growth of many organisms and widens the spectrum of bacteria producing beta hemolysis.

CHOCOLATE BLOOD AGAR

This medium is basically the same as blood agar but, by adding the blood to the base while the latter is still 80°C, the proteins precipitate, the red cells lyse, and the hemoglobin is converted to hematin, thereby making these nutrients more readily available for the growth of more fastidious organisms. Of course, the medium cannot demonstrate hemolytic properties of microorganisms.

SERUM BROTH

Various concentrations of serum from different species may be added to any of the basic broths. Sterile serum should be added aseptically to broth that has been cooled to below 65°C, to prevent protein from coagulating. Tryptic Soy-20% serum broth is particularly useful to preserve dehydrated cultures of fastidious organisms.

SERUM AGAR

Prepare as serum broth but add serum to a basic agar. If the serum concentration is to be high, one should take the dilution factor into consideration and increase the agar percentage accordingly.

LOEFFLER BLOOD SERUM

3 volumes of beef blood serum
1 volume of 1% dextrose

---

*Harris, H. H., and Coleman, M. B., eds.: *Diagnostic Procedures and Reagents.* 4th ed. New York, American Public Health Association, 1963, p. 133.

Adjust pH to 7.2. Dispense this mixture into tubes. Slant the tubes in wire baskets or on a special tray, and inspissate at 85°C for four hours. After the four hours, turn off the oven but let the tubes remain overnight. The next day, autoclave at 121°C for ten minutes. Be sure that the caps are on tight when you autoclave this medium, and exhaust the steam slowly. Loeffler blood serum allows luxuriant growth of *Corynebacterium diphtheriae*, producing characteristic morphology with different varieties of diphtheria species. Dehydrated Loeffler medium is commercially available.

SERUM SLOPES

Any medium that contains more than 5% serum may be solidified by inspissation and subsequently autoclaved, if necessary, in a manner similar to that described under Loeffler blood serum.

TRYPTOSE AGAR

Tryptose	20	g
Dextrose	1	g
NaCl	5	g
Agar	15	g
Thiamine hydrochloride	0.005	g
Distilled water	1000	ml

Prepare as nutrient agar, adjust pH to 7.2. This medium is particularly suited as a broth for the isolation of Brucellaceae from the blood.

BORDET GENGOU AGAR

Potato infusion from	125	g
NaCl	5.5	g
Agar	20	g

Dehydrated base media containing the above are available commercially.

Dissolve the above in 1000 ml of distilled water containing 10 ml of glycerol. Prepare further as blood agar, adding 15% to 25% blood.

This specially enriched medium is used for the isolation of *Bordetella pertussis* from cases of whooping cough by the so-called cough plate method. For primary isolation, the medium may be supplemented by selective antibiotics.

LEVINTHAL'S MEDIUM

Solution 1

Tryptic soy broth .... 500 ml
Sheep blood .... 50 ml

Boil at precisely 100°C for 20 minutes while stirring constantly. A deep brown clot will form. Filter until clear, then sterilize by filtration.

Solution 2

Agar .... 18 g
Distilled water .... 275 ml

Dissolve by boiling, then add 275 ml of tryptic soy broth.

Mix equal volumes of solutions 1 and 2 and pour into plates. This medium is useful in culturing *Haemophilus influenzae* without the need to supply additional hematin or NAD.

MUELLER-HINTON AGAR

Beef infusion .... 300 g
Peptone .... 17.5 g
Starch (soluble) .... 1.5 g
Agar .... 17 g
Distilled water .... 1000 ml

Dissolve ingredients by boiling, adjust to pH 7.4 and autoclave at 121°C for 15 minutes. Pour into plates. This medium is particularly useful for the assay of antibiotic susceptibilities and is recommended for the Kirby-Bauer method.

29-4 SELECTIVE, DIFFERENTIAL AND ENRICHMENT MEDIA

Selective media are usually basic or enriched agar media to which certain reagents have been added that will prevent the growth of the majority of bacteria, thereby allowing isolation of a selected few from specimens containing large numbers of organisms.

Differential media are basic or enriched media to which certain reagents have been added that will react with some specific types of bacteria in some observable way. For instance, when lactose and neutral red are added to nutrient agar, lactose-fermenting bacteria will be differentiated from non-lactose-fermenters by producing acid end-products demonstrable by a change in color (red at acid pH) of the neutral red. Of course, adding some inhibitory substances to differential media may render them selective as well as differential. Most so-called differential media are of this latter type.

Enrichment media usually are enriched, liquid media that contain some inhibitory substances, thereby creating an especially favorable environment for a rather narrow range of bacteria. Selenite F broth is one such medium, which reduces the growth of coliform bacilli, while simultaneously enhancing the growth of *Salmonella* and *Shigella*.

Because the ingredients that comprise selective, differential, and enrichment media are often similar, their definitions appear to overlap; thus, we discuss all three types of media in this section.

G. C. MEDIUM (THAYER-MARTIN MEDIUM)

Solution 1

Proteose peptone No. 3	15	g
Cornstarch	1	g
Dipotassium phosphate	4	g
Potassium dihydrogen phosphate	1	g
Sodium chloride	5	g
Agar	10	g
Distilled water	500	ml

Dehydrated base medium containing the above is available commercially. Dissolve by boiling, adjust pH to 7.2, autoclave at 121°C for 15 minutes. Cool to below 56°C and add 10 ml of supplement (Difco A or B).

Solution 2

Hemoglobin	10	g
Distilled water	500	ml

Dissolve, adjust the pH to 7.2, autoclave at 121°C for 15 minutes. Cool to below 56°C, mix equal volumes of solutions 1 and 2 and pour into plates. This medium is particularly useful for primary isolation of *Neisseria gonorrhoeae*.

The true Thayer-Martin medium would also contain 5 ml VCN and Isovitalex, added to the complete G.C. medium when it is cooled to about 50°C. Isovitalex is a complex mixture of several vitamins, amino acids and other ingredients that further enrich the medium; VCN is a mixture of the antibiotics vancomycin, colistin and nystatin, which renders the medium selective for *N. gonor-*

rhoeae. Both are available from Baltimore Biological Laboratories, Cockeysville, Md.

Recently, this medium has been further supplemented with 0.25 ml (20 mg/ml) of trimethoprim lactate. This antibiotic enhances the selectivity of the medium and reduces the spreading effect of *Proteus* species.

PHENYLETHANOL AGAR

Tryptose	10	g
Beef extract	3	g
NaCl	5	g
Agar	15	g
Phenylethanol	2.5	g
Distilled water	1000	ml

Prepare like nutrient agar. This medium may be further enriched by adding 5% blood. The phenylethanol inhibits most gram-negative bacilli, making this a selective medium for gram-positive organisms. Because the phenylethanol evaporates slowly, the plates should be stored for no longer than two weeks.

BILE BLOOD AGAR, 40%

Oxgall	43	g
Agar	40	g
Distilled water	1000	ml

Prepare like blood agar using 7.5% sheep blood. This is a highly selective medium useful to differentiate *Streptococcus faecalis* from other streptococci, as *S. faecalis* is the only species this medium will support.

BILE ESCULIN AGAR

Beef extract	3	g
Peptone	5	g
Oxgall	40	g
Esculin	1	g
Ferric citrate	0.5	g
Agar	15	g
Distilled water	1000	ml

Mix, boil, dispense into screwcapped tubes and autoclave at 121°C for 15 minutes. Cool in slanted position and store at 4°C.

This medium is useful to differentiate Group D streptococci from other streptococci, and *Listeria monocytogenes* from other corynebacteria. These organisms hydrolyse the esculin, to produce glucose and esculetin. These products react with the ferric citrate to form a dark brown salt, which is observable as a dark zone surrounding esculin positive cultures.

The addition of ferric ammonium citrate solution after culture allows one to detect esculin hydrolysis by some anaerobes.

TELLURITE BLOOD AGAR

Proteose peptone no. 3	20	g
Dextrose	2	g
NaCl	5	g
Agar	13	g
Distilled water	1000	ml

Prepare as nutrient agar, cool the sterile base down to just below 80°C, then add 20 ml of 1% potassium tellurite and 5% blood, heat to just over 80°C, until the medium turns to a brownish color. Cool and pour into plates.

This medium inhibits most bacteria but allows growth of the Corynebacteriaceae. Reduction of the inhibitor, tellurite, will further aid in the differentiation of *Corynebacterium diphtheriae*, since this will be demonstrated by a rather characteristic blackening of the colonies of the different varieties.

MODIFIED TINSDALE MEDIUM

Agar	20	g
Proteose peptone no. 3	20	g
NaCl	5	g
Distilled water	1000	ml

Mix, boil, and adjust pH to 7.4. Autoclave at 121°C for 15 minutes. Cool to 56°C and aseptically add each of the following ingredients in the order listed, mixing thoroughly before adding the next ingredient.

Horse, bovine, or rabbit serum	100	ml
N/10 NaOH	60	ml
0.4% L-cystine in N/10 HCl	60	ml
1% potassium tellurite (aqueous)	30	ml
2.5% sodium thiosulfate (anhydrous)	17	ml

All chemical solutions may be freshly prepared in sterile distilled water, and need not be sterilized thereafter. The serum should be fresh, free from hemolysis, and sterilized by filtration.

The complete medium is poured into petri dishes. This medium differentiates *Corynebacterium diphtheriae gravis* and *mitis* by stimulating the production of pronounced brown halos surrounding their colonies. *C. diphtheriae intermedius* and *C. xerosis* produce only faint halos. Other corynebacteria are suppressed or fail to produce a halo. Most other organisms are either completely inhibited or suppressed by the tellurite, but since the concentration of tellurite is reduced compared to tellurite blood agar, this medium usually results in a higher isolation rate of *C. diphtheriae* from carriers.

LOEWENSTEIN-JENSEN AGAR SLOPES

Asparagine	3.6 g
Magnesium citrate	0.6 g
Magnesium sulfate	0.24 g
Malachite green	0.4 g
Monopotassium phosphate	2.4 g
Potato flour	30 g
Distilled water	600 ml

Mix, dissolve by boiling, and autoclave at 121°C for 15 minutes. Often, 12 ml of glycerol are added to the water before the other ingredients, but should not be included if bovine strains of *Mycobacterium* are to be isolated, because these organisms are glycerophobic.

Cool this preparation to between 40° and 45°C and add 1000 ml of carefully blended whole eggs. The eggs should be scrubbed clean with soap, brush and lukewarm water, rinsed in tap water, sponged with 70% alcohol, broken aseptically, and the contents collected in a sterile container (preferably a Waring blender), and mixed gently to prevent stirring an excess of air bubbles into the egg mixture.

The first preparation can now be added slowly and aseptically to the egg mixture and the complete medium should be dispensed into suitable sterile tubes by the inverted or hooded pipette method. The tubes should then be slanted to obtain a maximal slant and placed in an inspissator set at 70° to 75°C for two to four hours. Remember, this medium is already sterile when dispensed, and inspissation is used only to coagulate the egg products. Caps should be tight to prevent escape of air and subsequent bubble formation on the surface of the medium.

This medium is an enriched selective medium used for the isolation of *Mycobacterium* species. The malachite green will inhibit most other organisms. Mycobacteria will produce fairly characteristic colonies on this medium, which permits some differentiation among the various species.

AZIDE BLOOD AGAR

Tryptose	10	g
Beef extract	3	g
Sodium chloride	5	g
Sodium azide	0.2	g
Agar	15	g
Distilled water	1000	ml

Prepare like blood agar. Sodium azide, at this concentration (1:5000) will inhibit most organisms other than *Streptococcus faecalis* and staphylococci and may be used to isolate these from spreading *Proteus* species.

SALT MANNITOL AGAR

Proteose peptone no. 3	10	g
Beef extract	1	g
Sodium chloride	75	g
d-Mannitol	10	g
Phenol red 1% solution	2.5	ml
Agar	15	g
Distilled water	1000	ml

Prepare as nutrient agar. The increased salt concentration makes this medium highly selective for staphylococci, and thus aids in the isolation of these organisms from stool specimens.

Mannitol fermentation, as affected by most *Staphylococcus aureus* strains, is also demonstrated by a change in color, from red to yellow, of the indicator phenol red.

MACCONKEY AGAR

Peptone	17	g
Proteose peptone	3	g
Lactose	10	g
Bile salts no. 3	1.5	g
Sodium chloride	5	g
Agar	13.5	g
Neutral red	0.03	g
Crystal violet	0.001	g
Distilled water	1000	ml

Prepare as nutrient agar; do not prolong the boiling period beyond the point required to dissolve all the ingredients. MacConkey agar is specifically designed for the isolation of organisms belonging to the family Enterobacteriaceae, and will allow differentiation between lactose-fermenting and nonlactose-fermenting members of this family. Lactose fermentation will be demonstrated by a change in color of the neutral red to purplish pink. Colonies will absorb this dye, and the bile salts, at acid pH, will precipitate to show off this color even more intensely. Nonlactose-fermenters appear as pale, smooth, opaque colonies. Bile salts, in combination with the crystal violet, will also inhibit most gram-positive organisms.

SALMONELLA-SHIGELLA AGAR

Beef extract	5	g
Proteose peptone	5	g
Lactose	10	g
Bile salts no. 3	8.5	g
Sodium citrate	8.5	g
Sodium thiosulfate	8.5	g
Ferric citrate	1	g
Agar	13.5	g
Brilliant green	0.00033	g
Neutral red	0.025	g
Distilled water	1000	ml

Prepare as MacConkey agar but do not autoclave. The lactose, bile salts and neutral red serve basically the same purpose here as they do in MacConkey agar. This medium, however, is highly selective for *Salmonella* and reasonably so for *Shigella* species, since most coliforms will be inhibited by the added citrate and brilliant green. Sodium thiosulfate aids in the H_2S production by many *Salmonella*, which may be detected by blackening of the colonies when the H_2S reacts with the ferric citrate to produce ferrous sulfite.

EOSIN METHYLENE BLUE AGAR (EMB)

Peptone	10	g
Lactose	5	g
Sucrose	5	g
Dipotassium phosphate	2	g
Agar	13.5	g
Eosin Y	0.4	g
Methylene blue	0.065	g
Distilled water	1000	ml

Prepare as MacConkey agar, if to be used immediately. Methylene blue, when reduced by autoclaving, may be reoxidized by shaking the medium before pouring plates. EMB agar is another differential medium for Enterobacteriaceae, showing lactose-fermenters as black or dark centered colonies; nonlactose-fermenters appear colorless.

Saccharose is added because some coliforms will ferment this sugar more readily than lactose. Inclusion of an additional sugar must put us on guard of course, since some of the nonlactose-fermenters could ferment the additional sugar and could thus be ironically mistaken for lactose-fermenters.

DESOXYCHOLATE CITRATE AGAR

Pork infusion	330	g
Proteose peptone no. 3	10	g
Lactose	10	g
Sodium citrate	20	g
Ferric ammonium citrate	2	g
Sodium desoxycholate	5	g
Agar	13.5	g
Neutral red	0.02	g
Distilled water	1000	ml

Prepare as MacConkey agar. The lactose, neutral red and sodium citrate serve the same purpose here as they do in *Salmonella-Shigella* agar.

Sodium desoxycholate and ferric ammonium citrate replace the bile salts and ferric citrate, serving similar purposes. Some differentiation between *Salmonella typhi*, *Salmonella* and *Shigella* may be ascertained from colonial morphology on this medium.

BISMUTH SULFITE AGAR

Beef extract	5	g
Peptone	10	g
Dextrose	5	g
Disodium phosphate	4	g
Ferrous sulfate	0.3	g
Bismuth sulfite	8	g
Agar	20	g
Brilliant green	0.025	g
Distilled water	1000	ml

Prepare as MacConkey agar, adjusting the pH to 7.7, but do not autoclave.

This medium is particularly useful in isolating S. *typhi*, which reduces the bismuth sulfite and shows it up as black. Bismuth sulfite also inhibits most gram-positive organisms, and brilliant green, of course, limits the growth of coliforms. Disodium phosphate acts as a buffer.

SELENITE F BROTH

Tryptone	5	g
Lactose	4	g
Disodium phosphate	10	g
Sodium selenite	4	g
Distilled water	1000	ml

Dissolve, adjust pH to 7.0, bring to a boil but do not autoclave, dispense in sterile tubes to a depth of at least two inches. Sodium selenite at this pH is toxic to coliforms, thereby allowing *Salmonella* a better chance to grow. The selenite will be slowly reduced, producing alkaline end products, which are counterbalanced by the acid end products produced by lactose fermentation. The disodium phosphate further aids to maintain the pH at 7.0, but a stable pH cannot be maintained for much longer than 12 hours.

XLD AGAR

Yeast extract	3	g
L-lysine	5	g
Xylose	3.75	g
Lactose	7.5	g
Sucrose	7.5	g
Sodium desoxycholate	2.5	g
Ferric ammonium citrate	0.8	g
Sodium thiosulfate	6.8	g
Sodium chloride	5	g
Agar	15	g
Phenol red	0.08	g

Dissolve by heat but do not boil, adjust to pH 7.4, and pour plates.

XLD agar provides another selective-differential medium for gram-negative bacilli. Lactose- or sucrose-fermenters produce yellow colonies, nonlactose-fermenters appear red. Hydrogen sulfide production is apparent by the production of black centers in the colonies. This medium appears to be more selective for *Shigella* than for other genera of the family Enterobacteriaceae.

29-5 SPECIAL MEDIA

Media that cannot be easily grouped under one of the foregoing headings will be discussed here. Most of these are used to ascertain one or more biochemical characteristics.

PHENOL RED-SUGAR BROTHS

Beef extract	1	g
Proteose peptone no. 3	10	g
Sodium chloride	5	g
Phenol red, 1% solution	1.8	ml
Distilled water	1000	ml

To this base, add 5 grams of the desired carbohydrate. Adjust the pH to 7.4, dispense in tubes containing inverted Durham tubes, and autoclave at 115°C for 10 minutes. When the organisms ferment the carbohydrate, acid production causes the phenol red to turn yellow, and gas is collected in the Durham tube. A simple medium such as this, of course, is useful only in the study of nonfastidious organisms.

FERMENTATION MEDIUM FOR CLOSTRIDIUM

Trypticase	40	g
Sodium chloride	10	g
Sodium thioglycolate	2	g
Agar	2	g
Distilled water	1000	ml

Dissolve by boiling, autoclave at 115°C for 10 minutes, add 20% of a filtered solution of the desired sugar, and dispense into sterile screwcapped tubes. Incubate inoculated tubes anaerobically for 72 hours, then test for acid production with a few drops of 0.5% neutral red. Indicators will be reduced under anaerobic conditions, thus losing their characteristics.

FERMENTATION MEDIUM FOR NEISSERIA*

Peptone	20	g
Agar	25	g
NaCl	5	g
Phenol red 1% solution	1.5	ml
Distilled water	900	ml

*Health Lab. Sc., 14:26–29, 1977.

Mix, boil, cool, adjust to pH 7.4, and autoclave at 121°C for 15 minutes. When the medium has cooled to 56°C, aseptically add 100 ml of 10% solution of carbohydrate and 50 ml of guinea pig serum, both of which have been sterilized by filtration. Aseptically dispense enough medium into suitable screwcapped tubes to allow a slant to form when placing the tube at a 45-degree angle. Cool tubes and store at 4°C. This medium gives the most consistent reactions with the fastidious *Neisseria* species.

CYSTINE TRYPTICASE AGAR (CTA)

Cystine	0.5	g
Trypticase	20.0	g
Agar	3.5	g
Sodium chloride	5.0	g
Sodium sulfite	0.5	g
Phenol red	0.017	g
Distilled water	1000	ml

Dissolve by boiling, adjust pH to 7.3, and dispense in tubes to form slants. Autoclave at 110°C for 10 minutes.

This is an excellent medium on which to maintain fastidious organisms at 25°C. With the addition of 0.5 or 1% carbohydrates, it also serves as a good medium to detect fermenting abilities of the genera *Corynebacterium* and *Neisseria*. The cystine and trypticase are extra nutrients; the sodium sulfite is a preservative.

TRIPLE SUGAR IRON AGAR (TSI)

Beef extract	3	g
Yeast extract	3	g
Peptone	15	g
Proteose	5	g
Dextrose	1	g
Lactose	10	g
Sucrose	10	g
Sodium chloride	5	g
Sodium thiosulfate	0.3	g
Ferrous sulfate	0.2	g
Agar	1.2	g
Phenol red, 1% solution	2.4	ml
Distilled water	1000	ml

Boil, adjust pH to 7.4, dispense in loose-capped culture tubes, just enough so that a slant as well as a one-inch butt will result when the tube is slanted at approximately 30 degrees. Autoclave tubes at 115°C for 10 minutes; slant tubes to solidify. This medium will detect an organism's ability to ferment dextrose, lactose, sucrose, or a combination of these, and to produce H_2S and gas. If only dextrose is fermented, oxygen seeping into the slope will revert the acid slant back to the alkaline state once all the dextrose has been fermented. Hence, dextrose is present in smaller proportions than the other sugars. Oxidation and subsequent reversion of the slant can occur only when air can enter the culture tube; loosely capped tops or cotton plugs are therefore mandatory for this medium. If either lactose or sucrose are fermented, large amounts of acid will continue to be produced and the slant as well as the butt will remain acid (yellow). Gas production will be indicated by the presence of bubbles or splitting of the medium in the butt of the tube.

Hydrogen sulfide will react with the ferrous sulfate as demonstrated by the appearance of a black precipitate. Table 15–4 indicates the usefulness of this medium.

SULFIDE INDOLE MOTILITY MEDIUM (SIM)

Peptone	30	g
Beef extract	3	g
Peptonized iron (Difco)	0.2	g
Sodium thiosulfate	0.025	g
Agar	3	g
Distilled water	1000	ml

Boil, adjust the pH to 7.4, dispense in culture tubes to a depth of about two inches, and autoclave at 121°C for 15 minutes. A semisolid medium will be produced from which the following bacterial characteristics may be ascertained:

   a. *Hydrogen sulfide* production from cystine in peptone and from the sodium thiosulfate is demonstrated by blackening of the medium by ferric sulfide formation.

   b. When the medium has been carefully stabbed with a straight inoculating wire, highly *motile* strains will grow away from the inoculation site.

   c. *Indole* may be readily produced from tryptophan in peptone and can be detected by adding a few drops of either Kovac's or Ehrlich's reagent (see p. 430).

MR-VP MEDIUM

Buffered peptone	7	g
Dextrose	5	g
Dipotassium phosphate	5	g
Distilled water	1000	ml

Dissolve, adjust the pH to 6.9, dispense in culture tubes (at least 5 ml per tube), and autoclave at 121°C for 15 minutes.

This medium is useful in the differentiation of lactose-fermenting organisms by means of two tests:

a. **Methyl red test.** Some organisms produce acid end-products when fermenting dextrose; these end-products are readily demonstrable by adding a few drops of a 1% solution of methyl red to a portion of a 48-hour culture. MR positive—red; MR negative—yellow.

b. **Voges-Proskauer test.** Other organisms produce acetyl-methylcarbinol from dextrose. This product may be detected by adding four drops of a 40% potassium hydroxide solution and 12 drops of a 5% solution of alpha naphthol in absolute ethanol to 1 ml of a 48-hour culture. A color reaction will occur near the surface of the mixture (which should therefore not be shaken) in anywhere from a few minutes to several hours. VP positive—red; VP negative—yellow.

Meat infusions contain acetylmethyl carbinol, and therefore cannot be used as a growth medium.

UREA AGAR SLOPES

Agar .... 15 g
Distilled water ....1000 ml

Dissolve by boiling, autoclave at 121°C for 15 minutes. Cool to below 55°C, then, aseptically add 1 ml of urea concentrate, dispense in sterile culture tubes and slant for maximum slopes. Members of the *Proteus* group, particularly, will rapidly produce urease, which hydrolyzes the urea to ammonia. Ammonia is detected by a change in color of the indicator phenol red from pale to a bright purplish pink in less than six hours.

Urea concentrate containing phenol red is available commercially.

PHENYLALANINE AGAR

Yeast extract .... 3 g
Dipotassium phosphate .... 1 g
Sodium chloride .... 5 g
dL-phenylalanine .... 2 g
Agar .... 12 g
Distilled water ....1000 ml

Dissolve by boiling, adjust the pH to 7.3, dispense in culture tubes so that maximal slants may be obtained, and autoclave for 15 minutes at 121°C. Some organisms, particularly those of the *Proteus* group, will deaminate phenylalanine to phenylpyruvic acid. This acid may be detected by running 1 ml of a 10% solution of ferric chloride over a 24-hour culture. Pyruvic acid combines with ferric chloride to produce the green compound, ferric phenyl pyruvate.

DECARBOXYLATION BROTH

Peptone	5	g
Beef extract	5	g
Bromcresol purple	0.01	g
Cresol red	0.005	g
Dextrose	0.5	g
Pyridoxal	5	ml
Distilled water	1000	ml

Dissolve, adjust the pH to 6.0, add 1% of the required L-amino acid or 2% when dL-amino acids are used. Dispense in culture tubes, and autoclave at 121°C for 15 minutes. A light floccular precipitate may form with ornithine; this may be disregarded. This medium is useful in differentiating among Enterobacteriaceae, since various amino acids may be decarboxylated by different members of that family.

All members of the family Enterobacteriaceae utilize the dextrose, producing small amounts of acid end-products until the small amount of dextrose is used up, thereby turning the indicator to a yellowish-green. Organisms that manufacture decarboxylase will decarboxylate the amino acid, thereby producing alkaline end-products and reverting the pH; this is demonstrated by a change in color from yellowish-green to purple. With a positive reaction, two color changes may occur; as the first change may often be missed by ill timing, a control base is often set up along with the test medium. This control base contains all the foregoing ingredients except the amino acid, and should therefore always demonstrate the acid reading. Pyridoxal provides an extra source of vitamin B_6.

SIMMON'S CITRATE AGAR

Sodium citrate	2	g
Sodium chloride	5	g
Magnesium sulfate	0.2	g
Monoammonium phosphate	1	g
Dipotassium phosphate	1	g
Agar	15	g
Bromthymol blue	0.08	g
Distilled water	1000	ml

Dissolve by boiling, adjust the pH to 6.9, dispense in scrupulously clean culture tubes, autoclave at 121°C for 15 minutes, cool in a slanted position so that a maximum slope will be obtained. Only those organisms that are capable of utilizing monoammonium phosphate as the sole source of nitrogen, and sodium citrate as the sole source of carbon will grow on this medium.

Bromthymol blue is incorporated to aid the detection of rapid growers; it changes from green to blue with a drop in pH. Note, however, that a positive citrate reaction is recorded whenever growth occurs on this medium, regardless of whether there is a color reaction or not.

KCN BROTH

Proteose peptone	3	g
Disodium phosphate	5.64	g
Monopotassium phosphate	0.225	g
Sodium chloride	5	g
Distilled water	1000	ml

Dissolve, adjust the pH to 7.6, autoclave at 121°C for 15 minutes. Cool to 20°C and aseptically add 15 ml of 0.5% KCN in sterile water. Dispense in tightly stoppered, sterile tubes. This medium should not be kept longer than four weeks.

This concentration of KCN will inhibit most *Salmonella* including *S. arizonae* species, but not *Citrobacter*. Because positives or negatives are recorded as growth or no growth, it is wise to include a control base that contains no KCN to check whether the base will support growth of the organisms under study.

MALONATE BROTH

Ammonium sulfate	2	g
Dipotassium phosphate	0.6	g
Monopotassium phosphate	0.4	g
Sodium chloride	2	g
Sodium malonate	3	g
Bromthymol blue	0.025	g
Distilled water	1000	ml

Dissolve, adjust the pH to 6.7, dispense in culture tubes, and autoclave at 121°C for 15 minutes. The medium contains ammonium sulfate as the sole source of nitrogen, and sodium malonate as a sole source of carbon. Utilization of these substances is ascertained in a manner similar to that described under Simmon's citrate agar. Only *Enterobacter-Klebsiella* and *Salmonella arizonae* are able to utilize these substances.

OF BASAL MEDIUM (HUGH-LEIFSON OXIDATION-FERMENTATION MEDIUM)

Tryptone	2	g
Sodium chloride	5	g
Agar	2.5	g
Phenol red, 1% solution	1.8	ml
Distilled water	1000	ml

Dissolve by boiling, adjust to a pH of 7.1, autoclave at 121°C for 15 minutes, aseptically add 10 ml of a 10% solution of the sugar to be studied, dispense into sterile cotton-plugged tubes, and store at 4°C for no longer than one week.

OF basal medium is useful in the examination of gram-negative bacilli that do not ferment any carbohydrate by using phenol red sugar broths. Two tubes of this medium must be used in conjunction. Both must be stabbed a few times with the culture under study on a straight inoculating wire. One of the tubes is then overlaid with a thin layer of hot paraffin oil. Both tubes must be incubated at 37°C for 24 hours.

If both tubes show acid formation (yellow), the organism under study does ferment that sugar. If only the tube without the paraffin shows acid formation (yellow), the organism does not ferment but oxidizes the sugar. Oxidation requires atmospheric oxygen, which is simply excluded by the paraffin.

Fermentation takes place both with or without oxygen. When both tubes remain unchanged (red), the organisms either did not grow or did not ferment or oxidize the sugar.

LITMUS MILK

Skim milk	100	g
Litmus-10%	30	ml
Distilled water	1000	ml

Dissolve, adjust the pH to 6.8, dispense in culture tubes, and autoclave at 121°C for 15 minutes.

This medium is mainly useful in the differentiation of *Clostridium* species in demonstrating lactose fermentation (changing the litmus to a red color), casein coagulation, gas production, and caseolysis, by which a renninlike enzyme produced by the organisms may completely hydrolyse the casein, resulting in a clear, purplish-brown solution. Rapid gas production, associated with casein coagulation by acid end-products, will result in a so-called stormy clot.

NITRATE BROTH

Beef extract	3	g
Peptone	5	g
Potassium nitrate	1	g
Distilled water	1000	ml

Dissolve, adjust the pH to 7.0, dispense in culture tubes, and autoclave at 121°C for 15 minutes. Several organisms are able to reduce nitrates to nitrites. Nitrites may be detected by adding to the broth a few drops of 0.8% sulfanilic acid in 5 N acetic acid and a few drops of 0.5% N, N-dimethyl-l-naphthylamine, also in 5 N acetic acid. Nitrites will demonstrate a pinkish-red color. Because some rapid growers may further reduce nitrites to nitrogen gas, it is wise to check all "negative" results by sprinkling a loopful of zinc dust onto the medium. Zinc will react with nitrate to produce a deep red color, indicating a true negative result.

THIOGLYCOLATE BROTH

Yeast extract	5	g
Casitone (Difco)	15	g
Dextrose	5	g
Sodium chloride	2.5	g
L-cystine	0.75	g
Thioglycolic acid	0.3	ml
Agar	0.75	g
Resazurin	0.001	g
Distilled water	1000	ml

Dissolve, adjust the pH to 7.1, dispense to a depth of about 2 inches in screwcapped culture tubes, and autoclave at 121°C for 15 minutes. Store in the dark at 25°C.

Agar at this concentration, and in the presence of the reducing agent thioglycolate, will reduce the convection currents to the extent that strict anaerobes will grow freely in the lower portion of this medium. Thioglycolic acid further aids in the initiation of growth of many anaerobes. Oxidation of the medium is demonstrated by a change in color of the resazurin to pink. When more than a third of the medium has changed to this color, the medium should be boiled to drive off the accumulated oxygen.

Methylene blue, 0.002 grams, may replace the resazurin but is more toxic. With this indicator, the medium will turn green when oxidized.

ROBERTSON'S COOKED MEAT

Beef heart, minced .... 450 g
Proteose peptone .... 20 g
Dextrose .... 2 g
Sodium chloride .... 5 g

A prepared, dehydrated medium of this formula is available commercially. Add a level teaspoon of the dehydrated kernels to large screwcap test tubes. Dispense 10 ml of distilled water in each tube. Refrigerate overnight, autoclave at 121°C for 15 minutes.

The unsaturated fatty acids in this medium will take up most of the oxygen, particularly when catalyzed by the hematin released from the meat, which permits the growth of strict anaerobes without the aid of anaerobic jars. If the medium is stored for over one week, excess oxygen may be driven off by boiling the medium prior to use.

STUART'S TRANSPORT MEDIUM

Sodium thioglycolate .... 0.9 g
Sodium glycerophosphate anhydrous .. 10 g
Calcium chloride .... 0.1 g
Methylene blue .... 0.002 g
Agar .... 3 g
Distilled water ....1000 ml

Dissolve by boiling, adjust pH to 7.4, dispense in screwcapped tubes to about ½ inch from the top of the tube, secure the caps tightly, and autoclave at 121°C for 15 minutes. This medium is non-nutritive, but will maintain even the more fastidious microorganisms during ordinary shipping practices. After charcoal-impregnated or rayon swabs have been used to collect the specimen, the swabs are stabbed into the medium, broken off, and the tube sealed again. In this manner, even such organisms as *Neisseria meningitidis, Haemophilus influenzae,* and *Bordetella pertussis* may be isolated following periods of 24 to 48 hours after collection of the specimens. Inoculate the swab onto suitable medium immediately upon arrival of the specimen by carefully and aseptically picking the swab from the transport medium with a pair of forceps.

The ingredients of this medium serve as reducing agents, collectively preserving the organisms.

LACTOSE-EGG YOLK-MILK AGAR

For approximately 15 plates:

Nutrient broth (see p. 387) .... 250 ml
Agar .... 2.2 g
Lactose .... 2.2 g
Skim milk   3   g
Neutral red, 1% solution .... 0.5 ml

Dissolve by boiling, autoclave at 121°C for 15 minutes. Cool to below 65°C, then add 10 ml of a 50-50 mixture of sterile saline and egg yolk. Mix carefully and pour into plates. This medium is particularly useful in the differentiation of *Clostridium* species.

The lactose and the neutral red allow detection of lactose fermentation, which will cause a deep red color to develop in and around the growth areas. Proteolytic enzymes will attack the milk, which causes the medium to become clear. Phospholipid enzymes (lecithinase) will split the lecithin in the egg yolk into diglyceride and phosphorylcholine. The diglyceride appears as a free fat and is demonstrated by an opalescence surrounding the inoculuation site.

Lecithinase activity may be selectively inhibited by inoculating one half of the plate with antitoxin before inoculating the plate with the culture under study.* Lecithinase activity is enhanced at 45°C. Following incubation at 37°C, the plates should be placed at 45°C for one hour before reading results.

ELEK'S MEDIUM

Preparation 1:

Proteose peptone   4   g
Maltose .... 0.6   g
Lactic acid .... 0.14 ml
Distilled water 100   ml

Dissolve and adjust pH to 7.8.

Preparation 2:

Agar   3   g
Sodium chloride   1   g
Distilled water 100   ml

---

*Nagler's reaction is an outmoded method employing serum instead of egg yolk, which does not react as readily in the presence of lecithinase.

Dissolve by heat, filter and adjust pH to 7.8. Mix equal parts of preparations 1 and 2, distribute 10 ml in screwcapped tubes, sterilize by flowing steam for 30 minutes on three successive days. Store indefinitely at 4°C.

For use, melt one tube, cool to below 55°C, add 2.0 ml of normal horse serum, pour into one plate. When solid, immediately apply a strip of filter paper that has been dipped and drip-dried into 1000 units/ml of diphtheria antitoxin. Dry the plate, and inoculate as indicated in Section 12–5.

EGG SALINE

Prepare a mixture containing three volumes of whole egg and one volume of saline. Wash the eggs with brush, soap and warm water, sponge them with 70% alcohol, and collect the contents carefully in a sterile blender jar. Add saline and mix gently.

Dispense this preparation by inverted flask-hooded pipette technique into suitable containers. Six large eggs will yield enough medium to fill 60 half-ounce bottles to a maximum slant. Secure caps tightly, autoclave at 121°C for 15 minutes. This medium will preserve all but the most fastidious organisms for at least three months when kept at 20°C.

PRESERVATION MEDIUM

Add three volumes of horse serum to one volume of nutrient broth containing 30% glucose.

This medium is extremely well-suited for preserving highly fastidious organisms in lyophilized state, and it readily supplies the reconstituted culture with an overly rich medium.

CHLAMYDOSPORE AGAR

Ammonium sulfate	1	g
Monopotassium phosphate	1	g
Biotin	5	μg
Trypan blue	0.1	g
Purified polysaccharide	20	g
Agar	15	g
Distilled water	1000	ml

Suspend the ingredients in the water and bring to a boil. The final pH should be 5.1. Autoclave at 121°C for 15 minutes and pour into plates. This medium is exceptionally suited for the demonstration of chlamydospore production by *Candida albicans* (see Chapter 22).

SUMMARY

This chapter contains only media commonly used in routine laboratories. Many hundreds of different media have been developed over the years, each serving some particular purpose. Once familiar with the media outlined here, the novice technologist should have little difficulty in choosing the medium most appropriate to whatever purpose. Such familiarity will also prepare him to evaluate adequately the many media that undoubtedly will be developed in the future.

FURTHER READING

1. Barry, A. L. and Fay, G. D.: A review of some common sources of error in the preparation of agar media. Amer. J. Med. Technol., 38:241-245, 1972.
2. Difco Manual, Difco Laboratories, Detroit, Mich. Reprinted 1971.
3. Prier, J. E., Bartok, J. T., and Friedman, H.: *Quality Control in Microbiology.* Baltimore, University Park Press, 1975.

chapter 30

Staining
and Related Methods

The efficacy of the examination of specimens and preparations from cultures depends on several factors:
  a. The type of specimen or preparation
  b. The type(s) of organisms under study
  c. The method of examination
  d. The data required
  e. The state of the organisms under study

In previous chapters, we have already discussed many of the factors under a through d. Here, we shall concern ourselves mainly with methods of studying living or nonliving organisms.

Live organisms must be examined in wet preparations in order to maintain their viability. Nonliving organisms may be fixed onto a glass slide and can then be stained with different dyes to emphasize special structures.

30-1 MOTILITY TEST OR WET-MOUNT

a. Cover all four edges of a coverslip with a small amount of petroleum jelly. This may be accomplished by first rubbing some petroleum jelly onto the palm of one hand, which may then be scraped off the hand onto the edges of the coverslip. The idea is to have the petroleum jelly serve as a seal between the coverslip and the surface of a microscope slide. An evenly applied narrow ridge that covers all four edges of the coverslip will be both neat and effective.

b. Place the coverslip on the bench, petroleum jelly uppermost.

c. In the square well now formed by the petroleum jelly, place a small drop of a broth culture, or a liquid or emulsified specimen.

d. Gently press a microscope slide onto the petroleum jelly so that it seals the drop between the slide and the coverslip.

e. Invert the slide quickly so that the liquid appears to float or hang from the coverslip.

f. Examine under low and high dry magnification; do not apply oil.

Remember that you are working with viable organisms that might be infectious. Prevent spillage onto bench or microscope stage, and discard the slides into a suitable disinfectant after examination.

By this method, morphologic features will not be distorted by drying or fixation. Motility also can be detected; it is demonstrated when some bacteria move in opposite or different directions from the majority. Beware of "Brownian movement," a phenomenon whereby all bacteria oscillate in the same spot.

30-2 PREPARATION OF SMEARS FOR STAINING

Before organisms can be stained, a satisfactory smear must be prepared from a culture of specimen. The simple method described here is useful.

a. Place a small drop of water on the surface of a precleaned slide.
b. With a sterile needle or loop, transfer a sufficient amount of the culture from the colony to the drop so that a thin film of organisms forms when the culture and the drop of water are mixed and spread out over 1 cm² of the slide.

    When examining broth cultures, combine steps a and b by simply spreading a loopful of culture over an equal area of the slide.
c. Allow the smear to dry by itself. Heating a wet smear will distort the structures of the organisms.
d. When dry, smears must be fixed onto the slide. This may be done by slowly passing the slide through the blue portion of a Bunsen flame, so that the slide will be heated to the extent that you can just tolerate it to rest on the back of your hand. Overheating will cause morphologic distortion if not complete destruction of the cells. Proper fixing "glues" the cell onto the slide, resulting in coagulation of proteins, and thus preserving morphologic details. The fixed smears are now ready for staining.

30-3 SIMPLE METHYLENE BLUE STAIN

Reagent. One percent methylene blue in distilled water.

Procedure
a. Prepare a smear and fix in the usual manner.
b. Apply methylene blue by flooding* the smear completely with the stain, so that a layer of the stain remains on the horizontal slide with the smear uppermost.
c. Leave for one minute.
d. Wash with tap water.
e. Blot and dry.
f. Examine.

Most organisms take up the methylene blue and will thus be easier to see under the microscope.

    The degree to which different types of organisms take up the dye varies. Also, certain structures, such as spores and volutin bodies, do not stain as readily as other parts of organisms, and thus may be differentiated from the organisms as a whole by this rather simple method.

---

*In the procedures described hereafter, "flooding" will be understood to mean the method as presented in b above.

30-4 GRAM'S STAINING METHOD

The gram stain was developed in 1883 by Christian Gram in Denmark. It serves as one of the most useful methods in bacteriology, and as such deserves our attention. By this method, it is possible to divide the bacteria into two large groups: gram-positive bacteria and gram-negative bacteria. When stained with crystal violet and treated with weak iodine solutions, all bacteria stain a deep dark purple. When subsequently treated with alcohol or acetone, gram-positive bacteria retain the dye much longer than gram-negative bacteria. This difference is attributed to the much higher lipid content of the cell walls of the so-called gram-positive bacteria. The alcohol removes most of the lipids of the cell wall of gram-negative bacteria quickly, thereby releasing the dye-iodine complexes that have formed.

You may have already surmised that differentiation by Gram's method centers around the rapidity of the alcohol treatment; this fact must always be remembered when carrying out this method. To distinguish further between gram-positive and gram-negative bacteria, a counterstain is employed to stain the decolorized gram-negative bacteria a contrasting color.

Reagents
a. *Crystal violet*

      Crystal violet 1   g

      Distilled water .... 100 ml

    Methyl violet and gentian violet may also be used but crystal violet is a purer stain. Gentian violet is a mixture of methyl violet and crystal violet.

b. *Gram's iodine*

    Dissolve 1 g of potassium iodide in 70 ml distilled water. Add 0.5 g of iodine and fill up to 100 ml with water. Shake until the iodine is dissolved.

c. *Acetone-alcohol* (decolorizer)

    Equal parts of acetone and 95% ethyl alcohol. Other proportions may also be used, but remember that more alcohol will retard and more acetone will advance decolorization.

d. *Safranin* (counterstain)

      Safranin .... 0.5 g

      Distilled water .... 100 ml

    In fact, any stain that stains differently from crystal violet could be used.

Procedure

    a. Prepare and fix a smear as usual.

    b. Flood the slide with crystal violet for 30 seconds.

    c. Rinse with water.

    d. Flood with Gram's iodine for one minute.

    e. Rinse with water and decolorize rapidly with acetone-alcohol. Remember that this is the most critical step in the reaction. Adequate decolorization is usually obtained when the slide is slanted, and the acetone-alcohol is run over the smear until no more "blue" appears to be emerging from the smear.

    f. Rinse immediately with water.

    g. Stain with the counterstain for 30 seconds.

    h. Rinse, blot and dry.

In the first step, all organisms are stained violet and all assume a dirty bluish-brown color after treatment with the iodine solution. The iodine serves as a mordant to fix the violet dye in certain types of organisms so it is not washed out by the decolorizer. The counterstain stains those organisms that have been decolorized.

    Organisms that retain the crystal violet-iodine combination are referred to as gram-positive; those that are decolorized and counterstained with the red dye are called gram-negative.

30-5 ZIEHL-NEELSEN STAINING

    Another useful method in medical diagnosis distinguishes between so-called acid-fast and nonacid-fast bacilli. In theory, this method is similar to Gram's method. Acid-fast bacilli are more resistant to decolorization by acid-alcohol than are other bacilli.

Reagents

    a. *Carbol fuchsin*

        Basic fuchsin .... 1 g

        95% ethanol .... 10 ml

        Phenol .... 5 g

        Distilled water ....100 ml

        Dissolve the basic fuchsin in the alcohol, the phenol in the water; then mix. Filter before use.

    b. *Decolorizer*

        Hydrochloric acid .... 5 ml

        95% ethanol .... 95 ml

    c. *Counterstain*

        Malachite green .... 0.3 g

        Distilled water ....100 ml

A knife's edge of sodium bicarbonate can be added to increase the staining rate of the malachite green.

Procedure
a. Prepare and fix a smear as usual.
b. Flood the smear with carbol fuchsin and heat over a flame until steam rises from the stain.* Reapply heat periodically for about five to ten minutes.
c. Rinse with water.
d. Flood the smear with acid-alcohol for one minute.
e. Rinse with water, flood again with acid-alcohol for 20 seconds.
f. Rinse with water.
g. Flood the smear with malachite green. Leave for one minute.
h. Rinse, blot, and dry.

Acid-fast bacilli stain red. Other bacilli or materials stain green with malachite green counterstain, or blue with methylene blue counterstain.

30-6 AURAMINE O STAINING

This fluorescent staining technique requires much less time in examining specimens for acid-fast bacilli than does the Ziehl-Neelsen method. It is also more specific for pathogenic acid-fast bacilli, since most rapid-growing strains of *Mycobacterium* will not react with this stain.

Reagents
a. *Auramine stain†*

Auramine O‡	1.5	g
Rhodamine B‡	0.75	g
Glycerol	75	ml
Phenol	10	ml
Distilled water	50	ml

Mix magnetically for 24 hours, or thoroughly after warming to about 70°C. Filter through glass wool and store

---

*Dried, stain-impregnated strips are available from Gugol Science Corp., Jersey City, N.J., 07304. The use of these strips obviates the need for the extra heat application.
† The prepared stain is available from Difco Laboratories, Detroit, Mich., and from Baltimore Biological Laboratories, Cockeysville, Md.
‡ Allied Chemical Co., Morris Township, New Jersey.

in glass-stoppered bottle at 4°C. A slight separation from solution may occur but is of no consequence. Discard the stain after four months.

b. *Decolorizer*

HCl	0.5 ml
Ethanol 70%	99 ml

c. *Counterstain*

Potassium permanganate	0.5 g
Distilled water	99.5 ml

Dissolve, filter, and store in a dark, glass-stoppered bottle.

Procedure

a. Prepare a smear in the usual manner.
b. Fix with gentle heat or on a slide warmer set at 65°C for two hours.
c. Remove from the warmer and flood with auramine stain for 20 minutes.
d. Rinse gently with water.
e. Flood slide with decolorizer for two minutes.
f. Rinse gently with water.
g. Flood with the counterstain for five minutes.
h. Rinse gently with water.
i. Blot lightly and air-dry.
j. Examine under a suitable fluorescence microscope. A compound microscope fitted with the following* should be adequate: an Osram HBO 200 maximum pressure mercury vapor lamp; an HBO-L2 bulb heat filter; a BG12 primary exciter filter; and an OG-1 yellow barrier filter. This filter combination will result in demonstrating auramine stained acid-fast bacilli as bright red-orange rods against a dark background. Nonspecific organic matter will show a pale yellow color.

It is recommended that positive results be corroborated by the Ziehl-Neelsen method, for which purpose the auramine-stained smear may be used.

30-7 ALBERT'S STAINING METHOD

This method is particularly suited to differentiate metachromatic granules and other features displayed by *Corynebacterium diphtheriae*.

---

*Truant, J. P., et al.: Henry Ford Hosp. Med Bull., **10**:287, 1962.

Reagents

a. *Albert's stain*

Toluidine blue	0.15 g
Malachite green	0.2 g
Acetic acid	1 ml
95% ethyl alcohol	2 ml
Distilled water	100 ml

Dissolve the dyes in the alcohol and then add to the acetic acid and water.

b. *Gram's iodine* (see Section 30–4)

Procedure

a. Prepare and fix a smear as usual.

b. Flood the smear with Albert's stain for about four minutes.

c. Rinse with water, shake off excess stain if necessary.

d. Flood with iodine for one minute.

e. Rinse with water, blot and dry.

The granules will appear black or dark blue, the bands or bars a light blue, and the cytoplasm a faint green.

30-8 LOEFFLER'S METHYLENE BLUE METHOD

This simple method serves the same purpose as Albert's stain.

Reagent

Methylene blue	0.3 g
Ethanol	30 ml

Dissolve and add 100 ml of water.

Procedure

a. Prepare and fix a smear as usual.

b. Flood with stain for about one minute.

c. Rinse with water, blot, and dry.

The granules will be a deep blue; the bands, a lesser blue; and the cytoplasm, a faint blue. Overstaining reduces the contrast, making Albert's method far superior.

30-9 SPORE STAINING

With simple staining methods and with Gram's method, the less penetrable spores usually remain as unstained refractile bodies. Several methods have been developed for those occasions when spores must also be stained. This method appears to be as satisfactory as some of the more complex methods.

Reagents
a. *Malachite green*

Malachite green	5	g
Distilled water	100	ml

b. *Fuchsin*

Basic fuchsin	0.05	g
Distilled water	100	ml

Procedure
a. Place a nonfixed, dry smear over a beaker of boiling water. With smear uppermost, rest the slide on the rim of the beaker.
b. Allow water of condensation to develop into large droplets on the bottom of the slide; then flood the slide with malachite green, leaving the slide on the boiling beaker.
c. Allow the stain to react for one to three minutes.
d. With forceps, remove the slide from the beaker and rinse with water.
e. Apply fuchsin for 30 seconds.
f. Wash with water, blot dry.

The spores should stain light green while the remainder of the organism should stain red. It is important not to fix the smear beforehand, because the steam loosens the spore to allow the malachite green to enter. Fixed spores will not yield to softening with steam.

30-10 FLAGELLAR STAINING

Reagent

Tannic acid	0.85	g
Sodium chloride	0.5	g
Pararosaniline acetate	0.55	g
Ethanol 95%	35	ml
Distilled water	65	ml

Dissolve the solids in the alcohol, then add the water. This stain is stable for a maximum of two weeks.

Procedure
a. Use only alcohol-washed new slides.
b. Use only fresh cultures, preferably a nutrient agar culture at 12 hours.
c. Gently suspend some of the culture in distilled water to give a milky suspension.
d. With a grease pencil, draw a heavy rectangle on the slide.

e. Allow a small drop of the culture to run over the long side of the enclosed area so that a thin film results.
f. Air-dry the film, do not apply heat.
g. Flood the slide gently with the stain for about eight to ten minutes.
h. Rinse gently with tap water without removing the slide from the rack.
i. Drain gently, and allow to dry in air. Do not blot.

Flagella will be stained red; the body of the organism will stain blue.

30-11 CAPSULE STAINING

This stain may be performed on smears of sputa, body fluids or fresh cultures.

Reagents

a. Crystal violet .... 1 g
Distilled water .... 100 ml

b. Copper sulfate .... 20 g
Distilled water .... 100 ml

Procedure
a. Prepare a smear but do not fix.
b. When dry, flood gently with the crystal violet and leave for about four minutes.
c. Wash off with the copper sulfate.
d. Allow to dry in air.

The organisms should be a deep purple; the capsule, a faint blue against a light purple background.

30-12 NEGATIVE STAINING

Particularly for the demonstration of capsules of *Cryptococcus* species, the following method is recommended over the previous one.

Procedure
a. Place a small drop or loopful of water on the surface of a microscope slide.
b. With a needle, suspend a small amount of a young culture in the water, but not enough to obtain a visibly dense suspension.

c. Add a small drop of India ink and cover immediately with a coverslip.

d. Examine by lowering the condenser to reduce the light intensity.

Capsules will appear as halos surrounding the unstained cell against a dark background.

30-13 LACTOPHENOL COTTON BLUE STAINING

This method is recommended for the examination of specimens and cultures for fungal elements.

Reagents

Phenol crystals	20	g
Lactic acid	20	ml
Glycerol	40	ml
Cotton blue	0.075	g
Distilled water	40	ml

Dissolve and mix the phenol and the liquids, then add and dissolve the dye by gentle heat.

Procedure

a. Place a small drop of the stain on a microscope slide.

b. Tease out a small portion of the culture or specimens into this drop.

c. Gently place a coverslip over the preparation.

d. Examine the slide in about ten minutes to allow the stain to penetrate some of the structures.

Septa, conidia and hyphal walls stand out nicely as dark blue features against a pale blue background.

30-14 D'ANTONI'S IODINE STAINING

This method is recommended for the examination of feces for parasitic ova and cysts.

Reagent

Potassium iodide	1	g
Distilled water	100	ml

Dissolve completely, then add 1.5 g of iodine crystals and dissolve.

Procedure

a. Place a small drop of the reagent on a microscope slide.

b. With a wooden applicator stick, emulsify in this drop some of the feces to be examined.

   c. Place a coverslip over the preparation and examine immediately.

When coarse particles are evident, remove them with the applicator stick before applying the coverslip. Features of ova and cysts will take on some of the iodine, appearing dark brown against a yellowish background.

FURTHER READING

1. Blair, J. E. et al.: *Manual of Clinical Microbiology.* 2nd ed. Bethesda, Md., American Society of Microbiology, 1974.

chapter 31
Biochemical and Related Methods

31-1 BACITRACIN AND OPTOCHIN TESTS

For best results, the plating procedure as outlined in Chapter 27 under the Kirby-Bauer method could be used, but less rigid procedures will also give reliable results.

425

a. Organisms to be tested for bacitracin or optochin susceptibility are spread evenly over the surface of a blood agar
   plate.
b. Aseptically apply discs containing two units of bacitracin or
   one drop of a 1:4000 dilution of optochin. Place at a distance
   of no less than one inch from one another.
c. Incubate the plates at 37°C for 18 to 24 hours.
d. A zone of inhibition of growth of 15 to 20 mm diameter,
   including the disc, indicates a positive result.

Streptococci of Group A are positive for bacitracin; *Streptococcus pneumoniae,* for optochin (see Chapter 10).

31-2 BILE SOLUBILITY TESTS

PLATE METHOD

Sparingly sprinkle some powdered bile (sodium taurocholate
or sodium desoxycholate) onto a few colonies growing on a blood
agar plate. Within a few minutes, the bile dissolves in the moisture
on the agar surface. Bile-soluble organisms dissolve completely in
this bile solution and are no longer recognizable. Fixed cells, or
ghost cells, remain as "greenish" areas on the agar surface. Doubtful results should be corroborated by the tube test.

TUBE METHOD

a. Add a few drops of 1/N NaOH to an overnight broth culture
   to be examined.
b. Divide the contents of the tube equally into two small test
   tubes.
c. Add an equal volume of 20% bile salt (see Plate Method) to
   one tube, and an equal volume of saline to the other.
d. Incubate both tubes at 37°C for 30 minutes.

Positive cultures will be clear in tube one only. Negative
cultures will be cloudy in both tubes. When both tubes are clear,
the culture is autolytic in saline, and a bile solubility test would
cause difficulty by any method.

Bile tests have fallen into disuse since the widespread use of
optochin for the identification of *Streptococcus pneumoniae.*

31-3 CAMP TEST*

In this test a beta-toxin producing strain of *Staphylococcus* is
streaked across the center of a sheep blood agar plate. Test cultures

---

*J. Clin. Microbiol., 1:171–174, 1975.

of streptococci are streaked perpendicularly to the staphylococcus streak without touching it. The plates are then incubated at 35°C for 18 hours in 5% CO_2. *Streptococcus agalactiae* (Group B) will produce a typical arrowhead-shaped zone of hemolysis in a zone surrounding the streptococcal culture.

31-4 CATALASE TESTS

FOR NON-MYCOBACTERIACEAE

Place a small drop of 10% to 30% hydrogen peroxide solution onto a colony on a nutrient agar plate. A positive reaction is indicated by immediate and violent effervescence.

It is wise to pretest an area of the plate on which no growth occurs, because some media contain small amounts of catalase which may give a delayed and weak reaction.

FOR MYCOBACTERIACEAE

This test may be performed on the portion of a *Mycobacterium* culture that remains after the niacin extract is removed (see Section 31–9).

Transfer a loopful of culture to the bottom of a small test tube. Add a few drops of a 50–50 mixture of a 30% hydrogen peroxide and a 10% Tween 80, both in aqueous solutions, to the culture. The degree of effervescence is measured from prompt and vigorous (4^+) to slow and feeble (1^+).

31-5 COAGULASE TESTS

SLIDE TEST

  a. Mark two sections on a microscope slide with a wax pencil.
  b. Place a drop of saline in each section.
  c. Emulsify some culture material taken from a nutrient agar plate in each drop of saline, using just enough culture to give a milky suspension.
  d. Add a drop of citrated rabbit plasma to the suspension to the right tube, stirring in the plasma with a wire loop.
  e. Check for clumping of the organisms.

Tube tests should also be done in the event of doubtful positive and, preferably, on all negative cultures.

TUBE TEST

  a. Place 0.5 ml of an overnight broth culture in a small test tube, or emulsify a few colonies in 0.5 ml of saline in a small test tube.

b. Add 0.5 ml of a 1:10 dilution of citrated rabbit plasma in saline.

c. Incubate at 37°C for 30 minutes.

d. Examine for clot formation, which is indicative of coagulase production by the culture. The clot may take up to four hours to form. However, since clots rapidly disintegrate once formed, periodic readings must be taken throughout the four-hour interval, in order not to miss a positive reagent.

31-6 CYTOCHROME OXIDASE TESTS

All aerobic respiratory bacteria produce the enzyme cytochrome oxidase. Some species also produce a reducing substance, "cytochrome c," and these are known as oxidase-positive bacteria. In the presence of either tetramethyl-p-phenylenediamine or dimethyl-p-phenylenediamine and alpha-naphthol, these bacteria cause a positive oxidase reaction. Two methods are practiced, the reagent and the disc methods. Only platinum wire loops should be used, because Nichrome may cause oxidation of the reagent.

REAGENT METHOD

Place a small drop of a fresh 1% solution of tetramethyl-p-phenylene-diamine dihydrochloride onto a colony of a culture to be tested. In the presence of oxidase, the reagent causes the colony to change colors from a light to deep purple to almost black.

Colonies tested by this method can be subcultured for future study if picked off within two minutes following this test. Organisms left longer in the reagent usually succumb. The reagent is labile and should be prepared daily. Allow it to stand for 15 minutes prior to use.

DISC METHOD

a. Place a disc* impregnated with para-amino-dimethylaniline near a colony to be tested.

b. With a loop, apply a drop of sterile distilled water to the disc.

c. Incubate the plate for 20–30 minutes at 37°C.

The reagent in the disc dissolves in the water, diffuses into the medium, and reacts with the oxidase produced. Oxidase-positive

---

*Taxodiscs, Baltimore Biological Laboratories, Cockeysville, Md.

colonies first turn red, then blue, purple, and finally black. Negative colonies remain unaltered.

With *Pseudomonas* species, best results are obtained by the reagent method; with *Neisseria*, by the disc method.

31-7   ESCULIN SPOT TEST*

Materials
 a. A filter-sterilized, 0.02% aqueous solution of esculin.† Store at 4°C for up to four weeks.
 b. Whatman filter paper No. 2 (F-2412), cut into strips the size of a microscope slide.
 c. Two glass rods, 7 cm long, Petri dishes, microscope slides, wooden applicators, and a Wood's lamp.

Procedure
 a. Place the glass rods side by side at the bottom of a Petri dish, spaced about 2 cm apart.
 b. With a pencil draw four to six circles of 1-cm diameter on a filter paper strip.
 c. Rest the strip on a microscope slide, and place the slide over the rods in the Petri dish.
 d. Flood the filter paper with esculin solution to wet it throughout without dripping.
 e. Touch the center of a colony of test culture (or the sediment of a broth culture) and rub the organisms gently onto the center of a circle on the impregnated filter strip.
 f. Close the Petri dish and place the dish in a moist chamber at 35°C for 30 minutes.
 g. Expose the opened Petri dish to a Wood's lamp (366 nm wavelength) in subdued light.
 h. At a distance of 15 cm, observe the spots in the center of the circles for fluorescence.

Positive cultures (those that hydrolyze the esculin) do not fluoresce and show a black spot in the center of the circle. Negative cultures appear bright throughout.

As controls, a known positive culture *(Klebsiella pneumoniae)* and negative culture *(Staphylococcus)* should be incorporated on each strip, or at least on one of a series of strips tested at the same time.

---

*J. Clin. Microbiol., 4:180–184, 1976.
†Nutritional Biochemical Corp., Cleveland, Ohio.

31-8 HYDROGEN SULFIDE TESTS

Many bacteria are capable of breaking down cystine with the production of H_2S. This H_2S production is easily detectable by either of two methods.

SPECIAL MEDIA

Media such as triple sugar iron and sulfide-indole-motility agar (SIM) contain cystine and some ferric compounds. When the cystine is broken down and H_2S is produced, the ferric compound is usually reduced, as demonstrated by blackening of the medium. *Salmonella-Shigella* agar, and some others, contain small amounts of ferric compounds. These media do not turn black, but colonies of H_2S-producing bacteria often display a black center when grown on such media.

LEAD ACETATE PAPER STRIPS

Some bacteria that do produce H_2S will not grow on media containing ferric compounds. Hydrogen sulfide production by these organisms may be detected by growing the organisms on an agar slant in a test tube. A paper strip impregnated with a 5% lead acetate solution may be hung from the lip of the tube over, but not touching, the slant. The paper strip blackens in the presence of H_2S. The paper strip method is more sensitive than the foregoing methods described under *Special Media*.

31-9 INDOLE TESTS

Indole is a by-product of the breakdown of tryptophan. It may be detected by testing a 24- or 48-hour broth culture (peptone, tryptone, or trypticase broth), or a culture on special medium (SIM), by one of two methods.

KOVAC'S METHOD

Reagent. Dissolve 10 g of paradimethylaminobenzaldehyde into 150 ml of amyl alcohol. When dissolved, slowly add 50 ml of concentrated hydrochloric acid. If stored in dark, glass-stoppered bottles at 4°C, it will remain stable for years.

Procedure. Add a few drops of Kovac's reagent to the culture to be tested. When indole is present, a deep red color appears within minutes.

EHRLICH'S METHOD

Reagent. Dissolve 2 g of paradimethylaminobenzaldehyde in 190 ml of 95% ethanol. When dissolved, slowly add 40 ml of concentrated hydrochloric acid. Store as Kovac's reagent.

Procedure

a. Add 1 ml of ether to a broth culture.

b. Shake the mixture and allow to rest until the ether rises to the top.

c. To the undisturbed layers, slowly add 0.5 ml of Ehrlich's reagent down the side of the tube, so that a ring forms between the ether and the broth.

d. In the presence of indole, the interphase ring turns a deep red.

31-10 MR-VP TESTS

Both the methyl red and the Voges-Proskauer tests may be performed on a 24- or 48-hour culture on MR-VP broth.

METHYL RED TEST

Reagent. Dissolve 0.1 g of methyl red into 300 ml of 95% ethanol. When dissolved, add distilled water to make 500 ml of solution. The reagent appears to be stable indefinitely.

Procedure. Add one drop of MR reagent to 1 ml of the culture. When large amounts of predominantly acid end-products have been formed, the indicator in the reagent turns red almost immediately, which is a positive result. Yellow represents a negative result.

VOGES-PROSKAUER TEST

To 1 ml of culture, add 0.6 ml of 5% alphanaphthol in absolute alcohol. To the mixture, add 0.2 ml of 40% KOH. Shake and leave at room temperature.

In the presence of acetyl-methyl-carbinol, a bright orange-red color will develop from the top downwards within 5 to 20 minutes. The tubes should be left undisturbed. A negative reaction results in an orange-brown color. Some reactions may be delayed for as much as two hours.

31-11 NEUTRAL RED TEST

This method is believed to differentiate between virulent and avirulent strains of *Mycobacterium tuberculosis*. The test must be performed on the culture before niacin is extracted.

a. Transfer a few loopfuls of culture to a small test tube containing 5 ml of 50% methanol.
b. Incubate the mixture at 37°C for one hour.
c. Carefully decant most of the alcohol and replace with fresh 50% methanol in equal volume.
d. Let the culture settle and decant the alcohol again.
e. Suspend the remaining culture in 5 ml of 5% NaCl in 1% barbitol, and add 1 ml of 20% aqueous neutral red.
f. In positive cultures, the dye becomes fixed to the bacteria, which appear red in a yellow supernatant. Virulent strains are usually positive; avirulent strains, negative.

31-12 NIACIN TESTS

Niacin (nicotinate) is a basic requirement for most organisms. *Mycobacterium* species are among the few organisms that actually synthesize niacin; of these, *M. tuberculosis* produces an excess of niacin. This excess niacin may be detected in actively growing cultures, which serves as a means of differentiating *M. tuberculosis* from other Mycobacteriaceae. Two methods are in common use:

WOLLINSKY'S METHOD

a. To a slant demonstrating prolific growth, add 1 ml of sterile distilled water.
b. Allow the water to stand on the slant for at least ten minutes. This period allows much of the niacin to be extracted from the culture.
c. Remove the extract from the culture, being careful not to remove any culture or medium, and place into a small test tube.
d. Add 1 ml of 4% aniline in 95% ethanol, and 1 ml of 10% cyanogen bromide in water.*
e. Read. Niacin reacts with the reagents to produce a yellow color. Without niacin, there is no color change.

BONICKE AND LISBOA'S METHOD

This method dispenses with the need for the dangerous cyanogen bromide. Instead, however, it requires the use of a special

*CAUTION: Cyanogen bromide gives off highly toxic fumes. It should be manipulated in a chemical fume cabinet only. Store in dark, glass-stoppered bottles at 4°C. A few milliliters of 10% ammonia may be added to the test tubes afterwards, to neutralize the cyanogen bromide before the tubes are autoclaved.

medium, which must be set up along with all other routine media when isolation attempts are begun.

 a. To 1 ml of a culture in Proskauer and Beck broth,† add 1 ml of 1% potassium cyanide and 1 ml of 5% chloramine T, both in aqueous solutions.
 b. Shake a few times and leave for about two minutes.
 c. Read. Niacin production is indicated by the development of a yellow color. No color change occurs in negative reactions.

31-13 ONPG TEST

Only when an organism produces both lactose permease and β-galactosidase can a culture demonstrate lactose fermentation by the conventional method. The ONPG test is designed to detect the production of β-galactosidase without the necessary presence of permease.

When O-nitrophenyl-1-β-D-galactoside (ONPG) is presented to β-galactosidase (also known as lactase), the ONPG is hydrolyzed. Although ONPG is a colorless substance, one of the end-products of ONPG hydrolysis is O-nitrophenol, which is yellow.

In the ONPG test, a tablet of ONPG* is dissolved in a small amount of sterile distilled water, and a heavy suspension of test culture is mixed into it with a sterile loop. The test is incubated for six hours at 35°C. Development of a yellow color is an indication of lactase production.

31-14 PHENYL PYRUVIC ACID TEST

Some organisms are capable of reducing phenylalanine to phenyl pyruvic acid.

 a. A slant of phenylalanine agar is seeded with the test culture and incubated at 37°C for 24 hours.
 b. A few drops of 10% (W/V) of ferric chloride in water are run over the growth on the slant.
 c. Read. When phenyl pyruvic acid has been produced, a deep green color will appear throughout the slant surface.

---

†J. Bact., **51**:703–710, 1946.
*Key Scientific Products Co., Los Angeles, Calif.

FURTHER READING

Blair, J. E. et al.: *Manual of Clinical Microbiology.* 2nd ed. Bethesda, Md., American Society Microbiology, 1974.

INDEX

Page numbers in italics refer to illustrations; those followed by n refer to footnotes, and those followed by t indicate tables or charts.